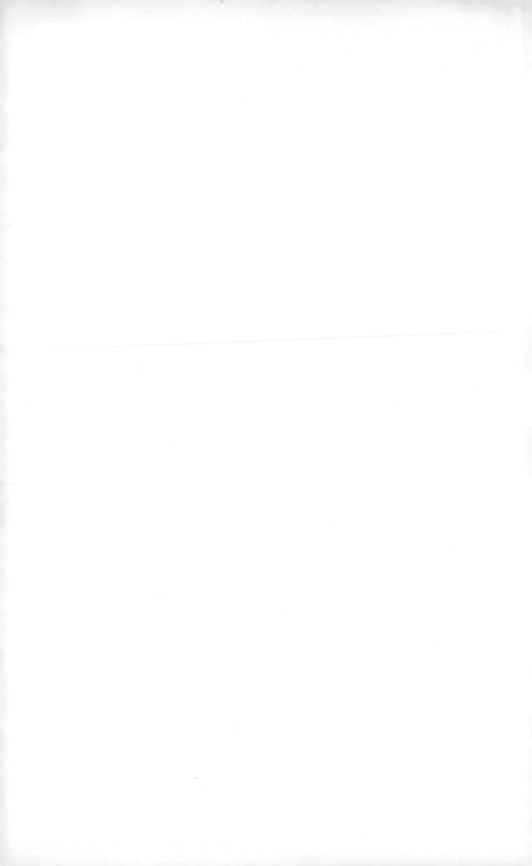

Emergency Pediatric Surgery

Editors

TODD A. PONSKY
AARON P. GARRISON

SURGICAL CLINICS
OF NORTH AMERICA

www.surgical.theclinics.com

Consulting Editor
RONALD F. MARTIN

February 2017 • Volume 97 • Number 1

ELSEVIER

1600 John F. Kennedy Boulevard • Suite 1800 • Philadelphia, Pennsylvania, 19103-2899

http://www.surgical.theclinics.com

SURGICAL CLINICS OF NORTH AMERICA Volume 97, Number 1
February 2017 ISSN 0039–6109, ISBN-13: 978-0-323-49677-3

Editor: John Vassallo, j.vassallo@elsevier.com
Developmental Editor: Colleen Dietzler

Surgical Clinics of North America (ISSN 0039–6109) is published bimonthly by Elsevier Inc., 360 Park Avenue South, New York, NY 10010-1710. Months of publication are February, April, June, August, October, and December. Business and Editorial Offices: 1600 John F. Kennedy Blvd., Suite 1800, Philadelphia, PA 19103-2899. Periodicals postage paid at New York, NY and additional mailing offices. Subscription prices are $386.00 per year for US individuals, $756.00 per year for US institutions, $100.00 per year for US students and residents, $469.00 per year for Canadian individuals, $958.00 per year for Canadian institutions, $525.00 for international individuals, $958.00 per year for international institutions and $250.00 per year for Canadian and foreign students/residents. To receive student/resident rate, orders must be accompanied by name of affiliated institution, date of term, and the *signature* of program/residency coordinator on institution letterhead. Orders will be billed at individual rate until proof of status is received. Foreign air speed delivery is included in all *Clinics* subscription prices. All prices are subject to change without notice. POSTMASTER: Send address changes to *Surgical Clinics*, Elsevier Health Sciences Division, Subscription Customer Service, 3251 Riverport Lane, Maryland Heights, MO 63043. **Customer Service (orders, claims, online, change of address): Telephone: 1-800-654-2452 (U.S. and Canada); 314-447-8871 (outside U.S. and Canada). Fax: 314-447-8029. E-mail: journalscustomerservice-usa@elsevier.com (for print support); journalsonlinesupport-usa@elsevier.com (for online support).**

Reprints. For copies of 100 or more, of articles in this publication, please contact the Commercial Reprints Department, Elsevier Inc., 360 Park Avenue South, New York, New York 10010-1710. Tel. 212-633-3874, Fax: 212-633-3820, E-mail: reprints@elsevier.com.

The Surgical Clinics of North America is also published in Spanish by McGraw-Hill Interamericana Editores S.A., P.O. Box 5-237 06500 Mexico D.F. Mexico; and in Portuguese by Interlivros Edicoes Ltda., Rua Comandante Coelho 1085, CEP 21250, Rio de Janeiro, Brazil; and in Greek by Paschalidis Medical Publications, Athens Greece.

The Surgical Clinics of North America is covered in *MEDLINE/PubMed (Index Medicus), EMBASE/Excerpta Medica, Current Contents/Clinical Medicine, Current Contents/Life Sciences, Science Citation Index*, and *ISI/BIOMED.*

Contributors

CONSULTING EDITOR

RONALD F. MARTIN, MD, FACS
Lead Surgeon, York Hospital, Maine; Colonel (ret.), United States Army Reserve, York Hospital, York, Maine

EDITORS

TODD A. PONSKY, MD, FACS
Associate Professor of Surgery and Pediatrics, Division of Pediatric Surgery, Akron Children's Hospital, Akron, Ohio

AARON P. GARRISON, MD, FACS
Division of Pediatric Surgery, Akron Children's Hospital, Assistant Professor of Surgery, Northeast Ohio Medical University, Akron, Ohio

AUTHORS

SOPHIA A. ABDULHAI, MD
Research Fellow, Division of Pediatric Surgery, Akron Children's Hospital, Akron, Ohio

MARY K. ARBUTHNOT, DO
Department of Surgery, Boston Children's Hospital, Boston, Massachusetts

KENNETH AZAROW, MD
Oregon Health and Science University, Portland, Oregon

ELIZABETH A. BERDAN, MD, MS
Pediatric Surgery Fellow, Children's Hospital of Wisconsin, Medical College of Wisconsin, Milwaukee, Wisconsin

PAUL R. BOWLIN, MD
Assistant Professor, Section of Urology, Department of Surgery, Children's Mercy Hospital, University of Missouri–Kansas City, Kansas City, Missouri

KRISTA J. CHILDRESS, MD
Fellow, Division of Pediatric and Adolescent Gynecology, Department of Obstetrics and Gynecology, Baylor College of Medicine, Houston, Texas

DYLAN R. CHILDS, MD, FACS
Division of Plastic Surgery, Summa Health System, Akron, Ohio

JOSEPH T. CHURCH, MD
Department of Surgery, University of Michigan Health System, Ann Arbor, Michigan

MATTHEW S. CLIFTON, MD
Associate Professor of Surgery and Pediatrics, Department of Surgery, Children's Healthcare of Atlanta, Emory University School of Medicine, Atlanta, Georgia

JENNIFER E. DIETRICH, MD, MSc
Associate Professor, Division of Pediatric and Adolescent Gynecology, Department of Obstetrics and Gynecology, Baylor College of Medicine, Houston, Texas

SABRINA DREXEL, MD
Oregon Health and Science University, Portland, Oregon

RICHARD A. FALCONE Jr, MD, MPH
Division of Pediatric and Thoracic Surgery, Cincinnati Children's Hospital Medical Center, Cincinnati, Ohio

IBRAHIM FARID, MD
Chair, Department of Anesthesia and Pain Medicine, Director, Pediatric Pain Center, Associate Professor of Anesthesia, NEOMED, Akron, Ohio

JOHN M. GATTI, MD
Associate Professor, Section of Urology, Department of Surgery, Children's Mercy Hospital, University of Missouri–Kansas City, Kansas City, Missouri

IAN C. GLENN, MD
Research Fellow, Division of Pediatric Surgery, Department of Surgery, Akron Children's Hospital, Akron, Ohio

MUBEEN A. JAFRI, MD
Oregon Health and Science University; Randall Children's Hospital, Portland, Oregon

MARCUS D. JARBOE, MD
Section of Pediatric Surgery, Department of Surgery, University of Michigan Health System, Ann Arbor, Michigan

PAUL T. KIM, MD
Department of General Surgery, University of Cincinnati Medical Center, Cincinnati Children's Hospital Medical Center, Cincinnati, Ohio

JACOB C. LANGER, MD
Professor of Surgery, Division of General and Thoracic Surgery, Hospital for Sick Children, University of Toronto, Toronto, Ontario

MARIA E. LINNAUS, MD
General Surgery Department, Mayo Clinic Hospital, Phoenix, Arizona

MATTHEW C. MITCHELL, DO
Anesthesiologist, Department of Anesthesia & Pain Medicine, Akron Children's Hospital, Akron, Ohio

DAVID P. MOONEY, MD, MPH
Department of Surgery, Boston Children's Hospital, Boston, Massachusetts

WILLIEFORD MOSES, MD
Resident, General Surgery, Department of Surgery, University of California, San Francisco, San Francisco, California

J. PATRICK MURPHY, MD
Professor, Section of Urology, Department of Surgery, Children's Mercy Hospital, University of Missouri–Kansas City, Kansas City, Missouri

ANANTH S. MURTHY, MD
Chief, Division of Plastic Surgery, Akron Children's Hospital, Akron, Ohio

DAVID M. NOTRICA, MD, FACS, FAAP
Trauma Medical Director, Department of Surgery, Phoenix Children's Hospital; Trauma Department, Phoenix Children's Hospital; Associate Professor, University of Arizona College of Medicine; Assistant Professor of Surgery, General and Thoracic Surgery, Mayo Clinic Hospital, Phoenix, Arizona

BENJAMIN E. PADILLA, MD
Assistant Professor, Division of Pediatric Surgery, University of California, San Francisco, San Francisco, California

ERIK G. PEARSON, MD
Department of Surgery, Emory University School of Medicine, Atlanta, Georgia

TODD A. PONSKY, MD, FACS
Associate Professor of Surgery and Pediatrics, Division of Pediatric Surgery, Akron Children's Hospital, Akron, Ohio

REBECCA M. RENTEA, MD
Department of Surgery, Children's Mercy Hospital, Kansas City, Missouri

THOMAS T. SATO, MD, FACS, FAAP
CEO Children's Specialty Group, Senior Associate Dean of Clinical Affairs, Professor of Surgery, Division of Pediatric Surgery, Children's Hospital of Wisconsin, Children's Corporate Center, Medical College of Wisconsin, Milwaukee, Wisconsin

SHAWN D. ST. PETER, MD
Director, Pediatric Surgical Fellowship and Scholars Programs; Director of Research, Department of Surgery, Children's Mercy Hospital, Kansas City, Missouri

Contents

> Indirect inguinal hernias are the most commonly incarcerated hernias in
> children, with a higher incidence in low birth weight and premature infants.
> Contralateral groin exploration to evaluate for a patent processus vaginalis
> or subclinical hernia is controversial, given that most never progress to
> clinical hernias. Most indirect inguinal hernias can be reduced nonopera-
> tively. It is recommended to repair them in a timely fashion, even in prema-
> ture infants. Laparoscopic repair of incarcerated inguinal hernia repair is
> considered a safe and effective alternative to conventional open hernior-
> rhaphy. Other incarcerated pediatric hernias are extremely rare and may
> be managed effectively with laparoscopy.

> Rotation abnormalities may be asymptomatic or may be associated with
> obstruction caused by bands, midgut volvulus, or associated atresia or
> web. The most important goal of clinicians is to determine whether the pa-
> tient has midgut volvulus with intestinal ischemia, in which case an emer-
> gency laparotomy should be done. If the patient is not acutely ill, the next
> goal is to determine whether the patient has a narrow-based small bowel
> mesentery. In general, the outcomes for children with a rotation abnormal-
> ity are excellent, unless there has been midgut volvulus with significant in-
> testinal ischemia.

> The pediatric patient presenting with acute scrotal pain requires prompt
> evaluation and management given the likelihood of testicular torsion as
> the underlying cause. Although other diagnoses can present with acute
> testicular pain, it is important to recognize the possibility of testicular tor-
> sion because the best chance of testicular preservation occurs with expe-
> ditious management. When testicular torsion is suspected, prompt
> surgical exploration is warranted. A delay in surgical management should
> not occur in an effort to obtain confirmatory imaging. When torsion is
> discovered, the contralateral testicle should undergo fixation to reduce
> the risk of asynchronous torsion.

> Relatively uncommon compared with the adult population, lower
> gastrointestinal bleeding in children requires expeditious evaluation and
> management because of the variety of causes ranging from benign to
> life-threatening conditions. The causes of lower gastrointestinal bleeding
> (LGIB) vary with patient age. This review focuses on the differential diag-
> nosis and management of LGIB in children. Because intussusception is
> one of the most common sources of LGIB, particular attention will be given
> to its diagnosis and management.

SURGICAL CLINICS
OF NORTH AMERICA

ISSUE OF RELATED INTEREST

Pediatric Clinics, August 2014 (Vol. 61, Issue 4)
Pediatric Hospital Medicine Pediatric Palliative Care
Mary C. Ottolini, Christina K. Ullrich, and Joanne Wolfe, *Editors*
Available at: http://www.pediatric.theclinics.com/

THE CLINICS ARE AVAILABLE ONLINE!
Access your subscription at:
www.theclinics.com

Foreword

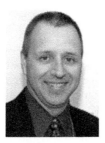

Ronald F. Martin, MD, FACS
Consulting Editor

To roughly paraphrase perhaps many people, the more one learns, the more one realizes how much one does not know. Surgery and medicine writ large are excellent disciplines to illustrate that point. Over the years, I have tried to focus more on understanding the questions in the belief that the answers may change, but the fundamental questions are more likely to endure. To what degree I have succeeded in that remains to be determined.

Of all the things that I thought I knew when I was younger that I am now convinced I know very little about is the degree to which doctors actually wish to be the solver of problems. When I was introduced to medicine, it seemed as if everyone was desirous of being someone who was able to take care of almost anything. There seemed a pride to it. Today, it is not that I think that our colleagues don't want to solve any problems, but rather, it seems that more and more of our colleagues only want to solve a specific subset of problems. More so, they may only want to solve a specific subset of problems that has a finite level of difficulty. I am certain my initial perceptions were less than accurate, and my perceptions today are also subjective.

This is hardly an observation that I alone have made. At least at the "Big Surgery" level, we have been discussing this for many years. It has been given lots of names: unable to be autonomous (the one I like the least), incomplete training, lack of ownership, to name a few. While all of those may be good concerns, I think the one that resonates best is that people feel compelled to only have to work within their "comfort zone." Somewhere along the line, we have conveyed that everybody should feel comfortable and safe all the time, including doctors dealing with very difficult situations. Perhaps it is a noble goal, but I doubt it is achievable. Even if it were achievable for many, it should not be achievable for everybody and definitively not for doctors. Of the many professions, we more than anybody deal routinely with the things that make people feel the least comfortable and the least secure. We have to deal with the most feared things that happen in many people's lives.

How we got to this era of "comfort entitlement" is unclear. Possibly it is a byproduct of helicopter parenting or of everybody being rewarded for participation. Maybe we

http://dx.doi.org/10.1016/j.suc.2016.11.002
0039-6109/17/© 2016 Published by Elsevier Inc.
surgical.theclinics.com

have reduced the incentive to do the "hard things" such that people simply won't invest the effort, or maybe we have just lowered the bar of expectation and enabled shifting of responsibility. It is hard to say.

Multiple structural and cultural factors have contributed as well. The change toward shift work, hyperspecialization, constant oversight, diminished willingness to accept variation (justified or unjustified), and constant threat of penalty for being below average or even average all have led many people to be risk averse in matters that they participate in. No doubt all of the above have also contributed to improvements in the system and may have shifted the needle in a positive direction to improve patient care under the right circumstances. However, out of context, many of the above have also had deleterious effects as well.

I can think of few categories in which this conundrum becomes more apparent than in the care of children. The physiology of children is different from adults in many regards and does vary rapidly as they grow. Such variation does not, however, make the care of children de facto outside the intellectual capacity of persons who do not exclusively care for children. Much of the basic physiology and operative issues are sufficiently similar if not identical.

I firmly believe that there are many issues in the care of children that significantly benefit from having the collective resources of a children's hospital. That said, not every disorder affecting every child rises to that level. The consequences of relying on a system in which every child's care is delivered in dedicated children's hospitals are substantial. Given the geographic distribution of hospitals that have dedicated services for children and the distribution of where children actually live, especially in the more rural parts of the United States, there is a built-in barrier to meeting families' needs for the care of their children without creating hardship for parents and families for just travel distance alone.

As we evolve to a system that inherently accepts the limits on what services providers are "comfortable" providing, whether real or perceived, we continue to endorse a system with geographic diminution of capacity built into the model. Ultimately, this shifts responsibility without necessarily shifting resources from the larger health care system to a smaller burdened subset. It also forces families to travel longer distances in many cases. For those families who also have responsibilities at home, it creates challenging tensions both socially and financially. While this will always be the case for some medical concerns, it should not be the case for all medical concerns of children.

Some facility requirements we cannot duplicate simply because of lack of resources: whether financial or in terms of human capital. We can increase our comfort zones for some things through better education and information. Dr Ponsky and his colleagues have amassed a great deal of information that should be useful to anybody who cares for children—either as a medical professional or as a concerned parent or loved one.

As I have written before, we are all going to continue to be asked to do more with less. The idea that we can narrow our comfort zones and expect others to find that of value is at best a fantasy. We must become more useful and more fluid in our response to challenges, especially as surgeons. Usable, reliable knowledge is the first step to expanding one's comfort zone. Knowledge alone will not be enough though; willingness to try to own the problem and solve it, within the boundaries of what is rational, is necessary for success. If not us, then who?

Growth in our profession requires spending time outside our comfort zones. At every level of our development, we need to find a way to reintroduce that set of opportunities. If we don't, we will have ever-narrowing and confining zones of comfort until we are of little use to anyone.

Ronald F. Martin, MD, FACS
Colonel (ret.), United States Army Reserve
York Hospital
16 Hospital Drive, Suite A
York, ME 03909, USA

E-mail address:
rmartin@yorkhospital.com

Preface

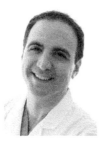
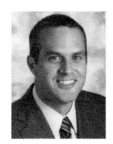

Todd A. Ponsky, MD, FACS   Aaron P. Garrison, MD, FACS
Editors

Pediatric surgery is a rapidly evolving field. When confronted with a difficult patient in the outpatient clinic, pediatric surgeons can refer to recent journal publications or textbooks to find the most current treatment options. Unfortunately, when patients present with certain emergency conditions, we may not have the luxury of time to review new treatment options. However, it has been said that "chance favors the prepared mind," which is why we have decided to publish this issue of the *Surgical Clinics of North America* on the treatment of pediatric surgical emergencies.

As you can see from the table of contents, pediatric surgical emergencies involve just about every organ system. To stay up-to-date with advances in a field as broad as ours is difficult. This issue of *Surgical Clinics of North America* addresses the major emergencies involving infants and children. Some of the approaches, such as a Ladd procedure for midgut volvulus, have not changed since 1941 when Ladd and Gross coauthored *Abdominal Surgery of Infancy and Childhood*. Others, such as the latest recommendations regarding the current management of the necrotic-appearing ovary, are not yet widespread in practice.

The issue begins with trauma, including the latest on nonoperative management of solid organ injury, head injury, and c-spine clearance. An important article on non-accidental trauma is a must-read for all who take care of children. The trauma section concludes with an update on minimally invasive approaches to the trauma patient. We then venture into some of the more controversial topics surrounding ovarian and testicular torsion, appendicitis, and esophageal/airway foreign bodies. This is followed by a nice review of intestinal rotation abnormalities and midgut volvulus, lower GI bleeding/intussusception, and the management of incarcerated pediatric hernias. Finally, we conclude with updates on the newest approaches to vascular access, an overview of wound healing, and a review of emergency anesthetic issues for the surgeon.

We believe this issue of the *Surgical Clinics of North America* will provide the reader with an update on the latest in pediatric surgical emergencies, so they can be prepared

Surg Clin N Am 97 (2017) xvii–xviii
http://dx.doi.org/10.1016/j.suc.2016.11.001
0039-6109/17/© 2016 Published by Elsevier Inc.

surgical.theclinics.com

when confronted with one of these situations. However, we hope this will also serve as a handy reference tool if time is available to prepare before heading to the operating room.

Todd A. Ponsky, MD, FACS
Division of Pediatric Surgery
Akron Children's Hospital
One Perkins Square
Akron, OH 44308, USA

Aaron P. Garrison, MD, FACS
Division of Pediatric Surgery
Akron Children's Hospital
One Perkins Square
Akron, OH 44308, USA

E-mail addresses:
TPonsky@chmca.org (T.A. Ponsky)
AGarrison2@chmca.org (A.P. Garrison)

Nonoperative Management of Blunt Solid Organ Injury in Pediatric Surgery

David M. Notrica, MD[a,b,c,d],*, Maria E. Linnaus, MD[e]

KEYWORDS

- Pediatric • Spleen injury • Liver injury • Kidney injury • Blunt trauma • Management
- Review

KEY POINTS

- Nonoperative management of blunt solid organ injury in children is achievable in a high percentage of injuries.
- Algorithms for management are important to improve care.
- Strategies for management of common complications associated with nonoperative management are reviewed.

BACKGROUND

Of the approximately 6 million children injured last year in the United States, an estimated 9600 sustained injury to the liver, spleen, or kidney.[1,2] The management of blunt solid organ injury (SOI; defined as liver, spleen, or kidney injury) in children has evolved and undergone numerous changes in a relatively short time.[3–8] Initially, the diagnosis of SOI was solely based on physical examination and clinical judgment; operative management was frequent. However, in the 1970s, pediatric surgeons in Toronto began advocating for nonoperative management (NOM) of splenic injuries based on clinical assessment; however, adoption was slow.[9] As computed tomography (CT) increased in sensitivity for identifying less severe injuries, an organ injury grading system was developed by the American Association for the Surgery of Trauma (AAST) in the 1990s[10] (Tables 1–3). With the advent of a new organ injury scale, CT grade of injury became incorporated into the management strategy of SOI in children and adults.

Disclosure Statement: The authors have no disclosures.
[a] Department of Surgery, Phoenix Children's Hospital, Phoenix, AZ, USA; [b] Trauma Department, Phoenix Children's Hospital, 1919 East Thomas Road, Phoenix, AZ 85006, USA; [c] Department of Child Health, University of Arizona College of Medicine, 550 East Van Buren Street, Phoenix, AZ 86004, USA; [d] General and Thoracic Surgery, Mayo Clinic Hospital, 5777 East Mayo Blvd, Phoenix, AZ 85054, USA; [e] General Surgery Department, Mayo Clinic Hospital, 5777 East Mayo Blvd, Phoenix, AZ 85054, USA
* Corresponding author. Trauma Department, Phoenix Children's Hospital, 1919 East Thomas Road, Phoenix, AZ 85006.
E-mail address: DNotrica@surgery4children.com

Surg Clin N Am 97 (2017) 1–20
http://dx.doi.org/10.1016/j.suc.2016.08.001
0039-6109/17/© 2016 Elsevier Inc. All rights reserved.

Table 1		
Organ injury scale for splenic injuries		
Grade	**Injury Type**	**Description of Injury**
I	Hematoma	Subcapsular, <10% surface area
	Laceration	Capsular tear, <1 cm parenchymal depth
II	Hematoma	Subcapsular, 10%–50% surface area; intraparenchymal <5 cm diameter
	Laceration	Capsular tear, 1–3 cm parenchymal depth that does not involve a trabecular vessel
III	Hematoma	Subcapsular, >50% surface area of expanding; ruptured subcapsular or parenchymal hematoma; intraparenchymal hematoma ≥5 cm or expanding
	Laceration	>3 cm parenchymal depth or involving a trabecular vessel
IV	Laceration	Laceration involving segmental or hilar vessels producing major devascularization (>25% of spleen)
V	Laceration	Completely shattered spleen
	Vascular	Hilar vascular injury with spleen devascularization

From Moore EE, Cogbill TH, Jurkovich GJ, et al. Organ injury scaling: spleen and liver (1994 revision). J Trauma 1995;38(3):323–4; with permission.

Outcomes, such as hospital length of stay, were then correlated with injury severity, and this led to evidence-based management strategies encouraging NOM.[11] The initial approach using hemodynamic status increasingly seemed to accurately determine which patients needed operation and which patients could undergo successful NOM.[5,12,13] This evolution continued as increased data demonstrated satisfactory outcomes for NOM even in high-grade injuries (**Fig. 1**). With the increasing evidence, NOM of SOI in pediatric trauma is achievable in a very high percentage of patients. This article reviews the nonoperative approach and the research supporting it.

Table 2		
Organ injury scale for liver injuries		
Grade	**Injury Type**	**Description of Injury**
I	Hematoma	Subcapsular, <10% surface area
	Laceration	Capsular tear, <1 cm, parenchymal depth
II	Hematoma	Subcapsular, 10% to 50% surface area, intraparenchymal <10 cm in diameter
	Laceration	Capsular tear 1–3 cm parenchymal depth, <10 cm in length
III	Hematoma	Subcapsular, >50% surface area of ruptured subcapsular or parenchymal hematoma; intraparenchymal hematoma >10 cm or expanding
	Laceration	>3 cm parenchymal depth
IV	Laceration	Parenchymal disruption involving 25% to 75% hepatic lobe or 1–3 Couinaud segments
V	Laceration	Parenchymal disruption involving >75% of hepatic lobe or >3 Couinaud segments within a single lobe
	Vascular	Juxtahepatic venous injuries; that is, retrohepatic vena cava or central major hepatic veins
VI	Vascular	Hepatic avulsion

From Moore EE, Cogbill TH, Jurkovich GJ, et al. Organ injury scaling: spleen and liver (1994 revision). J Trauma 1995;38(3):323–4; with permission.

Table 3
Organ injury scale for renal injuries

Grade	Injury Type	Description of Injury
I	Contusion	Microscopic or gross hematuria, urologic studies normal
	Hematoma	Subcapsular, nonexpanding without parenchymal laceration
II	Hematoma	Nonexpanding perirenal hematoma confined to renal retroperitoneum
	Laceration	<1.0 cm parenchymal depth of renal cortex without urinary extravasation
III	Laceration	>1.0 cm parenchymal depth of renal cortex without collecting system rupture or urinary extravasation
IV	Laceration	Parenchymal laceration extending through renal cortex, medulla, and collecting system
	Vascular	Main renal artery or vein injury with contained hemorrhage
V	Laceration	Completely shattered kidney
	Vascular	Avulsion of renal hilum with kidney devascularization

From Moore EE, Shackford SR, Pachter HL, et al. Organ injury scaling: spleen, liver, and kidney. J Trauma 1989;29(12):1664–6; with permission.

MANAGEMENT ALGORITHM FOR BLUNT SPLEEN AND LIVER INJURY

For trauma patients, treatment begins before diagnosis.[14] The critical principles of trauma and resuscitation—airway, breathing, and circulation—remain a priority regardless of injury or mechanism. In children, however, the evaluation and management of circulation presents unique challenges. Children in shock may not be hypotensive, and hypotension in a child may not indicate hypovolemic shock.[15,16] Unlike in the adult trauma population, hypotension secondary to isolated head injury in children occurs with nearly the same frequency as hypotension secondary to hemorrhage.[16,17]

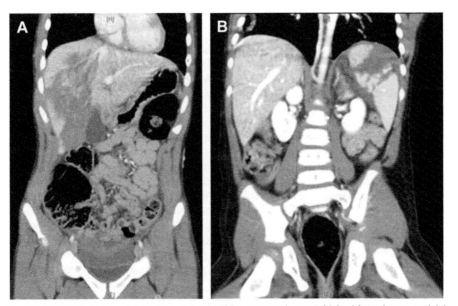

Fig. 1. (*A*) Grade V liver injury in a 13-year-old patient who was kicked by a horse and (*B*) Grade IV splenic injury in a 2-year-old patient who was hit by an all-terrain vehicle. Both patients were managed nonoperatively.

Therefore, identifying children with shock due to SOI and hemorrhage remains a challenge and requires a degree of clinical judgment.[5]

Management of Patients with Recent or Ongoing Bleeding

Management of pediatric blunt SOI is guided by clinical presentation (**Fig. 2**). Those with evidence of recent or ongoing bleeding are managed differently than those without signs of clinically significant bleeding.[5] Numerous prospective studies now support management based on hemodynamic status rather than severity of injury on CT.[13,18–20] For patients demonstrating hemodynamic instability, an initial attempt is made to achieve normotension with up to 20 mL/kg of isotonic fluid, followed by transfusion of blood.[5,20,21]

Patients who are nonresponsive to initial resuscitation

For children who do not stabilize after transfusion, care must be individualized based on the patient's identified injuries, and the resources available at the treating facility. These children cannot be managed through an algorithmic guideline. The clinician is then put into a very challenging position: managing the unstable injured child. Ongoing resuscitation with blood, plasma, and platelets in a 1:1:1 ratio should be undertaken. Crystalloid should be limited and a massive transfusion protocol should be instituted as soon as possible.[20] Tranexamic acid is also recommended as a component of the massive transfusion protocol.[22]

Options for intervention depend on local resources, identified injuries, and the geographic relationship of the trauma department, radiology department, and operating room; essentially, the child requires the resources of all 3 places at the same time. Absent these resources, operative exploration remains the default choice. Focused Abdominal Sonography in Trauma (FAST) may identify those benefiting from laparotomy; however, its lack of sensitivity and specificity, along with the addition of concomitant injuries, means clinical judgment remains a critical element of management.[23–27] More recently, minimally invasive techniques have been used, such as angioembolization (AE) (see later discussion).

Patients who are responsive to initial resuscitation

If the child responds to initial resuscitation fluids, imaging with CT allows an expeditious evaluation of the head, spinal cord, pelvic and abdominal injuries as indicated. The abdominal CT should be performed with intravenous (IV) contrast only. Once injuries are identified, management is contingent on a sustained response to the initial resuscitation. Those children with hemorrhage who develop a second episode of early hypotension are at high risk of death and intervention (operative or angiographic) should strongly be considered.[6,16]

Those who stabilize after clinically significant hypovolemia should be admitted to a pediatric-capable intensive care unit (ICU) or transferred to a facility with a pediatric ICU. Continuous hemodynamic monitoring is essential for these patients because a small portion of children with SOI will continue to bleed, and some of the early delayed bleeds (less than 48 hours after injury), may actually represent failure to identify continued bleeding.[15,28] Several studies, including a systematic review, suggest a transfusion threshold for a hemoglobin of 7.0 g/dL is safe and reasonable in injured children.[5,19,29] See later discussion of the role of frequent hemoglobin monitoring.

Defining failure

No published prospective studies have identified a maximum transfusion volume at which children fail NOM; however, significant consensus studies suggest that 40 mL/kg is a reasonable breakpoint at which failure of NOM is more likely.[30] In a

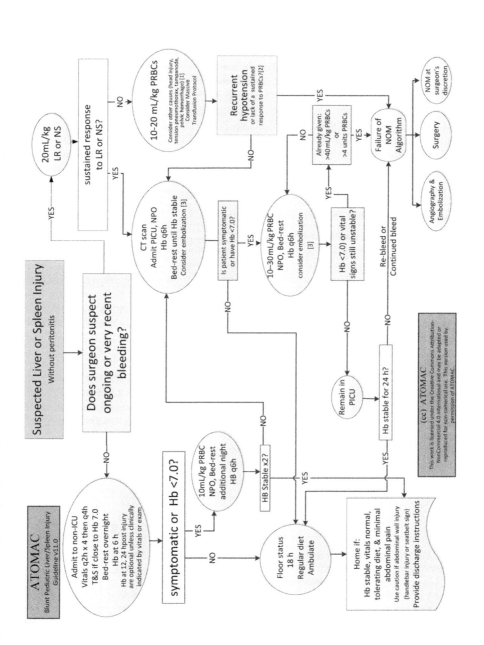

ATOMAC
Blunt Pediatric Liver/Spleen Injury
Guideline v11.0

Suspected Liver or Spleen Injury
Without peritonitis

Does surgeon suspect ongoing or very recent bleeding?

20mL/kg LR or NS

sustained response to LR or NS?

10-20 mL/kg PRBCs
Consider other causes (head injury, tension pneumothorax, tamponade, pelvic hemorrhage) [1]
Consider Massive Transfusion Protocol

Recurrent hypotension
or lack of a sustained response to PRBCs?[2]

CT scan
Admit PICU, NPO
Hb q6h
Bed-rest until Hb stable
Consider embolization [3]

Is patient symptomatic or have Hb <7.0?

10-30mL/kg PRBC
NPO, Bed-rest
Hb q6h
consider embolization [3]

Hb <7.0) or vital signs still unstable?

Already given:
>40 mL/kg PRBCs
or
>4 units PRBCs

Failure of NOM Algorithm

NOM at surgeon's discretion

Surgery

Angiography & Embolization

Remain in PICU

Re-bleed or Continued bleed

Hb stable for 24 h?

Admit to non-ICU
Vitals q2h x 4 then q4h
T&S if close to Hb 7.0
Bed-rest overnight
Hb at 6 h
Hb at 12, 24 hpost injury are optional unless clinically indicated by vitals or exam.

symptomatic or Hb <7.0?

10mL/kg PRBC
NPO, Bed-rest
additional night
HB q6h

HB Stable x2?

Floor status
18 h
Regular diet
Ambulate

Home if:
Hb stable, vitals normal, tolerating diet, & minimal abdominal pain
Use caution if abdominal wall injury (handlebar injury or seatbelt sign)
Provide discharge instructions

retrospective study from the US military regarding management of children injured in a combat zone, the investigators noted that a transfusion volume of 40 mL/kg of all blood products was associated with a significantly increased risk of death.[31] This threshold for failure was incorporated into recent treatment guidelines.[5,15]

Abbreviated hospital length of stay after bleeding

The previous American Pediatric Surgery Association (APSA) guideline from 2000 recommended the length of hospitalization following blunt SOI be equal to the radiographic grade of injury +1 (in days).[11] More recent data suggest very few children who stop bleeding will rebleed during this period.[5,15,28] In the current management algorithm, once the patient's hemoglobin has stabilized for 24 hours, the patient may leave the ICU. The following day, the child may be safely discharged if they have stable vital signs, minimal abdominal pain, and can tolerate a regular diet. Because a very small number of children (<0.3%) will rebleed and the median time to rebleeding is 10 days postinjury, specific discharge instructions and parental education are important (**Fig. 3**).[5,28]

Management of Stable Patients with Solid Organ Injury

Defining stable in a pediatric trauma patient presents challenges. Most surgeons can identify a stable patient when they see one; however, defining this is difficult. No single clinical parameter or test has perfect discrimination for identifying a child at risk of needing a blood transfusion or operation.[32] As previously noted, many children who are bleeding remain stable, whereas nearly half of those who are unstable are actually not bleeding.[5] In general, however, it seems that surgeon determination that a child has not bled recently seems to be accurate enough to guide therapy.[15]

Level of care

Ideally, ICU utilization should be reserved for children who require intervention or transfusion. Hemodynamic status, admission hemoglobin, and a pediatric-adjusted shock index at admission have shown some ability to discriminate children who need interventions.[5,19,33] In the recently published Arizona-Texas-Oklahoma-Memphis-Arkansas Consortium (ATOMAC) guideline, patients without clinical signs of recent or ongoing bleeding may be admitted to a non-ICU setting regardless of injury grade.[5] Many patients with low-grade SOI fit into this model. This is in contrast to previous decades in which CT injury grade determined the level of care for children; those with SOI grade IV or higher injuries were admitted to an ICU, resulting in

---

Fig. 2. ATOMAC guideline for management of pediatric BLSI. [1]More than 50% of injured children with hypotension have no significant intra-abdominal bleeding but do have severe traumatic brain injury. [2]Recurrent hypotension within the first hour because of intra-abdominal bleeding or systolic blood pressure of less than 50 mm Hg after transfusion is an ominous sign, and strong consideration should be given to operative or angiographic intervention. [3]Embolization of a CT contrast extravasation may be considered, but more than 80% of children with contrast extravasation do not require angiography for successful NOM. [4]Interventional modalities such as ERCP, laparoscopy, angiography, or percutaneous drainage may be required to manage complications of bile leak or hemobilia. Hb, hemoglobin; NPO, "non per os" or nothing per mouth; PICU, pediatric ICU; PRBC, packed red blood cell; q6h, every 6 hours; SBP, systolic blood pressure. Licensed under Creative Commons Attribution NonCommercial 4.0 International. Used by permission of ATOMAC.

ATOMAC

Pediatric Trauma

ATOMAC Guideline Discharge Instructions

- Return to Emergency Room (ER) for increasing pain, paleness, dizziness, shortness of breath, vomiting, worsening shoulder pain, intestinal bleeding, or black tarry stools.
- Call trauma surgeon's office for fever (temp >101°F) or jaundice (yellow eyes, yellow skin)
- Restricted activity for (grade +2) weeks
    - Your child's injury grade was a grade _____ .
    - Your child may return to sports in _____ weeks.
- No ibuprofen (Motrin, etc), aspirin, or other NSAIDS. Acetaminophen (Tylenol) is okay.
- Child may go back to school when off pain meds, but no gym classes or sports.
- The patient is granted medical permission to change class 5 min early (to prevent re-injury between classes).
- Follow-up:
    - Grade 1–2 Injury: Phone call follow-up at 2 wk and again at 2 months after injury.
    - Grade 3–5 injury: Office visit at 2 wk. Phone call follow-up at 2 months after injury
- No routine follow-up imaging is required. Imaging is recommended for patients with increasing pain, or symptoms.

Your Surgeon's Name:_____ office telephone _____

I understand the above instructions. I understand there is a small, but important risk of bleeding up to several weeks after injury.

Guardian Name:_____

Guardian Signature:_____

Fig. 3. ATOMAC discharge instructions for blunt SOI in children.

unnecessary resource utilization without identifiable benefit in some series.[11,19,33] AAST's organ injury scales for liver, spleen, and kidney are shown in **Tables 1–3**. In clinical practice, grade V injuries without recent or ongoing bleeding at admission are rarely seen; however, given the small numbers and high failure rates of NOM, grade V patients may warrant ICU admission.[34]

Length of stay for patients without signs of significant bleeding
Despite the initial APSA guidelines recommending grade +1 in days of hospitalization for monitoring signs of rebleeding, the national data have shown a trend toward shorter hospitalization throughout the United States.[1] This has been supported by studies showing children with isolated low-grade injuries seem to be at very low risk of rebleeding. Discharge after a short period of hospitalization (less than 24 hours in some cases) seems safe in a selected population.[3,12,19] A recent literature review by the ATOMAC group also found that several prospective observational studies supported an abbreviated protocol for length of hospitalization and ultimately recommended that children without clinical signs of bleeding from SOI may be safely discharged after 24 hours of observation.[5]

Serial hemoglobin measurements
Once the stable patient is admitted, serial vital signs with clinical examination, initial hemoglobin, and pediatric-adjusted shock index seem to reliably identify the children in need of transfusion, obviating frequent serial hemoglobin rechecks.[18,32,35] Hemoglobin checks, therefore, can be performed as indicated by the patient's clinical parameters. Moreover, several studies now support either a single 6-hour postinjury hemoglobin or no serial hemoglobin checks after the initial value is obtained.[15,18,35]

FAILURE OF NONOPERATIVE MANAGEMENT IN SPLEEN AND LIVER INJURY: WHO, WHAT, WHEN, WHERE, WHY

Understanding the characteristics of failure of NOM can significantly improve outcome and also allows for better benchmarking between centers. Only 1 study thus far has looked at the characteristics and timing of failure of NOM in children with detail.[34]

Who Fails Nonoperative Management?

Very few children with blunt SOI fail NOM. Nationally, it is estimated that fewer than 400 children per year undergo splenectomy for trauma, with even fewer laparotomies for liver or kidney injury.[7,34] The splenic NOM failure rate in the early 2000s was around 15% but in a downward trend.[36] More recently, the prospective Pediatric Emergency Care Applied Research Network (PECARN) study published early in 2016 identified a splenectomy rate at children's hospitals of 7.4%, a laparotomy rate of 3.2% (5/157) for liver injuries and 0% for renal injuries.[7] In a retrospective study by Holmes and colleagues,[34] the rate of failure for NOM of isolated injuries at pediatric trauma centers was 3% for liver and kidney, each respectively, and 4% for spleen.

Risk factors for failure at pediatric trauma centers included higher Injury Severity Scale, lower Glasgow Coma Scale (GCS) at presentation, higher organ injury grade, and/or multiple organs injured. Isolated grade I or II isolated injuries have extremely low rates of failure.[7] In this same study, age did not seem to be a risk factor for failure at children's hospitals; however, older children are significantly more likely to fail according to national data.[34,36] Although few prospective studies look at the characteristics of those who fail NOM of blunt SOI, the authors are current participants in a large, multi-institutional study, and additional data should be available soon.

What Causes Failure of Nonoperative Management?

In the multicenter, retrospective study done at children's hospitals, hypovolemic shock or persistent hemorrhage accounted for 48% of failures. Another 42% failed for peritonitis or hollow visceral injury and 1% failed for a ruptured diaphragm.[34] In the PECARN data, hemorrhage was also the main cause of failure.[7]

When Do Children Fail Nonoperative Management?

In the rare event that an injured child fails NOM of SOI, the timing of failure seems to be early.[6] In the Holmes and colleagues[34] study, the median time to failure was 2 hours, with 76% of failures determined by 12 hours postinjury. This was also consistent with a large retrospective study using the Kids' Inpatient Database (KID), a national discharge dataset, which showed failure of NOM occurred within 48 hours postinjury in the overwhelming majority (85%) of children requiring splenectomy for blunt splenic injury in the United States.[37]

Where Do They Fail?

Failure of NOM occurs at different rates at different centers.[37] Another study using the KID demonstrated that most children suffering from traumatic injury are cared for at nonchildren's hospitals.[37] Comparative studies have suggested that the type of hospital affects the rate of failure, with not-for-profit hospitals and pediatric trauma centers more likely achieve NOM than other centers, even after adjusting for severity of injury and grade.[37–40] Bowman and colleagues[37] found that children cared for at nonpediatric general hospitals were 5 times more likely to undergo splenectomy than those cared for at a children's hospital.

Why Do Children Fail Nonoperative Management?

As previously discussed, hemorrhage is a common cause of failure. The difference in failure rates between centers may be related to differences in comfort level for continued NOM between general surgeons and pediatric surgeons, as well as familiarity with clinical practice guidelines.[41,42] In a survey sent to general surgeons and pediatric surgeons, there were clear differences in how different types of surgeons would handle identical scenarios.[41] Overall, general surgeons seem less likely to pursue NOM in pediatric patients. Implementation of a SOI pathway has been shown to improve NOM success.[43] In 1 state, the inclusion of a pediatric trauma center within a statewide trauma system was temporarily associated with a significant decrease in NOM failure rates; this finding was consistent with other data showing the impact of pediatric trauma centers on a statewide level.[44,45] As more children's hospitals become verified trauma centers,[46] a similar trend of increased NOM at all centers might be expected.

NONOPERATIVE MANAGEMENT OF BLUNT RENAL TRAUMA

The management of blunt renal injury has evolved similarly to liver and spleen injury, and high rates of NOM are now frequently reported.[4,6,34] Although randomized studies do not exist, strong prospective studies support NOM.[47,48] Conservative management for renal injury grades I through III is well-accepted. Operative intervention in low-grade renal injuries is mainly incidental to cases of surgical intervention for concomitant injuries.[49] For high-grade injuries, evidence is even less available but surgeons seem to have adopted NOM in high-grade renal injuries with successful outcomes.[50–56] The only evidence-based absolute indication for operative management is persistent hemodynamic instability.[47]

NOM of renal injury generally follows the same guidelines as liver or spleen injury but little evidence is available regarding recommendations for ICU, antibiotics, routine urinary catheter placement, or bedrest.[47,48] Prolonged bedrest contributes to increased length of hospitalization without demonstrated benefit.[4] A prospective series of blunt renal injury subjects treated without strict bedrest did not demonstrate a negative impact on subject outcomes and resulted in shortened hospitalizations.[4]

Children with High-Grade Renal Injuries

In a meta-analysis assessing NOM in grade IV renal injuries, 73% of subjects achieved NOM without any required intervention.[51] In this report, at least partial renal preservation was successful in 95% of subjects.[51] A systematic review by LeeVan and colleagues[47] reported NOM in grade IV and V renal injuries was 80% to 100% successful.

Factors associated with failure of NOM include collecting duct system hematoma, increased urinoma size, interpolar extravasation, and dissociated renal fragments.[57] Lacerations to the anteromedial or medial portion of the kidney have also been associated with an increased need for urologic intervention.[58,59] The study investigators hypothesize laceration in this area is related to the pliability of the overlying peritoneum resulting in increased capability of urinoma expansion.[58] Large perinephric hematoma, intravascular contrast extravasation (CE), and increased transfusion requirement were also associated with higher rates of required intervention in those with attempted NOM.

Adjunctive procedures, such as stenting, percutaneous drainage, and AE, may assist in avoiding laparotomy.[7,47] Transcatheter arterial embolization has been advocated as a first step in management of active renal bleeding to maximally preserve parenchyma and renal function.[60]

CONTRAST EXTRAVASATION AND ANGIOEMBOLIZATION
Angioembolization for Splenic Injury

With improved CT scanning, active CE was identified as a defined entity, and initially associated with failure of NOM.[61,62] In the adult population, the treatment of CE with AE revolutionized management; however, in the pediatric population, NOM had already become so successful that the significance of CE was questioned.[63-66] CE is seen in approximately 5% to 15% of children with splenic injury usually in the high-grade injuries.[65-67] Most children with CE related to splenic injury do not need AE.[65,66] Evidence suggests the decision for AE should be based on physiologic response and/or reserved for those children who are otherwise failing NOM.[68-71]

Angioembolization for Liver Injury

Unlike AE for splenic injury, only a handful of cases of pediatric hepatic artery embolization have been reported.[72,73] Very few liver injuries demonstrate CE and these are mainly high-grade injuries.[74] AE may be beneficial in appropriately selected cases of bleeding.

Angioembolization for Renal Injury

AE for bleeding from renal injury (**Fig. 4**) is generally accepted and is associated with improved success of NOM[48] and subsequent decreased morbidity. Indications for AE in the setting of blunt renal injury include continued clinically significant bleeding.[75,76]

SPECIAL SITUATIONS
Spleen

Splenic artery pseudoaneurysm

Splenic artery pseudoaneurysms result from blunt abdominal trauma in approximately 5% to 9% of splenic injuries, with an increased incidence in high-grade injuries.[67,77] Symptoms typically include abdominal pain followed by hematochezia or hemetemesis.[78] Additional symptoms may include back pain, chest pain, or nausea.[78] Unless diagnosed at initial CT scan, splenic artery pseudoaneurysm is most commonly identified on reimaging for symptoms.[77] AE may be beneficial in the setting of symptoms, with AE successful in more than 85% of cases.[78] In research studies identifying

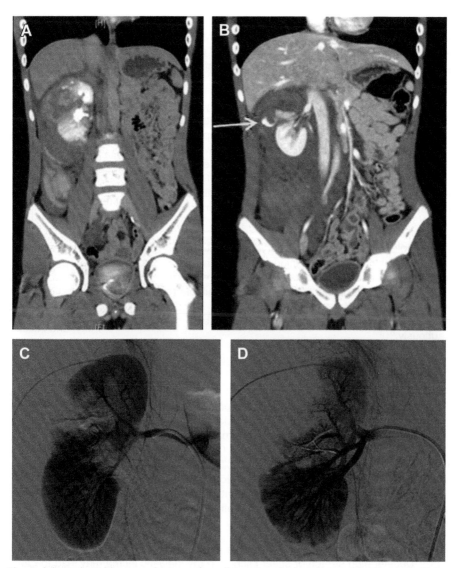

Fig. 4. (*A*) Grade IV blunt renal injury after all-terrain vehicle collision. (*B*) CT reveals CE (*arrow*). (*C*) Angiography confirming active extravasation. (*D*) Renal vasculature after angiographic embolization.

asymptomatic splenic artery pseudoaneurysms, 89% of cases underwent spontaneous thrombosis, thus supporting a selective approach to reimaging.

Liver

Biloma

Biloma after blunt hepatic trauma is an uncommon occurrence in the pediatric literature, seen in approximately 2% of retrospective studies.[79] Patients may present with increasing abdominal pain, poor feeding tolerance, and elevated liver function tests after a history of blunt abdominal trauma.[79] Most of these cases are managed with percutaneous drainage and bile duct stenting via endoscopic retrograde cholangio-pancreatography (ERCP).[80] In patients who require surgery for another indication, laparoscopic drainage or open drainage may also be performed.[81] Antibiotics may also be required after drainage in the case of infection from bacterial dissemination.[81]

Major bile duct injury

Few series have identified major bile duct injury after SOI; however, a recent study of ERCP in pediatric trauma identified 2 patients with major duct injuries who were managed with stenting and percutaneous or laparoscopic drainage on a semielective basis.[80] Many major duct injuries in the past were probably bilomas that underwent drainage or hepatorrhaphy without specific identification of the duct injury by magnetic resonance cholangiopancreatography (MRCP) or ERCP. Infrequent ductal imaging has contributed to the relative paucity of literature surrounding this topic. Direct operative management is rarely required to control bile leaks.

Hepatic artery pseudoaneurysm

Unlike splenic artery pseudoaneurysm, hepatic artery pseudoaneurysms are rare, occurring only in high-grade injuries (IV or higher).[67] These pseudoaneurysms seem less likely to undergo spontaneous thrombosis and may be at a higher risk of bleeding.[82] Unfortunately, limited data are available to make recommendations.[83] In these situations, AE has been recommended by some investigators; however, this recommendation is based on very small numbers of subjects and should be taken cautiously.[67,83]

Kidney

Renal artery pseudoaneurysms

Traumatic creation of a pseudoaneurysm of the main renal artery can occur in high-grade blunt renal injuries although less frequently than in penetrating renal injuries. Patients may present after a history of blunt renal trauma with hematuria, hypertension, or abdominal pain with or without a mass. Conservative attempts with interventional radiologic techniques, such as AE and coiling, should be attempted first and have been successful in small reports.[50,84] Surgical intervention may be required if the patient is hemodynamically unstable at presentation or if AE is unsuccessful. This should be of rare occurrence with the modern proficiency of interventional radiologists.

Renal artery thrombosis

Traumatic renal artery thrombosis is a rare event, especially in the pediatric population.[85] Deceleration stretch or sheer injuries to the inelastic intima may lead to damage, followed by impaired flow and thrombus formation.[85] Injuries are typically identified on contrast-enhanced CT scan, with nonopacification of the effected kidney. Complete arterial thrombus formation leads to renal ischemia and operative repair has historically had a low success rate, even when surgically patent and done as early as within 5 hours.[85] NOM has been advocated by some investigators, particularly before the availability of catheter-based therapy.[85]

Currently, minimally invasive techniques, such as arterial thrombolysis and stenting, in the case of renal artery occlusion may be used. These provide benefits of avoiding laparotomy and potentially restoring flow more quickly. In addition, some reports of successful catheter-based reestablishment of flow well after injury have also been published.[86] Additional considerations should include the presence of other abdominal or nonabdominal injuries that may preclude the ability to anticoagulate after stent placement, further complicating management. Suction and aspiration of thrombus have been also described.[87] If interventional radiology techniques are unsuccessful, operative revascularization may be performed; however, success rates are typically low.

Urinoma

High-grade renal injuries may be associated with progressive urinoma, often with ongoing hematuria. Management of persistent or increasing urinoma is controversial, often because the injuries are concerning for ureteropelvic junction disruption. Symptomatic urinoma occurs in approximately 17% of patients with a high-grade renal injury.[51] However, more than three-fourths of these patients can be managed with percutaneous drainage of the urinoma and cystoscopic placement of ureteral stents.[7,50–53,88] Operative intervention is not as well supported by evidence in the literature; however, rarely, surgical pyeloplasty may be required.

CONCOMITANT INJURIES
Blunt Intestinal Injury

Blunt intestinal injury led to laparotomy almost as often as bleeding in the Holmes and colleagues[34] multicenter prospective study. One of the initial concerns with endorsing NOM of SOI included missing intestinal injury.[89] However, Bensard and colleagues,[90] and later Letton and colleagues,[91] showed that reasonable delays in identification of intestinal injury (up to 48 hours) were not associated with adverse outcomes, thus allowing time for clinical decision-making to determine the need for exploration.

Traumatic Brain Injury

Concomitant traumatic brain injury (TBI) complicates NOM.[34] As noted previously, children may become hypotensive due to TBI without significant hemorrhage, and failure of NOM is clearly associated with decreasing GCS.[16,34] However, the interaction between the 2 factors is unclear at best. Hemodynamic instability worsens brain outcome in TBI, so less tolerance for bleeding causing instability may be a prudent course.[92] In the absence of such bleeding, however, there is no evidence to suggest patients with TBI and SOI cannot undergo successful NOM of their abdominal injuries.[5,15]

Pelvic Fracture in Unstable Children

The relative contribution of a pelvic fracture to hemodynamic instability is difficult to ascertain in pediatric trauma. Most pelvic fractures in younger children are not associated with significant bleeding. In older children, significant bleeding may occur. In these cases, fracture geometry may help predict bleeding.[93] In rare cases with significant pelvic fractures, children may fail NOM of their SOI at presentation because they are too unstable for CT and a positive FAST examination suggests SOI bleeding. Clinical judgment is important to limit the frequency of minimally therapeutic laparotomy; however, some cases still seem to be unavoidable.[7]

Pancreatic Injury

NOM of pancreatic injury is complicated and controversial.[6,94] In cases of major duct transection requiring surgery for the pancreas, splenorrhaphy or hepatorrhaphy may be required to reduce bleeding in an injury that might have otherwise ceased spontaneously. The presence of a minor, nonoperative pancreatic injury should not preclude NOM of other injuries, nor should minor SOI preclude necessary pancreatic surgery.

DISCHARGE AND FOLLOW-UP CARE
Activity Restriction

The APSA guidelines recommend activity restriction equal to the grade of injury +2 in weeks. No evidence is available to support or refute this recommendation, which continues to be in general use currently. However, nothing in the original recommendations would prevent return to school on hospital discharge, and many centers now allow return to school on hospital discharge. However, the child may not participate in gym class, competitive sports, activities with wheels, or any activities in which both feet leave the ground at the same time.

Reimaging After Liver or Spleen Injury

Since the original APSA guideline, no routine imaging is recommended for blunt liver or spleen injury. For children who develop symptoms such as dizziness, lightheadedness, jaundice, or increasing abdominal or shoulder pain, reimaging with ultrasound may be prudent.[5]

Reimaging After Renal Injury

Unlike liver and spleen injuries, adjunctive studies in the follow-up period after severe renal injury may be used to determine renal function and to document complete healing.[58] An assessment of renal function using technetium-99m dimercaptosuccinic acid scan (DMSA) may be used in the early postinjury period and at long-term follow-up; however, there are limited data in its current application and, therefore, it is not strongly recommended.[48] Some centers have elected to perform follow-up ultrasound on injuries involving the collecting duct or resulting in urinoma, although low-grade injuries involving only the parenchyma may not require any repeat imaging.[48] There does not seem to be a strong consensus on imaging because other reports recommend routine follow-up with ultrasound at 3 months postinjury or CT or MRI as well.[95] Regardless, the consensus seems to be consistent that postinjury imaging of some sort should be used around the 3-month period to document healing in severe injuries.[95]

Follow-up

In clinical practice, many children with low-grade injuries do not follow-up in a surgery or trauma clinic. The ATOMAC guideline recommends a telephone call follow-up for low-grade injuries, and an office follow-up for grade III or higher injuries.[5] A telephone call follow-up at 2 months may be prudent; however, it is unlikely to detect clinically significant problems.

After renal injury, most patients successfully managed with NOM do well without long-term sequelae.[96,97] Postinjury hypertension after nonvascular injury seems to be very rare in the pediatric population. In follow-up studies, the risk of long-term complications seems to be correlated with increased grade of injury and is not significantly different from early functional outcomes.[98]

SUMMARY

Overall, NOM of blunt SOI in children is highly successful. With the increasing wealth of evidence supporting NOM, several important changes have occurred. These include adoption of standardized treatment algorithms, shortened hospitalization in stable patients, management based on hemodynamic status at admission rather than CT grade of injury, and overall decreased resource utilization for these patients.

REFERENCES

1. Dodgion CM, Gosain A, Rogers A, et al. National trends in pediatric blunt spleen and liver injury management and potential benefits of an abbreviated bed rest protocol. J Pediatr Surg 2014;49(6):1004–8.
2. CDC WISQARS Nonfatal. Available at: http://webappa.cdc.gov/sasweb/ncipc/nfirates2001.html. Accessed April 28, 2016.
3. St Peter SD, Sharp SW, Snyder CL, et al. Prospective validation of an abbreviated bedrest protocol in the management of blunt spleen and liver injury in children. J Pediatr Surg 2011;46(1):173–7.
4. Graziano KD, Juang D, Notrica D, et al. Prospective observational study with an abbreviated protocol in the management of blunt renal injury in children. J Pediatr Surg 2014;49(1):198–200 [discussion: 200–1].
5. Notrica DM, Eubanks JW 3rd, Tuggle DW, et al. Nonoperative management of blunt liver and spleen injury in children: Evaluation of the ATOMAC guideline using GRADE. J Trauma Acute Care Surg 2015;79(4):683–93.
6. Notrica DM. Pediatric blunt abdominal trauma: current management. Curr Opin Crit Care 2015;21(6):531–7.
7. Wisner DH, Kuppermann N, Cooper A, et al. Management of children with solid organ injuries after blunt torso trauma. J Trauma Acute Care Surg 2015;79(2):206–14.
8. Davies DA, Pearl RH, Ein SH, et al. Management of blunt splenic injury in children: evolution of the nonoperative approach. J Pediatr Surg 2009;44(5):1005–8.
9. Aronson DZ, Scherz AW, Einhorn AH, et al. Nonoperative management of splenic trauma in children: a report of six consecutive cases. Pediatrics 1977;60(4):482–5.
10. Moore E, Shackford S, Pachter H, et al. Organ injury scaling: spleen, liver, and kidney. J Trauma 1989;29(12):1664–6.
11. Stylianos S. Evidence-based guidelines for resource utilization in children with isolated spleen or liver injury. The APSA Trauma Committee. J Pediatr Surg 2000;35(2):164–7 [discussion: 167–9].
12. Mehall JR, Ennis JS, Saltzman DA, et al. Prospective results of a standardized algorithm based on hemodynamic status for managing pediatric solid organ injury. J Am Coll Surg 2001;193(4):347–53.
13. St Peter SD, Aguayo P, Juang D, et al. Follow up of prospective validation of an abbreviated bedrest protocol in the management of blunt spleen and liver injury in children. J Pediatr Surg 2013;48(12):2437–41.
14. Advanced Trauma Life Support for Doctors (ATLS). 8th edition. Chicago (IL): American College of Surgeons; 2008.
15. Notrica DM. Pediatric Blunt Solid Organ Injury: Beyond the APSA Guidelines. Curr Surg Rep 2015;3(4):1–6.
16. Partrick DA, Bensard DD, Janik JS, et al. Is hypotension a reliable indicator of blood loss from traumatic injury in children? Am J Surg 2002;184(6):555–9 [discussion: 559–60].
17. Gardner AR, Diz DI, Tooze JA, et al. Injury patterns associated with hypotension in pediatric trauma patients: a national trauma database review. J Trauma Acute Care Surg 2015;78(6):1143–8.
18. Golden J, Dossa A, Goodhue CJ, et al. Admission hematocrit predicts the need for transfusion secondary to hemorrhage in pediatric blunt trauma patients. J Trauma Acute Care Surg 2015;79(4):555–62.

19. McVay M, Kokoska E, Jackson R, et al. Throwing out the "grade" book: management of isolated spleen and liver injury based on hemodynamic status. J Pediatr Surg 2008;43(6):1072–6.

20. Duchesne JC, Heaney J, Guidry C, et al. Diluting the benefits of hemostatic resuscitation: a multi-institutional analysis. J Trauma Acute Care Surg 2013; 75(1):76–82.

21. Acker SN, Ross JT, Partrick DA, et al. Injured children are resistant to the adverse effects of early high volume crystalloid resuscitation. J Pediatr Surg 2014;49(12): 1852–5.

22. Eckert MJ, Wertin TM, Tyner SD, et al. Tranexamic acid administration to pediatric trauma patients in a combat setting: the pediatric trauma and tranexamic acid study (PED-TRAX). J Trauma Acute Care Surg 2014;77(6):852–8 [discussion: 858].

23. Soundappan SV, Holland AJ, Cass DT, et al. Diagnostic accuracy of surgeon-performed focused abdominal sonography (FAST) in blunt paediatric trauma. Injury 2005;36(8):970–5.

24. Scaife ER, Rollins MD, Barnhart DC, et al. The role of focused abdominal sonography for trauma (FAST) in pediatric trauma evaluation. J Pediatr Surg 2013; 48(6):1377–83.

25. Ben-Ishay O, Daoud M, Peled Z, et al. Focused abdominal sonography for trauma in the clinical evaluation of children with blunt abdominal trauma. World J Emerg Surg 2015;10:27.

26. Schonfeld D, Lee LK. Blunt abdominal trauma in children. Curr Opin Pediatr 2012;24(3):314–8.

27. Carter JW, Falco MH, Chopko MS, et al. Do we really rely on fast for decision-making in the management of blunt abdominal trauma? Injury 2015;46(5):817–21.

28. Davies DA, Fecteau A, Himidan S, et al. What's the incidence of delayed splenic bleeding in children after blunt trauma? An institutional experience and review of the literature. J Trauma 2009;67(3):573–7.

29. Lacroix J, Hebert PC, Hutchison JS, et al. Transfusion strategies for patients in pediatric intensive care units. N Engl J Med 2007;356(16):1609–19.

30. Olthof DC, van der Vlies CH, Joosse P, et al. Consensus strategies for the nonoperative management of patients with blunt splenic injury: A Delphi study. J Trauma Acute Care Surg 2013;74(6):1567–74.

31. Neff LP, Cannon JW, Morrison JJ, et al. Clearly defining pediatric massive transfusion: Cutting through the fog and friction with combat data. J Trauma Acute Care Surg 2015;78(1):22–9.

32. Acker SN, Ross JT, Partrick DA, et al. Pediatric specific shock index accurately identifies severely injured children. J Pediatr Surg 2015;50(2):331–4.

33. Fremgen HE, Bratton SL, Metzger RR, et al. Pediatric liver lacerations and intensive care: evaluation of ICU triage strategies. Pediatr Crit Care Med 2014;15(4): e183–91.

34. Holmes JH, Wiebe DJ, Tataria M, et al. The failure of nonoperative management in pediatric solid organ injury: a multi-institutional experience. J Trauma 2005;59(6): 1309–13.

35. Golden J, Mitchell I, Kuzniewski S, et al. Reducing scheduled phlebotomy in stable pediatric patients with blunt liver or spleen injury. J Pediatr Surg 2014;49(5): 759–62.

36. Bowman SM, Zimmerman FJ, Christakis DA, et al. The role of hospital profit status in pediatric spleen injury management. Med Care 2008;46(3):331–8.

37. Bowman SM, Zimmerman FJ, Christakis DA, et al. Hospital characteristics associated with the management of pediatric splenic injuries. JAMA 2005;294(20): 2611–7.
38. Liu S, Bowman SM, Smith TC, et al. Trends in pediatric spleen management: Do hospital type and ownership still matter? J Trauma Acute Care Surg 2015;78(5):935–42.
39. Densmore J, Lim H, Oldham K, et al. Outcomes and delivery of care in pediatric injury. J Pediatr Surg 2006;41(1):92–8.
40. Safavi A, Skarsgard ED, Rhee P, et al. Trauma center variation in the management of pediatric patients with blunt abdominal solid organ injury: a national trauma data bank analysis. J Pediatr Surg 2016;51(3):499–502.
41. Sims CA, Wiebe DJ, Nance ML. Blunt solid organ injury: do adult and pediatric surgeons treat children differently? J Trauma 2008;65(3):698–703.
42. Bowman SM, Bulger E, Sharar SR, et al. Variability in pediatric splenic injury care: results of a national survey of general surgeons. Arch Surg 2010;145(11): 1048–53.
43. Dervan LA, King MA, Cuschieri J, et al. Pediatric solid organ injury operative interventions and outcomes at Harborview Medical Center, before and after introduction of a solid organ injury pathway for pediatrics. J Trauma Acute Care Surg 2015;79(2):215–20.
44. Notrica DM, Weiss J, Garcia-Filion P, et al. Pediatric trauma centers: correlation of ACS-verified trauma centers with CDC statewide pediatric mortality rates. J Trauma Acute Care Surg 2012;73(3):566–70 [discussion: 570–62].
45. Murphy EE, Murphy SG, Cipolle MD, et al. The pediatric trauma center and the inclusive trauma system: Impact on splenectomy rates. J Trauma Acute Care Surg 2015;78(5):930–3 [discussion: 933–4].
46. Johnson KN, Harte M, Garcia-Filion P, et al. Fate of the combined adult and pediatric trauma centers: impact of increased pediatric trauma requirements. Am Surg 2014;80(12):1280–2.
47. LeeVan E, Zmora O, Cazzulino F, et al. Management of pediatric blunt renal trauma: A systematic review. J Trauma Acute Care Surg 2016;80(3):519–28.
48. Fraser JD, Aguayo P, Ostlie DJ, et al. Review of the evidence on the management of blunt renal trauma in pediatric patients. Pediatr Surg Int 2009;25(2):125–32.
49. Nance ML, Lutz N, Carr MC, et al. Blunt renal injuries in children can be managed nonoperatively: outcome in a consecutive series of patients. J Trauma 2004; 57(3):474–8 [discussion: 478].
50. Eassa W, El-Ghar MA, Jednak R, et al. Nonoperative management of grade 5 renal injury in children: does it have a place? Eur Urol 2010;57(1):154–61.
51. Umbreit EC, Routh JC, Husmann DA. Nonoperative management of nonvascular grade IV blunt renal trauma in children: meta-analysis and systematic review. Urology 2009;74(3):579–82.
52. Salem HK, Morsi HA, Zakaria A. Management of high-grade renal injuries in children after blunt abdominal trauma: experience of 40 cases. J Pediatr Urol 2007; 3(3):223–9.
53. Russell RS, Gomelsky A, McMahon DR, et al. Management of grade IV renal injury in children. J Urol 2001;166(3):1049–50.
54. Rogers CG, Knight V, MacUra KJ, et al. High-grade renal injuries in children–is conservative management possible? Urology 2004;64(3):574–9.
55. Okur MH, Arslan S, Aydogdu B, et al. Management of high-grade renal injury in children. Eur J Trauma Emerg Surg 2016. [Epub ahead of print].
56. Mohamed AZ, Morsi HA, Ziada AM, et al. Management of major blunt pediatric renal trauma: single-center experience. J Pediatr Urol 2010;6(3):301–5.

57. Reese JN, Fox JA, Cannon GM Jr, et al. Timing and predictors for urinary drainage in children with expectantly managed grade IV renal trauma. J Urol 2014;192(2):512–7.
58. Lee JN, Lim JK, Woo MJ, et al. Predictive factors for conservative treatment failure in grade IV pediatric blunt renal trauma. J Pediatr Urol 2016;12(2)(93):e91–7.
59. Bartley JM, Santucci RA. Computed tomography findings in patients with pediatric blunt renal trauma in whom expectant (nonoperative) management failed. Urology 2012;80(6):1338–43.
60. Lin WC, Lin CH. The role of interventional radiology for pediatric blunt renal trauma. Ital J Pediatr 2015;41:76.
61. Schurr MJ, Fabian TC, Gavant M, et al. Management of blunt splenic trauma: computed tomographic contrast blush predicts failure of nonoperative management. J Trauma 1995;39(3):507–12 [discussion: 512–3].
62. Alarhayem AQ, Myers JG, Dent D, et al. "Blush at first sight": significance of computed tomographic and angiographic discrepancy in patients with blunt abdominal trauma. Am J Surg 2015;210(6):1104–10 [discussion: 1110–1].
63. Nwomeh BC, Nadler EP, Meza MP, et al. Contrast extravasation predicts the need for operative intervention in children with blunt splenic trauma. J Trauma 2004; 56(3):537–41.
64. Davis KA, Fabian TC, Croce MA, et al. Improved success in nonoperative management of blunt splenic injuries: embolization of splenic artery pseudoaneurysms. J Trauma 1998;44(6):1008–13 [discussion: 1013–5].
65. Eubanks JW 3rd, Meier DE, Hicks BA, et al. Significance of 'blush' on computed tomography scan in children with liver injury. J Pediatr Surg 2003;38(3):363–6 [discussion: 363–6].
66. Davies DA, Ein SH, Pearl R, et al. What is the significance of contrast "blush" in pediatric blunt splenic trauma? J Pediatr Surg 2010;45(5):916–20.
67. Safavi A, Beaudry P, Jamieson D, et al. Traumatic pseudoaneurysms of the liver and spleen in children: is routine screening warranted? J Pediatr Surg 2011; 46(5):938–41.
68. Bansal S, Karrer FM, Hansen K, et al. Contrast blush in pediatric blunt splenic trauma does not warrant the routine use of angiography and embolization. Am J Surg 2015;210(2):345–50.
69. Lutz N, Mahboubi S, Nance ML, et al. The significance of contrast blush on computed tomography in children with splenic injuries. J Pediatr Surg 2004; 39(3):491–4.
70. van der Vlies CH, Saltzherr TP, Wilde JC, et al. The failure rate of nonoperative management in children with splenic or liver injury with contrast blush on computed tomography: a systematic review. J Pediatr Surg 2010;45(5):1044–9.
71. Gross JL, Woll NL, Hanson CA, et al. Embolization for pediatric blunt splenic injury is an alternative to splenectomy when observation fails. J Trauma Acute Care Surg 2013;75(3):421–5.
72. Fallon SC, Coker MT, Hernandez JA, et al. Traumatic hepatic artery laceration managed by transarterial embolization in a pediatric patient. J Pediatr Surg 2013;48(5):E9–12.
73. Brunelle F, Maurage C, Lacombe A, et al. Emergency embolization in posttraumatic hemobilia in a child. J Pediatr Surg 1985;20(2):172–4.
74. Bertens KA, Vogt KN, Hernandez-Alejandro R, et al. Non-operative management of blunt hepatic trauma: does angioembolization have a major impact? Eur J Trauma Emerg Surg 2015;41(1):81–6.

75. Vo NJ, Althoen M, Hippe DS, et al. Pediatric abdominal and pelvic trauma: safety and efficacy of arterial embolization. J Vasc Interv Radiol 2014;25(2):215–20.
76. Stewart AF, Brewer ME Jr, Daley BJ, et al. Intermediate-term follow-up of patients treated with percutaneous embolization for grade 5 blunt renal trauma. J Trauma 2010;69(2):468–70.
77. Durkin N, Deganello A, Sellars ME, et al. Post-traumatic liver and splenic pseudoaneurysms in children: Diagnosis, management, and follow-up screening using contrast enhanced ultrasound (CEUS). J Pediatr Surg 2016;51(2):289–92.
78. Tessier DJ, Stone WM, Fowl RJ, et al. Clinical features and management of splenic artery pseudoaneurysm: case series and cumulative review of literature. J Vasc Surg 2003;38(5):969–74.
79. Giss SR, Dobrilovic N, Brown RL, et al. Complications of nonoperative management of pediatric blunt hepatic injury: Diagnosis, management, and outcomes. J Trauma 2006;61(2):334–9.
80. Garvey EM, Haakinson DJ, McOmber M, et al. Role of ERCP in pediatric blunt abdominal trauma: A case series at a level one pediatric trauma center. J Pediatr Surg 2015;50(2):335–8.
81. Soukup ES, Russell KW, Metzger R, et al. Treatment and outcome of traumatic biliary injuries in children. J Pediatr Surg 2014;49(2):345–8.
82. Saad DF, Gow KW, Redd D, et al. Renal artery pseudoaneurysm secondary to blunt trauma treated with microcoil embolization. J Pediatr Surg 2005;40(11):e65–7.
83. Ong CC, Toh L, Lo RH, et al. Primary hepatic artery embolization in pediatric blunt hepatic trauma. J Pediatr Surg 2012;47(12):2316–20.
84. Halachmi S, Chait P, Hodapp J, et al. Renal pseudoaneurysm after blunt renal trauma in a pediatric patient: management by angiographic embolization. Urology 2003;61(1):224.
85. Haas CA, Dinchman KH, Nasrallah PF, et al. Traumatic renal artery occlusion: a 15-year review. J Trauma 1998;45(3):557–61.
86. Vidal E, Marrone G, Gasparini D, et al. Radiological treatment of renal artery occlusion after blunt abdominal trauma in a pediatric patient: is it never too late? Urology 2011;77(5):1220–2.
87. Rha SW, Wani SP, Suh SY, et al. Images in cardiovascular medicine. Successful percutaneous renal intervention in a patient with acute traumatic renal artery thrombosis. Circulation 2006;114(20):e583–5.
88. Philpott JM, Nance ML, Carr MC, et al. Ureteral stenting in the management of urinoma after severe blunt renal trauma in children. J Pediatr Surg 2003;38(7):1096–8.
89. Cocanour CS. Blunt splenic injury. Curr Opin Crit Care 2010;16(6):575–81.
90. Bensard DD, Beaver BL, Besner GE, et al. Small bowel injury in children after blunt abdominal trauma: is diagnostic delay important? J Trauma 1996;41(3):476–83.
91. Letton RW, Worrell V, APSA Committee on Trauma Blunt Intestinal Injury Study Group. Delay in diagnosis and treatment of blunt intestinal injury does not adversely affect prognosis in the pediatric trauma patient. J Pediatr Surg 2010;45(1):161–5 [discussion: 166].
92. Adelson PD, Bratton SL, Carney NA, et al. Guidelines for the acute medical management of severe traumatic brain injury in infants, children, and adolescents. Chapter 11. Use of hyperosmolar therapy in the management of severe pediatric traumatic brain injury. Pediatr Crit Care Med 2003;4(3 Suppl):S40–4.
93. McIntyre RC Jr, Bensard DD, Moore EE, et al. Pelvic fracture geometry predicts risk of life-threatening hemorrhage in children. J Trauma 1993;35(3):423–9.

94. Potoka DA, Gaines BA, Leppaniemi A, et al. Management of blunt pancreatic trauma: what's new? Eur J Trauma Emerg Surg 2015;41(3):239–50.
95. Canon S, Recicar J, Head B, et al. The utility of initial and follow-up ultrasound reevaluation for blunt renal trauma in children and adolescents. J Pediatr Urol 2014;10(5):815–8.
96. Barera G, Bazzigaluppi E, Viscardi M, et al. Macroamylasemia attributable to gluten-related amylase autoantibodies: a case report. Pediatrics 2001;107(6):E93.
97. Keller MS, Eric Coln C, Garza JJ, et al. Functional outcome of nonoperatively managed renal injuries in children. J Trauma 2004;57(1):108–10 [discussion: 110].
98. Keller MS, Green MC. Comparison of short- and long-term functional outcome of nonoperatively managed renal injuries in children. J Pediatr Surg 2009;44(1): 144–7 [discussion: 147].

Nonaccidental Trauma in Pediatric Surgery

Paul T. Kim, MD[a], Richard A. Falcone Jr, MD, MPH[b],*

KEYWORDS

- Nonaccidental trauma • Child abuse • Abusive head trauma

KEY POINTS

- Children younger than 5 years account for 81.5% of all child abuse with those younger than 1 year being the most vulnerable group.
- Abusive head trauma is the leading cause of fatality in children younger than 2 years old and early detection can be lifesaving.
- Abdominal injuries are uncommon but are the second most common cause of death following nonaccidental trauma (NAT).
- Burns in NAT are commonly caused by immersion or contact with hot objects and are characterized by uniform depth and sharp demarcation or clear outline of the object.
- Careful and consistent screening for nonaccidental trauma is crucial in allowing early detection and prevention of more serious injuries.

INTRODUCTION/EPIDEMIOLOGY

Child abuse/neglect is a significant cause of morbidity and mortality in the pediatric population, with 702,000 confirmed cases in the United States in 2014, including 1580 fatalities. Approximately 17% of the cases were physical abuse or nonaccidental trauma (NAT) and an additional 8.3% suffered sexual abuse.[1] More importantly, the number of admissions and deaths secondary to physical abuse has not decreased since the 1970s despite increased efforts in child protection, not only in the United States but also in other developed countries.[2] In a recent study at a large level 1 pediatric trauma center, patients with NAT had higher injury severity score, rate of intensive care unit stay, and mortality. There was also a delay in the diagnosis of NAT in 20% of the cases.[3] Thus it is critical to recognize and properly evaluate patients with NAT.

[a] Department of General Surgery, University of Cincinnati Medical Center, Cincinnati Children's Hospital Medical Center, 231 Albert Sabin Way ML 0558, Cincinnati, OH 45267-0558, USA;
[b] Division of Pediatric and Thoracic Surgery, Cincinnati Children's Hospital Medical Center, MLC 2023, 3333 Burnet Avenue, Cincinnati, OH 45229-3026, USA
* Corresponding author.
E-mail address: Richard.Falcone@cchmc.org

Surg Clin N Am 97 (2017) 21–33
http://dx.doi.org/10.1016/j.suc.2016.08.002
0039-6109/17/© 2016 Elsevier Inc. All rights reserved.
surgical.theclinics.com

Younger children are at a higher risk of child abuse, as 81.5% of the cases occurred in children younger than 5 years. Children younger than 1 year are the most vulnerable group, representing 24.4% of all cases. Additionally, younger children suffer more significant injuries, as 70% of the child fatalities were in those younger than 3 years.[1] Other risk factors include prior history of abuse in victims as well as perpetrators; medical conditions in victims, such as intellectual disability, or in perpetrators, such as various psychiatric disorders or substance abuse; and other stress factors within the home environment, including financial and relationship issues.[1,4,5] In more than 80% of the cases, biological parents were the perpetrators and nonbiological parents or partners accounted for 12%.[1]

CLINICAL PRESENTATION
Head Trauma

Abusive head trauma (AHT) or shaken baby syndrome is the leading cause of severe brain injury and death in children younger than 2 years.[6,7] AHT is also associated with a significant increase in morbidity compared with nonabusive head trauma (nAHT).[8] Unfortunately, often there is no history of head trauma and only vague clinical symptoms and signs, making the diagnosis difficult. However, early recognition of AHT can be lifesaving.[9] After AHT, children can be asymptomatic or can have lethargy, irritability, decreased appetite, poor sucking or swallowing, nausea, emesis, headache, or seizures. Most minor head injuries are accidental, but significant findings, such as skull fracture or intracranial injuries, especially in a child younger than 1 year, should prompt detailed evaluation looking for other nonaccidental injuries.[6,7]

AHT can result in primary and secondary injuries. Primary injuries are damage directly related to the traumatic rotational and translational forces applied to the child's head. Secondary injuries occur subsequently as complications of primary injuries due to hypoxia and/or ischemia. Secondary injuries occur an estimated 3 times more often in AHT compared with severe nAHT.[10]

Primary injuries include retinal hemorrhages, skull fractures, intracranial hemorrhages, parenchymal injuries, and spinal cord injuries. Retinal hemorrhages are present much more frequently in AHT than nAHT. In one literature review, retinal hemorrhages occurred in 78% of AHT versus only 5% in nAHT. The odds ratio of AHT and retinal hemorrhage was 14.7 with probability of 91%. Characteristically in AHT, hemorrhage is bilateral and involves multiple layers of the retina.[11] Ophthalmology should be consulted for children younger than 1 year with intracranial injuries to fully and accurately document ophthalmologic findings as part of the evaluation for AHT.

Skull fractures are another common finding in AHT but are also frequent in nonintentional trauma. In both AHT and nAHT, linear, parietal fractures are the most common and require careful analysis of the history and overall clinical findings. On the other hand, complicated skull fractures (multiple, bilateral, stellate, crossing suture lines, depressed, or diastatic) strongly suggest AHT, although specificity varies depending on studies.[6,7]

Intracranial hemorrhage (ICH) is common and characteristic of AHT. In low-impact trauma, such as a short vertical fall, ICH is rare.[12] ICH can be divided into subdural, epidural, and subarachnoid hemorrhages. Subdural hemorrhage (SDH) is a result of bleeding bridging veins from shearing and rotational forces and is more common in AHT. Usually, blood is reabsorbed without further issues if only SDH is present.[6] However, in some patients with AHT, hemispheric hypodensity can be seen on imaging in one or both hemispheres. These patients undergo rapid progressive atrophy with elevated intracranial pressures and have mortality rates up to 70%. Survivors are usually left with permanent neurologic disabilities. This progression and poor outcome are thought to be secondary to hypoxic-ischemic injuries after the initial insult.[13]

Epidural hemorrhage (EDH) is the result of tears in dural sinus or diploic veins from direct impact (ie, falls) and as such is more common in nAHT. Because EDH in children is venous in nature, hemorrhage tends to be small and may resolve without significant morbidity and mortality when no other concomitant injuries are present.[6]

Subarachnoid hemorrhage (SAH) results from tearing or shearing of the subarachnoid vessels. It is found much less commonly in pediatric head trauma. SAH is present in nearly all fatal cases of AHT, but overall incidence is equal in AHT and nAHT.[6] In one retrospective study, SAH was associated with worse overall prognosis and disposition showing higher mortality, increased length of stay, greater infection rates, and fewer ventilator-free days.[14]

Parenchymal injuries from direct impact, inertial forces, and hypoxia/ischemia can manifest in various ways. Direct-impact forces result in cerebral contusions or lacerations usually in frontal or temporal regions. Inertial forces result in axonal injuries, gliding contusions, and parenchymal tears commonly in subcortical white matter, corpus callosum, internal capsule, and brainstem. Hypoxic-ischemic injuries can be caused by multiple factors, including direct damage of brainstem with resulting apnea and hypoxia, secondary hypotension, prolonged seizure activity, and/or infection. These injuries are seen more commonly with AHT and are associated with poor prognosis.[6,7,10]

AHT also can result in various spinal injuries, such as spinal cord injury, ligamentous injury, extra-axial hemorrhage, and trauma to paraspinal tissues. Most injuries are clinically silent and these findings also can be seen in nAHT.[15] However, in the absence of traumatic history, any spinal-related injuries should raise suspicion for abuse.

Although it is not difficult to diagnose children with significant head injuries, in cases of mild to moderate injuries, a high index of suspicion is needed to take the proper steps to make the correct diagnosis. Cerebrospinal fluid analysis or ophthalmologic examination can hint at an intracranial injury in children with nonspecific symptoms.[6,11] But with suspicion of abuse, imaging is the key to timely identification of AHT. Computed tomography (CT) scan without intravenous (IV) contrast is the modality of choice, as it is readily available in most hospitals and can rapidly demonstrate subdural, epidural, subarachnoid, and intraparenchymal hemorrhages, as well as cortical contusion and ischemia with high sensitivity and specificity. With any positive intracranial findings, neurosurgery should be consulted, and repeat imaging may be needed. CT, however, may not demonstrate brain edema or diffuse axonal injury in an acute setting. Thus, MRI still is an important study for fully assessing intracranial injury and can help diagnose subtle injuries as well as edema and diffuse axonal injury. MRI should be obtained in children who had a normal CT but continue to display neurologic symptoms. MRI also may be considered in asymptomatic patients with suspected head trauma if it can be obtained in a timely manner.[16–18]

In summary, AHT can result in a variety of injuries. Infants with head injuries ranging from skull fractures to ICHs should therefore be carefully evaluated for the possibility of NAT.

Abdominal Injuries

Abdominal injuries, although uncommon, are the second most common cause of death after NAT. Prevalence is estimated to be 3% to 4%, but mortality can be as high as 45%.[19] Motor vehicle collision is the most common overall cause of abdominal trauma, but in children younger than 2 years, abusive trauma is unfortunately the leading cause.[20] Abdominal injuries can be difficult to diagnose due to lack of traumatic history and examination findings, such as bruises. In addition, most of these patients present in a delayed fashion because of attempts to hide the injury or failure to recognize the severity.[19,20] In one retrospective study, patients with NAT were more likely to have multiple and severe injuries compared with patients with accidental trauma.[21]

Injuries are variable but can be largely divided into solid organ and hollow viscus injuries.

As in accidental trauma, solid organ injuries are more common than hollow viscus injuries. The liver is most frequently affected and injuries include contusion, laceration, or hematoma. The spleen is also commonly damaged, resulting in laceration or hematoma. Pancreatic injuries are uncommon but are seen more often with NAT compared with accidental trauma. It is also associated with other abdominal injuries, such as duodenal tear, perforation, or hematoma. Rarer organs affected are kidneys, adrenal glands, stomach, and bladder.[22,23] Like with accidental trauma, most solid organ injuries can be managed nonoperatively.[24]

Hollow viscus injuries are more common in NAT and include bowel and mesenteric injuries secondary to shearing mechanism (**Fig. 1**).[21–23,25] In particular, duodenal perforation or hematoma in children younger than 4 years should be especially concerning for child abuse.[26] Hollow viscus injuries account for most emergent surgeries in abdominal NAT. Often there is a delay in diagnosis as well as treatment because bowel injuries are difficult to diagnose.[27]

If history or physical examination reveal concerning findings, such as abdominal pain, bruising, or distension, abdominal CT scan with IV contrast should be performed. In a study by Hilmes and colleagues,[22] children who showed abdominal-related symptoms or signs had a significantly higher rate of abnormal CT findings as well as subsequent surgical intervention. Oral contrast can be given, which can better highlight bowel injuries, but it does put children at higher risk of aspiration. Abdominal ultrasound may be considered for screening, but high false-negative rates limit its usefulness and CT should remain the gold standard for delineating occult abdominal injuries.[17] In asymptomatic children, liver function tests can be helpful. Lindberg and colleagues[27] showed hepatic transaminases ≥80 IU/L had sensitivity of 83.8% and specificity of 83.1% for abdominal injuries. Thus, for transaminases ≥80 IU/L, CT scan should be obtained if there is suspicion of NAT.

In short, abdominal injuries in NAT are difficult to identify, and there can be significant delay in diagnosis. Therefore, if there is a concern for abuse and possible abdominal symptoms, there should be a low threshold for obtaining an abdominal CT scan.

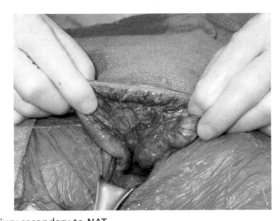

Fig. 1. Bowel injury secondary to NAT.

Fractures

Fractures are the second most common manifestation of NAT after bruises. NAT is the most prevalent cause of fractures in children younger than 2 years.[28,29] Nevertheless, presence of suspicious fractures alone is never pathognomonic for abuse. As with any other injuries, there are multiple suggestive factors in the history and physical examination that should be considered as a whole.

Although there is no pathognomonic fracture for NAT, there are findings that have high specificity for abuse, which include classic metaphyseal lesion, posteromedial rib, scapular, spinous process, and sternal fractures.[30–32] Additionally, femur fractures in children younger than 3 years should also raise suspicion.[33] Metaphyseal fractures are the most common long-bone fracture resulting from forceful pulling or twisting of the extremity. They can be seen as corner or bucket handle fractures on radiographs. However, it can be difficult to radiographically detect an acute fracture. Rib fractures, especially posteromedial location, result from anteroposterior compression of the chest. Unfortunately, again, acute rib fractures are difficult to diagnose on plain radiographs and may warrant a repeat radiograph in a few weeks. Scapular, spinous process, and sternal fractures are rare in other conditions, making these findings highly specific for abuse. In addition, multiple fractures of different healing stages are specific for NAT.[30–32]

There are multiple medical conditions that predispose patients to pathologic fractures, but those conditions like metabolic bone disorders (rickets) or various connective tissue disorders (osteogenesis imperfecta, Ehlers-Danlos syndrome) are rare and likely to have family history or other features consistent with the disease process.[32] If there is any uncertainty of the fracture etiology, a multidisciplinary approach to a full workup should be considered.

When children present with suspicious fractures (<6 months old with any fracture, classic metaphyseal lesion, posteromedial rib, scapular, spinous process, sternal or femur fractures) or findings concerning for NAT (head injury, suspicious bruising), full NAT evaluation should be performed, including a skeletal survey to rule out occult fractures.[34–37]

Integumentary Injuries: Bruises/Bites, Burns

Bruises are the most common manifestation of NAT but are not very specific for NAT. However, location and pattern of the bruising can suggest abuse rather than unintentional trauma. Accidental trauma usually results in bruising on bony prominences and extremities. On the other hand, bruising in NAT commonly occurs centrally: face, ear, neck, torso, back, genitourinary area, and buttocks (**Fig. 2**). Suspicious patterns include linear bruises, belt marks, handprints, or loop marks (**Fig. 3**). Bruises with such characteristics without an appropriate history should raise suspicion for abuse. Nonetheless, in children with multiple bruises, appropriate coagulopathy workup should be performed.[38–40]

Human bites are usually superficial and circular or oval in nature. They may or may not have discernable teeth marks or associated bruising. Any suspected bite wounds should be swabbed for DNA testing and also followed and documented serially as the wound becomes more prominent after few days.[41]

Burns occur in approximately 8% to 12% of NAT cases. Like accidental burns, most common etiologies are scald and contact burns. Other mechanisms, such as flame, electric, or chemical burns, are more unusual. Scald burn secondary to forced immersion is the most common mechanism characterized by a sharp line of demarcation and uniform depth in the buttocks and stocking or glove distribution with sparing of

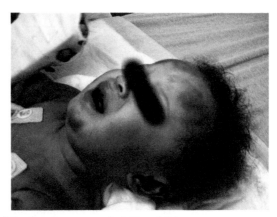

Fig. 2. Bruising of the face in a nonambulating child.

flexed skin folds, palms, and soles (**Fig. 4**). It lacks drip or splash marks that would be present if the injury was caused by spilled liquid. Branding with hot object such as iron, hot plate, or cigarettes is also common. The wounds are characterized by clear imprinting of the object in a uniform depth compared with accidental contact, which leaves only a shallow partial outline due to withdrawal reflex.[42,43]

In conclusion, children with central bruising, especially in face and neck, human bites without an appropriate history, or burns consistent with immersion or branding should raise red flags and NAT workup should be performed.

EVALUATION/DIAGNOSIS

Despite increased child protection efforts, child abuse remains a large and significant issue in the United States. Children suffering NAT have complex injury patterns spanning multiple organ systems, and timely diagnosis and management of each injury are critical to their outcome. Pediatric surgeons have an important role as they are experienced in polytrauma and can help expedite diagnosis and treatment as well as coordinate care among multiple disciplines. Nonetheless, a study at a level 1 pediatric trauma center showed that pediatric surgeons were consulted in only 56% of the

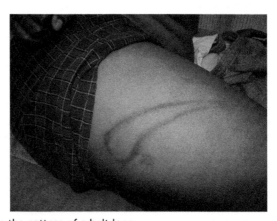

Fig. 3. Bruising in the pattern of a belt loop.

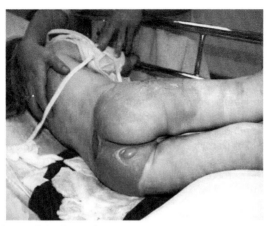

Fig. 4. Immersion burn of the buttock.

cases, possibly delaying diagnosis of occult injuries.[44] So, no matter the size or resources available at the hospital, it is important to have a concerted, coordinated effort among multiple disciplines to correctly address a complicated issue such as NAT.

As with any trauma, Advanced Trauma Life Support (ATLS) principles should be followed to stabilize the patient as needed. Evaluation then starts with a thorough history and physical examination. If any red flags arise, a complete investigation should be performed involving a multidisciplinary team familiar with child abuse to ensure correct documentation and reporting. Because children often present with nonspecific findings, more data are needed so as not to miss subtle injuries by obtaining imaging and laboratory studies. As mentioned in the previous section, imaging studies can include CT and/or MRI of the head, CT abdomen, and skeletal survey. General laboratory studies include complete blood count, coagulation studies, electrolytes, and liver function tests. Other tests can be added more specific to types of injury suspected. Unfortunately, due to the complex nature of NAT and unfamiliarity of many health care providers, many of these critical evaluations can be easily missed without a proper screening protocol.

Nonetheless, there remains significant variations of screening patterns among major US hospitals as well as in other developed countries, highlighting the need for a consensus protocol in screening.[36,45,46] In addition, there are other factors, such as race, that can influence and bias providers, complicating the matter even further. National data show that black children were 2 times more likely to be investigated for abuse. Multiple studies have examined the reason for the disparity, and it is likely multifactorial: economic, social, and environmental factors.[47–49] But this is precisely why a consensus screening protocol would help eliminate any biases or misconceptions that may exist.

Multiple studies have inspected the effects of implementing a consensus screening protocol. Louwers and colleagues[50] in 2 separate studies showed that having a systematic screening protocol in place increased the detection rate of child abuse in Dutch emergency departments.[51] Also, the rate of screening significantly rose with training of the nursing staff and legal requirement.[51] Escobar and colleagues,[52] in a retrospective study at a single level II pediatric trauma center, showed that there was poor documentation of relevant history, such as caregiver's alcohol or drug use, history of mental illness, and criminal history before implementation of a systematic protocol. Moreover, standardized screening can eliminate disparity, as shown in our study, where application of head injury screening guideline resulted in equal screening between black and white children.[53] Similar findings were noted in the study by Higginbotham and colleagues,[54] which demonstrated elimination of screening bias toward children of lower socioeconomic status and overall significant increase of important screening studies, such as skeletal survey and liver function tests.

So how do we go about implementing a screening protocol? The study by Wilkins and colleagues[55] suggests information sharing among hospitals and increasing public and health care provider awareness are important in improving NAT screening. The study examined the effects of implementing systematic screening protocol following a sentinel event in North Carolina where an undiagnosed NAT led to child abuse within the hospital after admission. The data from 2 states, North Carolina and Delaware, were compared. The screening rate in North Carolina from in all hospitals increased significantly from 40% to 81%, but such change did not occur in Delaware (23.9% to 29.7%). The investigators attributed the increase to the efforts of the index hospital where the sentinel event occurred to share its screening protocol with other hospitals, as well as promoting awareness of NAT within the health care community and media publicity. So increasing awareness is crucial in identifying NAT cases, and putting a standardized screening protocol in place can achieve that goal.

Even so, for the health care providers and institutions less familiar with NAT, setting up a screening protocol can seem like a tall order. Fortunately, there are several studies that devised tools and guidelines that can minimize the missed abuse cases. In a recent study, Louwers and colleagues[56] validated a 6 variable screening instrument that detected abuse with 80% sensitivity and 98% specificity when ≥ 1 variable was positive. The 6 variables were inconsistent history, delay in seeking care, injury mechanism inconsistent with child's developmental level, inappropriate behavior between caretaker and child, physical findings inconsistent with history, and presence of other suspicious signals detected by the health care provider. These variables can be a good starting guideline for inexperienced providers.

For head trauma specifically, a study by Hymel and colleagues[57] validated a 4-variable clinical prediction rule for AHT in pediatric intensive care patients that demonstrated 96% sensitivity with a negative predictive value of 93% in detecting abuse when at least one variable was positive. Those 4 variables were acute respiratory compromise; bruising of torso, ears, or neck; bilateral or interhemispheric subdural hemorrhages; and any skull fractures. In another study, Cowley and colleagues[58] validated a 6-variable prediction tool that showed 72.3% sensitivity and 85.7% specificity when ≥ 3 features were present. Those 6 features included head or neck bruising, seizures, apnea, rib fracture, long-bone fracture, and retinal hemorrhage. Although not perfect, these tools may aid in decreasing the missed AHT cases.

Although there have been studies to develop prediction tools for abdominal injuries in accidental trauma, there has not been one in NAT. Nonetheless, some of the data may be extrapolated especially for solid organ injuries. Streck and colleagues[59] showed 4 variables were significant predictors in patients with accidental trauma: elevated transaminases, decreased hematocrit, abnormal abdominal examination, and abnormal chest radiograph. Two of which also are significant predictors in NAT populations. Decreased hematocrit and abnormal chest radiograph may also have significance in NAT but should be taken with a grain of salt. Other commonly obtained laboratory tests, such as amylase and urinalysis, were not predictive of abdominal injuries.

In terms of occult fractures, Wood and colleagues[33–36] described children who require detailed skeletal survey: children younger than 6 months old with any bruises, children younger than 12 months old with suspicious bruising (eg, face, neck, torso, buttock) or any fracture, children 12 to 24 months old with suspicious fractures (classic

Table 1
Findings concerning for nonaccidental trauma

History	Head	Abdomen	Musculoskeletal	Skin
No trauma history or history inconsistent with findings	Retinal hemorrhage	Abdominal pain, distension, bruise	Classic metaphyseal lesion	Bruises in face, ear, neck, torso, back, buttocks, genitals
Delay in seeking care	Complex skull fractures	Hollow viscus injuries	Posterior rib fractures	Patterned bruises (belt, hand, loop)
Prior emergency department visits	Subdural hemorrhage	Mesenteric hematoma	Scapular fracture	Bite marks
Domestic violence	Hypoxic-ischemic injuries	LFTs >80 IU/L	Spinous process fracture	Immersion burn
Caretaker with alcohol/ drug abuse	Spine-related injuries without traumatic history		Sternal fracture	Branding burn
Caretaker with mental illness			Femur fracture in children <3 y old	
Chronic medical condition			Fractures with different healing stages	

Abbreviation: LFT, liver function tests.

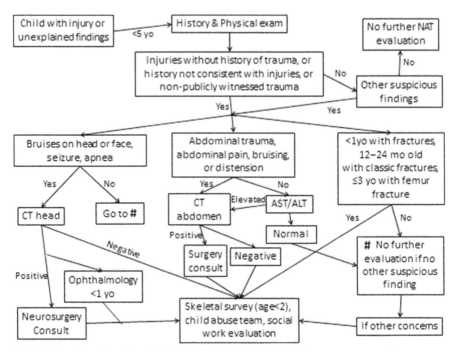

Fig. 5. Evaluation algorithm for NAT. AST, aspartate transaminase; yo, year old.

metaphyseal lesion, posteromedial rib, etc), and children younger than 2 years old with suspicion for abuse. Skeletal survey includes at least 16 images focused on specific anatomic areas in appendicular and axial skeletons to detect any occult fractures.[17] In one large retrospective study, skeletal survey detected approximately 11% of children with occult fractures consistent with NAT.[37] Some occult fractures are difficult to identify in an acute setting and may need a repeat imaging in 2 weeks. Radionuclide bone scan is occasionally used as an adjunct to skeletal survey, as it can be more sensitive in detecting rib fractures and subtle shaft fractures. However, the study is expensive and often requires sedation. Also, all positive areas must be additionally imaged with radiography. Therefore, it is not recommended routinely.[17]

Table 1 and **Fig. 5** give a brief summary of concerning findings that should prompt NAT workup and potential evaluation algorithm for NAT.

SUMMARY

Child abuse/NAT is a complicated issue that demands a multidisciplinary approach, especially in screening and diagnosis. Each institution should have a set protocol in place to standardize how children are evaluated to minimize the number of missed cases. In addition, ongoing education of health care providers as well as the public will improve the overall identification and care.

REFERENCES

1. Child maltreatment 2014. Report, Children's Bureau. Washington, DC: U.S. Department of Health and Human Services; 2014. Available at: http://www.acf.hhs.gov/sites/default/files/cb/cm2014.pdf.

2. Gilbert R, Fluke J, O'Donnell M, et al. Child maltreatment: variation in trends and policies in six developed countries. Lancet 2012;379(9817):758–72.

3. Estroff JM, Foglia RP, Fuchs JR. A comparison of accidental and nonaccidental trauma: it is worse than you think. J Emerg Med 2015;48(3):274–9.

4. Falcone RA Jr, Brown RL, Garcia VF. The epidemiology of infant injuries and alarming health disparities. J Pediatr Surg 2007;42(1):172–6 [discussion: 176–7].

5. Vinchon M, Defoort-Dhellemmes S, Desurmont M, et al. Accidental and nonaccidental head injuries in infants: a prospective study. J Neurosurg 2005;102(4 Suppl):380–4.

6. Chiesa A, Duhaime A-C. Abusive head trauma. Pediatr Clin North Am 2009;56(2):317–31.

7. Parks SE, Kegler SR, Annest JL, et al. Characteristics of fatal abusive head trauma among children in the USA, 2003-2007: an application of the CDC operational case definition to national vital statistics data. Inj Prev 2011;18(3):193–9.

8. Keenan HT, Runyan DK, Nocera M. Child outcomes and family characteristics 1 year after severe inflicted or noninflicted traumatic brain injury. Pediatrics 2006;117(2):317–24.

9. Jenny C, Hymel KP, Ritzen A, et al. Analysis of missed cases of abusive head trauma. JAMA 1999;281(7):621–6.

10. Ichord RN, Naim M, Pollock AN, et al. Hypoxic-ischemic injury complicates inflicted and accidental traumatic brain injury in young children: the role of diffusion-weighted imaging. J Neurotrauma 2007;24(1):106–18.

11. Maguire SA, Watts PO, Shaw AD, et al. Retinal haemorrhages and related findings in abusive and non-abusive head trauma: a systematic review. Eye (Lond) 2013;27(1):28–36.

12. Tarantino CA, Dowd MD, Murdock TC. Short vertical falls in infants. Pediatr Emerg Care 1999;15(1):5–8.

13. Foster KA, Recker MJ, Lee PS, et al. Factors associated with hemispheric hypodensity after subdural hematoma following abusive head trauma in children. J Neurotrauma 2014;31(19):1625–31.

14. Hochstadter E, Stewart TC, Alharfi IM, et al. Subarachnoid hemorrhage prevalence and its association with short-term outcome in pediatric severe traumatic brain injury. Neurocrit Care 2014;21(3):505–13.

15. Choudhary AK, Ishak R, Zacharia TT, et al. Imaging of spinal injury in abusive head trauma: a retrospective study. Pediatr Radiol 2014;44(9):1130–40.

16. Kemp AM, Jaspan T, Griffiths J, et al. Neuroimaging: what neuroradiological features distinguish abusive from non-abusive head trauma? A systematic review. Arch Dis Child 2011;96(12):1103–12.

17. Section on Radiology, American Academy of Pediatrics. Diagnostic imaging of child abuse. Pediatrics 2009;123(5):1430–5.

18. Foerster BR, Petrou M, Lin D, et al. Neuroimaging evaluation of non-accidental head trauma with correlation to clinical outcomes: a review of 57 cases. J Pediatr 2009;154(4):573–7.

19. Lane WG, Dubowitz H, Langenberg P, et al. Epidemiology of abusive abdominal trauma hospitalizations in United States children. Child Abuse Negl 2012;36(2):142–8.

20. Trokel M, DiScala C, Terrin NC, et al. Blunt abdominal injury in the young pediatric patient: child abuse and patient outcomes. Child Maltreat 2004;9(1):111–7.

21. Wood J, Rubin DM, Nance ML, et al. Distinguishing inflicted versus accidental abdominal injuries in young children. J Trauma 2005;59(5):1203–8.

22. Hilmes MA, Hernanz-Schulman M, Greeley CS, et al. CT identification of abdominal injuries in abused pre-school-age children. Pediatr Radiol 2011;41(5):643–51.
23. Trokel M, Discala C, Terrin NC, et al. Patient and injury characteristics in abusive abdominal injuries. Pediatr Emerg Care 2006;22(10):700–4.
24. Roaten JB, Partrick DA, Bensard DD, et al. Visceral injuries in nonaccidental trauma: spectrum of injury and outcomes. Am J Surg 2005;190(6):827–9.
25. Barnes PM, Norton CM, Dunstan FD, et al. Abdominal injury due to child abuse. Lancet 2005;366(9481):234–5.
26. Gaines BA, Shultz BS, Morrison K, et al. Duodenal injuries in children: beware of child abuse. J Pediatr Surg 2004;39(4):600–2.
27. Lindberg DM, Shapiro RA, Blood EA, et al. Utility of hepatic transaminases in children with concern for abuse. Pediatrics 2013;131(2):268–75.
28. Loder RT, Feinberg JR. Orthopaedic injuries in children with nonaccidental trauma: demographics and incidence from the 2000 kids' inpatient database. J Pediatr Orthop 2007;27(4):421–6.
29. Leventhal JM, Martin KD, Asnes AG. Incidence of fractures attributable to abuse in young hospitalized children: results from analysis of a United States database. Pediatrics 2008;122(3):599–604.
30. Flaherty EG, Perez-Rossello JM, Levine MA, et al. Evaluating children with fractures for child physical abuse. Pediatrics 2014;133(2):e477–89.
31. Pandya NK, Baldwin K, Wolfgruber H, et al. Child abuse and orthopaedic injury patterns: analysis at a level I pediatric trauma center. J Pediatr Orthop 2009;29(6):618–25.
32. Servaes S, Brown SD, Choudhary AK, et al. The etiology and significance of fractures in infants and young children: a critical multidisciplinary review. Pediatr Radiol 2016;46(5):591–600.
33. Wood JN, Fakeye O, Mondestin V, et al. Prevalence of abuse among young children with femur fractures: a systematic review. BMC Pediatr 2014;14(1):169.
34. Wood JN, Fakeye O, Feudtner C, et al. Development of guidelines for skeletal survey in young children with fractures. Pediatrics 2014;134(1):45–53.
35. Wood JN, Fakeye O, Mondestin V, et al. Development of hospital-based guidelines for skeletal survey in young children with bruises. Pediatrics 2015;135(2):e312–20.
36. Wood JN, French B, Song L, et al. Evaluation for occult fractures in injured children. Pediatrics 2015;136(2):232–40.
37. Duffy SO, Squires J, Fromkin JB, et al. Use of skeletal surveys to evaluate for physical abuse: analysis of 703 consecutive skeletal surveys. Pediatrics 2011;127(1):e47–52.
38. Maguire S, Mann MK, Sibert J, et al. Are there patterns of bruising in childhood which are diagnostic or suggestive of abuse? A systematic review. Arch Dis Child 2005;90(2):182–6.
39. Pierce MC, Kaczor K, Aldridge S, et al. Bruising characteristics discriminating physical child abuse from accidental trauma. Pediatrics 2010;125(1):67–74.
40. Kemp AM, Dunstan F, Nuttall D, et al. Patterns of bruising in preschool children–a longitudinal study. Arch Dis Child 2015;100(5):426–31.
41. American Academy of Pediatrics Committee on Child Abuse and Neglect, American Academy of Pediatric Dentistry, American Academy of Pediatric Dentistry Council on Clinical Affairs. Guideline on oral and dental aspects of child abuse and neglect. Pediatr Dent 2008;30(7 Suppl):86–9.
42. Wibbenmeyer L, Liao J, Heard J, et al. Factors related to child maltreatment in children presenting with burn injuries. J Burn Care Res 2014;35(5):374–81.

43. Dissanaike S, Wishnew J, Rahimi M, et al. Burns as child abuse: risk factors and legal issues in West Texas and Eastern New Mexico. J Burn Care Res 2010;31(1): 176–83.

44. Larimer EL, Fallon SC, Westfall J, et al. The importance of surgeon involvement in the evaluation of non-accidental trauma patients. J Pediatr Surg 2013;48(6): 1357–62.

45. Hulson OS, Rijn RRV, Offiah AC. European survey of imaging in non-accidental injury demonstrates a need for a consensus protocol. Pediatr Radiol 2014; 44(12):1557–63.

46. Hoytema Van Konijnenburg EM, Teeuw AH, Zwaard SA, et al. Screening methods to detect child maltreatment: high variability in Dutch emergency departments. Emerg Med J 2013;31(3):196–200.

47. Drake B, Jolley JM, Lanier P, et al. Racial bias in child protection? A comparison of competing explanations using national data. Pediatrics 2011;127(3):471–8.

48. Putnam-Hornstein E, Needell B, King B, et al. Racial and ethnic disparities: a population-based examination of risk factors for involvement with child protective services. Child Abuse Negl 2013;37(1):33–46.

49. Lanier P, Maguire-Jack K, Walsh T, et al. Race and ethnic differences in early childhood maltreatment in the United States. J Dev Behav Pediatr 2014;35(7): 419–26.

50. Louwers ECFM, Korfage IJ, Affourtit MJ, et al. Detection of child abuse in emergency departments: a multi-centre study. Arch Dis Child 2011;96(5):422–5.

51. Louwers ECFM, Korfage IJ, Affourtit MJ, et al. Effects of systematic screening and detection of child abuse in emergency departments. Pediatrics 2012; 130(3):457–64.

52. Escobar MA, Pflugeisen BM, Duralde Y, et al. Development of a systematic protocol to identify victims of non-accidental trauma. Pediatr Surg Int 2016;32(4):377–86.

53. Rangel EL, Cook BS, Bennett BL, et al. Eliminating disparity in evaluation for abuse in infants with head injury: use of a screening guideline. J Pediatr Surg 2009;44(6):1229–35.

54. Higginbotham N, Lawson KA, Gettig K, et al. Utility of a child abuse screening guideline in an urban pediatric emergency department. J Trauma Acute Care Surg 2014;76(3):871–7.

55. Wilkins GG, Ball J, Mann NC, et al. Increased screening for child physical abuse in emergency departments in a regional trauma system. J Trauma Nurs 2016; 23(2):77–82.

56. Louwers EC, Korfage IJ, Affourtit MJ, et al. Accuracy of a screening instrument to identify potential child abuse in emergency departments. Child Abuse Negl 2014; 38(7):1275–81.

57. Hymel KP, Armijo-Garcia V, Foster R, et al. Validation of a clinical prediction rule for pediatric abusive head trauma. Pediatrics 2014;134(6):e1537–44.

58. Cowley LE, Morris CB, Maguire SA, et al. Validation of a prediction tool for abusive head trauma. Pediatrics 2015;136(2):290–8.

59. Streck CJ Jr, Jewett BM, Wahlquist AH, et al. Evaluation for intra-abdominal injury in children after blunt torso trauma: can we reduce unnecessary abdominal computed tomography by utilizing a clinical prediction model? J Trauma Acute Care Surg 2012;73(2):371–6 [discussion: 376].

Head and Cervical Spine Evaluation for the Pediatric Surgeon

 CrossMark

Mary K. Arbuthnot, DO[a],*, David P. Mooney, MD, MPH[a],
Ian C. Glenn, MD[b]

KEYWORDS

• Pediatric trauma • Cervical spine • Traumatic brain injury • Imaging • Evaluation

KEY POINTS

- Head Evaluation
  - Traumatic brain injury (TBI) is the most common cause of death among children with unintentional injury.
  - Patients with isolated loss of consciousness and Glasgow Coma Scale (GCS) of 14 or 15 do not require a head CT.
  - Maintenance of normotension is critical in the management of the severe TBI patient in the emergency department (ED).
- Cervical spine evaluation
  - Although unusual, cervical spine injury (CSI) is associated with severe consequences if not diagnosed.
  - The pediatric spine does not complete maturation until 8 years and is more prone to ligamentous injury than the adult cervical spine.
  - The risk of radiation-associated malignancy must be balanced with the risk of missed injury during.

HEAD EVALUATION
Introduction

The purpose of this article is to guide pediatric surgeons in the initial evaluation and stabilization of head and CSIs in pediatric trauma patients. Extensive discussion of the definitive management of these injuries is outside the scope of this publication.

Conflicts of Interest: None.
Disclosures: None.
[a] Department of Surgery, Boston Children's Hospital, 300 Longwood Avenue, Fegan 3, Boston, MA 02115, USA; [b] Department of Surgery, Akron Children's Hospital, 1 Perkins Square, Suite 8400, Akron, OH 44308, USA
* Corresponding author. Department of General Surgery, Boston Children's Hospital, 300 Longwood Avenue, Fegan 3, Boston, MA 02115.
E-mail address: mary.thorpe@childrens.harvard.edu

The diagnostics and management strategies contained within this text are written in the context of the ED or trauma bay.

TBI is a broad term and refers to an acquired condition that results in temporary or permanent alteration in brain function. GCS is frequently used to classify TBI as mild (14–15), moderate (9–13), and severe (3–8).[1] The GCS is not as well validated for pediatric populations nor does it hold the same prognostic value as for adults.[2,3]

In the United States, the primary cause of death for individuals aged 0 to 14 years of age is unintentional injury, with TBI the injury most often associated with death.[4,5] This population group is estimated to experience more than 500,000 TBI events per year, the majority caused by falls and being struck by or against an object.[6,7] From the 2001 to 2002 to 2009 to 2010, the number of TBI-related ED visits doubled for patients aged 0 to 4 years of age.[8]

Nonaccidental trauma (NAT) was responsible for 80% of serious or fatal TBIs.[9] Nationwide, this leads to approximately 800 deaths annually.[10] (For more information regarding NAT, see Paul Kim and Richard A Falcone's article, "Non-accidental Trauma in Pediatric Surgery," in this issue).

Relevant Anatomy and Pathophysiology

Commonly used nomenclature for TBI includes intra-axial and extra-axial. Intra-axial lesions refer to injuries of the brain parenchyma and include diffuse axonal injury (DAI), contusions, infarctions, and cerebral edema. Extra-axial injuries are outside the brain parenchyma and contain skull/facial fractures and hemorrhage (epidural, subdural, and subarachnoid).[11,12]

Although contusions and infarctions are more discrete injuries, DAI (also referred to as traumatic axonal injury) involves larger portions of the brain, although not necessarily uniformly. DAI occurs when the brain experiences angular, or rotational, forces causing a shearing effect on neurons.[11,12]

A few interrelated concepts must be discussed to understand normal brain physiology and the perturbations that are associated with TBI. The Monro-Kellie doctrine states that the cranial vault contains a fixed volume, and the sum of the volumes of the brain, intracranial blood, and intracranial cerebrospinal fluid is constant. The brain is relatively incompressible and the blood and cerebrospinal fluid volumes vary. In children, prior to fusion of the fontanels, there is some expansion in the cranial volume.[13,14] Furthermore, newer research suggests that in intracranial hypertension (ICH), excessive pressure is not equally exerted on all portions of the brain.[15]

Damage to the brain may occur not only as a result of the primary injury but also from postinjury factors, such as hypotension, hypoxemia, pyrexia, hypoglycemia, and cerebral edema (secondary injury). Secondary insults vary in both preventability and reversibility and may result from both systemic and intracranial factors.[16,17]

Cerebral perfusion pressure (CPP) is defined as the difference between the mean arterial pressure and the intracranial pressure (ICP). Generally, the ideal CPP is 70 mm Hg for an adult patient.[18] Children are known, however, to have greater tolerance of low CPP and the ideal CPP is unclear for children. The youngest children tolerate the lowest values off CPP, with the ideal value falling between 30 mm Hg and 40 mm Hg.[19]

Cerebral blood flow (CBF) is maintained over a wide range of both CPP and ICP. As a function of systolic blood pressure, CBF is maintained when SBP ranges from 60 mm Hg to 150 mm Hg through autoregulation. Autoregulation of CBF may be perturbed by trauma, hypoxia, or hypercarbia.[17,20]

Important physiologic differences between adults and children include greater elasticity of the cranial vault and tolerance of lower CPP in the pediatric population.

Clinical Presentation and Examination

The initial evaluation of all trauma patients, including patients with suspected head or cervical spine trauma, should adhere to the American College of Surgeons Advance Trauma Life Support algorithm and begin with a primary survey of the airway, breathing, circulation, and neurologic disability, followed by a secondary survey. During the secondary survey, a full neurologic examination should be performed, including calculation of the GCS. **Box 1** summarizes the common signs and symptoms seen in children with a TBI.[21] In addition, a thorough history of present illness and past medical history should be taken with attention paid to factors that are associated with clinically significant TBI (**Box 2**).[21]

Diagnostic Evaluation

Computed tomography scan

The noncontrast head computed tomography (CT) scan is the default imaging modality in TBI because it is an excellent tool to evaluate for both intra-axial and extra-axial hemorrhage, brain herniation, and skull and facial fractures. The short period of time required to perform a head CT allows for rapid identification and treatment of life-threatening lesions.[12] **Fig. 1** depicts a right-sided epidural hematoma that is easily identified on CT scan in a 2-year-old who sustained a fall from height onto a tile floor.

For patients with severe TBI, there is strong evidence supporting the use of head CT to rule out serious intracranial pathology.[22,23] For patients with mild or moderate TBI, however, the data are less clear and at times conflicting. There is considerable debate as to the significance of historical features, such loss of consciousness and amnesia, and physical examination as well as what role these should play in the decision to order a head CT.[12,24–28]

That said, Lee and colleagues[28] conducted a multicenter prospective study of more than 40,000 children aged 0 to 18 years who presented to the ED with minor, blunt head trauma and a GCS of 14 or 15 with no other physical examination findings. Those with loss of consciousness did not have a statistically significant higher rate of clinically significant TBI and thus routine head CT for this patient population was not recommended. The American College of Radiology has generated guidelines that recommend a noncontrast head CT in cases of suspected or confirmed NAT.[29]

All these considered, reasonable indications for head CT are listed:

- GCS less than 13
- Minor trauma combined with neurologic deficits or evidence of basilar skull fracture

---

Box 1
Signs and symptoms of traumatic brain injury

Clinical findings in traumatic brain injury

Altered mental status

Loss of consciousness

Headache

Emesis

Neurologic deficit

Skull fracture

Data from National Clinical Guideline Centre (UK). Head injury: triage, assessment, investigation and early management of head injury in children, young people and adults 2014.

Box 2
Prognostic factors associated with clinically significant traumatic brain injury

Loss of consciousness

Amnesia

Preceding drug/alcohol use

Anticoagulant use

History of bleeding diathesis

Mechanism of injury (high vs low energy)

Emesis

History of neurosurgery

Data from National Clinical Guideline Centre (UK). Head injury: triage, assessment, investigation and early management of head injury in children, young people and adults 2014.

- High-energy mechanism
- Suspected or confirmed NAT

Repeat head computed tomography

It is common practice at many institutions for routine, serial head CT scans to be obtained on patients with head injuries. Whether as inpatient, or in the ED, repeat head CT scan should be reserved for patients who have experienced a change in their

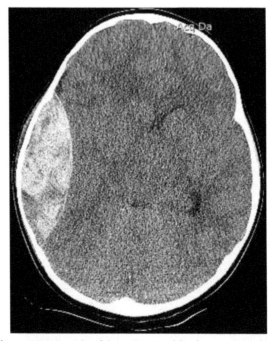

Fig. 1. Epidural hematoma sustained in a 2-year-old who presented with lethargy and emesis following a fall from standing height.

neurologic examination.[30–32] For those with diagnosed intracranial injury, it is recommended to collaborate with a neurosurgeon for the timing of any additional imaging.

Magnetic resonance imaging

Indications for MRI include TBI with symptoms that are not explained by head CT findings, in particular DAI, as well as subacute injuries with neurocognitive deficits.[11,12,29] Rapid-sequence MRI may be used to supplant follow-up head CT in brain injured children, to decrease the radiation burden. Again, imaging studies should be ordered only after consultation with neurosurgery or neurology.

Management

As discussed previously, the definitive management of TBI typically is not undertaken by a pediatric surgeon in the trauma setting. Pediatric surgeons should, however, initiate management of the brain injury awaiting arrival of a neurosurgeon should the occasion arise. This section briefly covers management of 2 extremes of TBI: (1) those with minor injuries warranting discharge and (2) those with severe injuries that may require immediate intervention on the part of the pediatric surgeon to minimize secondary injuries as well as death or serious disability due to ICH and the risk of subsequent herniation.

Minor traumatic brain injury

In the absence of concern for NAT, asymptomatic patients may be safely discharged home from the ED if imaging reveals the following[33–39]:

- Normal imaging
- An isolated, linear, nondisplaced skull fracture not involving the skull base

These patients, however, likely benefit from neurocognitive evaluation both prior to ED discharge and as an outpatient.[40]

Severe traumatic brain injury

A major cause of secondary brain injury in trauma patients is brain hypoperfusion and hypoxia due to systemic hypotension. Although CPP goals for pediatric patients have been established, it is unlikely that an ICP monitor will have been placed when the patient is first evaluated by a pediatric surgeon. Therefore, maintenance of normal blood pressure is the goal. Adult literature has suggested that traditional SBP goals are inadequate, and target SBP should be approximately 120 mm Hg.[41,42] Unfortunately, equivalent values are not available for pediatric patients. Therefore, the recommendation is to maintain SBP near the upper limit of normal for a patient's age group.

Furthermore, ICH can raise the ICP and is another significant cause of secondary brain injury, herniation, and death. The gold standard for measurement of ICP is the placement of an invasive monitor into one of the lateral ventricles.[14] This luxury is often not afforded in the trauma bay and, therefore, presumptive diagnosis, and subsequent treatment, of ICP is initially based on physical examination, imaging, and clinical suspicion. The brain herniation syndromes (subfalcine, tonsillar, and uncal) are traditionally associated with increased ICP and may occur independently of ICH.[43] There are no rigorous criteria or thresholds for treatment of suspected ICH in the ED or trauma bay setting; however, initial management includes the following[44]:

- Intubation for children with severe TBI or GCS less than 8
- Avoiding hypoxia
- Avoiding hypercarbia
- Avoiding hypotension

- Avoiding hypothermia
- Pediatric ICU admission

There is no consensus on ICP treatment thresholds, even in children who have an invasive monitor; however, level 3 recommendations were made to support an ICP treatment threshold of 20 mm Hg and a CPP threshold greater than 40 mm Hg in children.[45,46] A survey of ED physicians demonstrated that a majority would administer a hyperosmotic solution for severe TBI with reactive mydriasis, midline shift on head CT, or compression of the skull base cisterns on head CT.[47]

In adult patients, hypertonic saline in is the first-line pharmacologic therapy for management of ICH. Unfortunately, solution concentrations (3%–23.4%) and doses vary and pediatric experience is more limited.[43,48–51] If treatment is administered in the setting of impeding herniation, hypertonic saline (3% saline 3–10 mL/kg bolus) should be the first-line agent administered in addition to 30° head of bed elevation and midline head placement.[44] Emergent neurosurgical consultation should be obtained and the use of additional hyperosmolar agents, sedatives, analgesics, and anticonvulsant therapy should be discussed with the neurosurgeons and intensivists involved in a patient's care.

A Cochrane Library review of the literature concerning adults with TBI recommends against the routine use of corticosteroids in patients with TBI.[52] Pediatric guidelines also recommend against the use of steroids for ICP management, because it has been demonstrated that they have no effect on ICP, CPP, or outcome and are associated with an increase in infections.[44]

Clinical Outcomes

Clinical outcomes in pediatric TBI are clouded by varied study methodologies and limited standardization for categorizing postinjury function. Furthermore, few studies were conducted in a longitudinal fashion and publications have drawn conflicting conclusions.

A meta-analysis from Babikian and Asarnow[53] of 28 pediatric TBI publications revealed that patients who experienced mild TBI tend to not suffer any neurocognitive impairments in the short term or long term (24 months or greater). Those with moderate TBI tended to have persistent deficits and had worse outcomes than those with mild TBI but fared better than the severe TBI group. The analysis did not capture a difference in outcomes based on age at injury. There were studies included, however, in the meta-analysis that demonstrated worse outcome in those suffering TBI at an earlier age. Compared with adults, children 15 years of age or younger who suffered a TBI had improved mortality and functional outcomes.[3]

A longitudinal study conducted by Rivara and colleagues[54] demonstrated that patients who have persistent disability at 24-month postinjury follow-up do not show interval improvement at 36-month evaluation.

Several studies have demonstrated the impact of home life and background on patient outcome, independent of injury severity. Negative prognostic factors include low household income, lack of parent formal education, Medicaid insurance, Hispanic ethnicity, mental health of the caregiver, and functionality of the family.[55,56]

Not only are pediatric TBI patients at risk for failing to return to their preinjury baseline neurologic function, they also are at risk for development of postinjury psychiatric disorders.[57] Severity of illness is correlated with the likelihood of development of psychiatric disorder, but even children with mild TBI were at risk of psychiatric disorder development compared with a cohort of patients with an orthopedic injury.

Finally, patients who suffered TBI as a result of NAT experienced higher morbidity and mortality than those injured via unintentional mechanisms.[58,59]

Summary

- TBI is a significant source of morbidity and mortality in children.
- Indications for noncontrast head CT in the ED to evaluate for TBI include GCS less than 13, lower-energy mechanisms when combined with neurologic deficits or evidence of basilar skull fracture, high-energy mechanisms, and suspected or confirmed NAT.
- Patients with normal imaging and examination may be discharged from the ED and do not require observation.
- Immediate management of severe TBI includes maintenance of normal P_{CO_2}, normal oxygenation, and normal blood pressure with possible administration of hypertonic saline for signs of ICH. Corticosteroids should not be given.
- Outcomes in pediatric TBI patients are related to injury severity, presence of NAT, and socioeconomic background.

CERVICAL SPINE EVALUATION
Introduction

CSIs are estimated to occur in 1% to 2% of all pediatric trauma patients.[60–62] The incidence in very young patients, less than or equal to 5 years old, is estimated to be much less (0.4%).[63] Although unusual, CSIs can have serious consequences, including death and permanent disability[64]; 5% to 10% of patients with missed injuries develop worsening of neurologic symptoms or complete disability, reinforcing the importance of accurate diagnosis of CSI.[65] Anatomic differences between the adult and pediatric cervical spine pose a unique challenge during the evaluation and management of CSIs in children. In children without neurologic deficits, clearance of the cervical spine is not an emergency and, if unable to be cleared on arrival, children should be maintained in a properly fitted cervical collar, awaiting resolution of the urgent atmosphere that accompanies a trauma evaluation prior to reexamination. This strategy allows clinical clearance of many children without imaging. This article examines the characteristics of pediatric CSIs and an approach to the diagnostic evaluation of the pediatric cervical spine.

Relevant Anatomy and Pathophysiology

Pediatric anatomy

The cervical spine is the most common location for spinal injuries in children, accounting for 60% to 80% of spinal injuries compared with 30% to 40% of spinal injuries in adults.[60,66] Patient age also affects the location of injury. Injuries to the cervical spine in children less than 8 years of age are more likely to occur in the upper cervical spine, from the occiput to C3, and are more likely to be ligamentous as opposed to bony fractures.[67,68] In younger patients, the hypermobile and elastic cervical vertebral column can stretch as much as 2 inches without fracturing, whereas the spinal cord can only stretch 0.25 inches, predisposing children to a greater proportion of dislocations and spinal cord injury without radiographic abnormality (SCIWORA).[69,70] After the age of 8 to 10 years, the pediatric spine completes its maturation process and begins to take on adult characteristics and patterns of injury, including fractures and injuries to the lower cervical spine.[60,70,71] **Table 1** illustrates the unique characteristics of the pediatric cervical spine.[60,67,68,72,73] Certain conditions, including Down syndrome, mucopolysaccharidosis, achondrodysplasia, and os odontoideum (a congenital abnormality where the odontoid process is separated from the body of the axis by a transverse gap), are associated with spine abnormalities and an increased risk of CSI.[66,74]

Table 1 Unique characteristics of the pediatric cervical spine injuries	
Structure	Anatomic Considerations in Children Greater Than 8 y of Age
Occiput	Larger occiput-to-body ratio, smaller occipital condyles, more horizontal orientation of atlanto-occipital joints
Musculature	Weak nuchal muscles
Fulcrum	Fulcrum of motion at C2–C3 in comparison to C5–C6 in mature cervical spine
Ligaments, joints, and joint capsules	Incomplete ossification, more lax and stretchable ligaments and joints, susceptible to pseudosubluxation
Facets	Shallow and angulated facet joints
Vertebral bodies	Physiologic anterior wedging of vertebral bodies
Uncinate processes	Absent uncinate processes
Spinous processes	Underdeveloped spinous processes

Data from Refs.[60,67,68,72,73]

Normal variants

Familiarity with the pediatric vertebral architecture is important to differentiate fusion abnormalities or incomplete ossification from pathologic fracture. Common ossification sites and time to normal fusion are presented in **Table 2**.[67] Unlike epiphyseal plates, which appear sclerotic, smooth, and in predictable locations, fractures are irregular in appearance, nonsclerotic, and in unusual locations.[67]

Clinical Presentation and Examination

Mechanism of injury

Adults and children less than 8 years old with CSI are more frequently injured in motor vehicle crashes (MVCs) and falls, whereas sports-related injuries predominate in older children.[60,61,75,76]

Table 2 Embryologic considerations in imaging the developing pediatric spine		
Level	Ossification Centers	Time to Maturation
C1	3 Ossifications sites: anterior arch and 2 neural arches	Anterior arch ossification: 1 y Posterior fusion of neural arches: 3 y Anterior arch and neural arch fusion: 7 y
C2	4 Ossification sites: 2 odontoid and 2 neural arches, 1 body	Odontoid process: fuses midline in 7th fetal month. Second ossification center at apex (os terminale) appears between 3 y and 6 y and fuses by age 12 Posterior fusion of neural arches: 2–3 y Fusion of neural arches and body: 3–6 y
C3-7	3 Ossifications sites: 1 body and 2 neural arches	Posterior fusion of neural arches: 2–3 y Fusion of neural arches and body: 3–6 y Secondary ossification sites: tips of transverse processes and at the superior and inferior vertebral bodies may persist into adulthood

Data from Lustrin ES, Karakas SP, Ortiz AO, et al. Pediatric cervical spine: normal anatomy, variants, and trauma. Radiographics 2003;23(3):539–60.

NAT must be in the differential diagnosis when evaluating young patients with CSI. Abuse should be suspected in any child with a whiplash mechanism of injury.[61] In a retrospective review of 342 children with spinal injuries admitted to a level 1 trauma center, Knox and colleagues[77] evaluated the characteristics associated with spinal trauma secondary to NAT. NAT accounted for 3.2% of spinal trauma, and all children with spinal injuries secondary to NAT were under the age of 2 years. In this series, NAT and MVC were equally common mechanisms of injury in children less than 2 years old. A majority of these children (73%) sustained injuries to the cervical spine, and ligamentous injuries predominated. In addition, 91% had at least 1 other significant injury, with head injuries predominating.[77] It is important that NAT is not overlooked as a potential cause of CSI in very young patients, and other injuries are investigated in the evaluation of these patients.

Prehospital management
All unconscious children, children with injuries cephalad to the clavicles, or children involved in a high-speed MVC, are assumed to have a CSI.[72] Proper immobilization of the cervical spine is of key importance in the prehospital management of children with suspected CSI to prevent further injury. Children should be placed in a cervical collar and backboard immobilization and have their torso elevated or the head placed in a cervical recess to maintain neutral cervical alignment (see **Fig. 1**).[73,75,78]

Clinical examination
It is essential to perform a thorough history and physical examination, including a complete neurologic examination, in any child who presents with concerns of a CSI. Patel and colleagues[69] emphasized the importance of the physical examination in a retrospective review of 1098 children with CSIs. In this series, 50% of children with symptomatic spinal cord injury identified on physical examination had no radiographic findings (SCIWORA), highlighting the importance of a timely and complete neurologic examination to identify spinal cord injury early and prevent the extension of a partial neurologic deficit to a complete one. Furthermore, certain history and physical examination findings may alert a physician to the possibility of CSI in children. Leonard and colleagues[79] reviewed 540 cases of children less than 16 years of age across 17 hospitals in the Pediatric Emergency Care Applied Research Network and identified 8 factors associated with CSI, which are detailed in **Box 3**. The presence of 1 or more factors had a 98% sensitivity (95% CI, 96%–99%) in detecting CSI.[79]

Box 3
Risk factors associated with pediatric cervical spine injury

Altered mental status

Focal neurologic findings

Neck pain

Torticollis

Substantial torso injury

Preexisting conditions predisposing to CSI

Diving mechanism

High-risk MVC

Data from Leonard JC, Kuppermann N, Olsen C, et al. Factors associated with cervical spine injury in children after blunt trauma. Ann Emerg Med 2011;58(2):145–55.

Diagnostic Evaluation

Clinical prediction rules

There are several well-validated clinical prediction rules in adult cervical spine trauma that, when applied correctly, can identify patients that are at low risk for a CSI and do not need additional imaging. Applying these decision-making tools to children, especially very young children, poses a unique challenge to the examining physician. Fear and anxiety may be confused with pain, and a child may not be developmentally able to follow instructions or communicate with a provider, further complicating the picture. Additionally there is no single, well-defined clinical prediction rule for children.

The most commonly cited clinical adult decision tools are the National Emergency X-Radiography Utilization Study (NEXUS) decision tool and the Canadian C-Spine Rule (CCR). NEXUS consists of 5 low-risk criteria that, when absent, make CSI unlikely and usually obviate additional imaging in adult patients, with a sensitivity of 99% (95% CI, 98%–99.6%).[80] The CCR asks 3 questions, none of which relies on physical examination findings and, when applied in hemodynamically stable and alert adult patients, had a 100% sensitivity (95% CI, 98%–100%) in detecting clinically significant CSI.[81] A comparison of the NEXUS low-risk criteria and the CCR is presented in **Table 3**. Stiell and colleagues[82] compared the NEXUS decision tool to the CCR and found that the CCR was more sensitive (99.4% compared with 90.7%) and specific (45.1% compared with 36.8%) than the NEXUS criteria when applied to stable, alert adults. Furthermore, the CCR was superior to NEXUS on secondary analysis of indeterminate patients.

In 2001, Viccellio and colleagues[83] applied the NEXUS decision tool to children less than 18 years old. Of the 3065 patients examined, 30 were found to have a CSI. Of the 603 patients who met the low-risk criteria, none had a CSI, resulting in a sensitivity of 100% (95% CI, 87.8%–100%). Unfortunately, when further examining the sensitivity of the tool, the CI was wide, and, in addition, there were only 4 injured children who were less than 9 years old and none less than 2 years old. The investigators cautioned the application of this tool in infants and children, despite the initial apparent success in the pediatric population.

Table 3
A comparison of the National Emergency X-Radiography Utilization Study low-risk criteria and the Canadian C-Spine Rule

National Emergency X-Radiography Utilization Study Criteria	Canadian C-Spine Rule
No midline cervical tenderness	Is there any high-risk factor present that mandates radiography (ie, dangerous mechanism)?
No focal neurologic deficit	Is there any low-risk factor present that allows safe assessment of range of motion (ie, position in ED, ambulatory at any time since injury)?
Normal alertness	Is the patient able to actively rotate neck 45° to the left and right?
No intoxication	
No painful distracting injury	

Data from Hoffman JR, Mower WR, Wolfson AB, et al. Validity of a set of clinical criteria to rule out injury to the cervical spine in patients with blunt trauma. National Emergency X-Radiography Utilization Study Group. N Engl J Med 2000;343(2):94–9; and Stiell IG, Wells GA, Vandemheen KL, et al. The Canadian C-spine rule for radiography in alert and stable trauma patients. JAMA 2001;286(15):1841–8.

Several years later, Ehrlich and colleagues[84] applied the NEXUS low-risk criteria and the CCR to case-matched patients less than 10 years old. They concluded that neither rule was sensitive or specific enough for that age group.

To address the challenge of clinical clearance in young patients, Lee and colleagues[85] recruited a multidisciplinary team to design a cervical spine clearance algorithm for children less than 8 years old. Ten criteria were defined:

1. Unconscious patient or patient with abnormal neurologic examination
2. High-risk mechanism of injury (high-speed motor vehicle collisions [MVC], falls greater than body height, and so forth)
3. Neck pain
4. Focal neck tenderness or inability to assess secondary to distracting injury
5. Abnormal neurologic examination findings after complete examination
6. Transient neurologic symptoms suggestive of SCIWORA
7. Physical signs of neck trauma
8. Unreliable examination secondary to substance abuse
9. Significant trauma to the head or face
10. Inconsolableness

Presence of 1 or more of these criteria resulted in cervical spine imaging. The application of the clearance algorithm resulted in no missed injuries and a reduction in the time to cervical spine clearance in both intubated and nonintubated children.[85]

Nonverbal infants and toddlers pose an even greater challenge when it comes to clinical clearance. Pieretti-Vanmarcke and colleagues[86] sought to determine if there were any clinical indicators of CSI in children less than 3 years old and were able to identify 4 independent predictors, which are presented in **Table 4**. Each predictor was assigned a score, and a total score of 0 or 1 had a negative predictive value (NPV) of 99.93% (95% CI, 99.85%–99.97%) and a sensitivity of 92.9% (95% CI, 85.1%–97.3%) in ruling out CSI without additional imaging. CSI were identified in 83 of the 12,537 patients in this study. Of these, 5 children with significant injuries scored less than 2, which would have been missed with this prediction model; however, all children with missed injuries had neck splinting or evidence of facial or skull fractures on physical examination.[86] This study reinforced that well-applied clinical prediction rules are efficacious, even in infants and toddlers, but they cannot take the place of a well-performed clinical examination.

In summary, it is possible to rule out CSI clinically in many but not all children. A combination of the NEXUS and CCR can be used. At minimum, screening cervical

---

Table 4
Independent clinical predictors of cervical spine injury in children less than 3 years of age and assigned score*

Clinical Finding	Score
GCS <14	3 Points
$GCS_{EYE} = 1$	2 Points
Motor vehicle accident	2 Points
Age 2 y or older (24–36 mo)	1 Point

* A score of 0–1 points was associated with a low risk of CSI.
Data from Pieretti-Vanmarcke R, Velmahos GC, Nance ML, et al. Clinical clearance of the cervical spine in blunt trauma patients younger than 3 years: a multi-center study of the american association for the surgery of trauma. J Trauma 2009;67(3):543–9. [discussion: 549–50].

spine imaging should be obtained in all unconscious children and conscious children who present with the following[78,84,86]:

- After a fall from 10 feet or greater (or body height if <8 years)
- MVC
- Suspected NAT
- GCS <14 (GCS_{EYE} = 1 if <3 years)
- Neurologic deficit
- Significant head, face, or neck trauma
- Neck pain or torticollis
- Distracting injury or intoxication

Plain radiographs

After clinical stratification, the ideal imaging strategy in pediatric CSI identifies injuries while minimizing cumulative radiation dose and subsequent risk of malignancy. Plain radiographs are the initial screening tool of choice for children who cannot be clinically cleared. There is controversy over what films should be obtained. In small children, the sensitivity of a lateral film alone is 73% but increases to 93% in children over 8 years of age.[70] Because of this, the anteroposterior (AP) film is often included and has resulted in an increase in sensitivity to greater than 90%, although other reports indicate that the addition of the AP film is unlikely to increase sensitivity.[68,70,87] The role of the odontoid view is also controversial and likely unnecessary in children less than 9 years of age, because most dens fractures in this age group re visible on the lateral film.[68] It is important to visualize the entire cervical spine on lateral film (C1–C7) to avoid delays and the associated untoward consequences of a missed CSI. There is little role for oblique or flexion/extension films acutely in the setting of normal lateral and AP films.[64,68,70]

Computed tomography

The use of CT to screen for CSI is associated with high doses of ionizing radiation, and the risk of malignancy is not inconsequential. Children, especially girls, are disproportionally more sensitive to the adverse effects of ionizing radiation, and this risk decreases linearly with age.[88,89] Although CT has been reported to be more sensitive in detecting CSI compared with plain films, most clinically significant injuries in children found on CT are also noted on plain film.[70] Additionally, young children are more likely to have ligamentous injury, which is not identified on CT. A focused CT can limit radiation and may be indicated to clarify abnormalities identified on plain films.[90] MRI may be the imaging modality of choice for children less than 8 years of age, because the incidence of identifying a clinically significant fracture on CT not present on radiograph is low, and there is an increased risk of developing radiation-induced cancer, particularly to the thyroid gland.[76,91,92] **Fig. 2**A depicts a C2 fracture in a 16-month-old who was involved in an MVC. The patient then underwent MRI (see **Fig. 2**B), which revealed an unstable C2 fracture with disruption of the interspinal ligament and the anterior and posterior longitudinal ligaments from C2 to C3 as well as cord contusion from C2 to C7, which was not apparent on CT. The patient was placed in halo traction and review of the postoperative lateral film (see **Fig. 2**C) reveals the C2 fracture that would have easily been identifiable had this patient had an initial screening lateral cervical spine film.

MRI

MRI of the cervical spine is the best imaging modality for the diagnosis of soft tissue injuries, such as ligamentous injuries, cord edema or hematoma, cord transections, and cord compression.[93] In a meta-analysis of adult blunt trauma patients, Muchow and colleagues[94] demonstrated a high sensitivity (97.2%, 95% CI, 89.5%–99.35%)

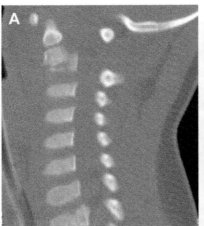
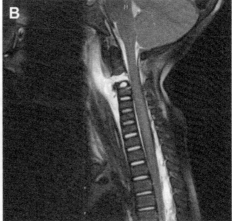
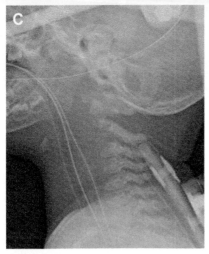

Fig. 2. (A) C2 cervical spine fracture depicted on initial CT obtained in a 16-month old girl after a motor vehicle accident. (B) An MRI was obtained in this child that further revealed an unstable C2 fracture with disruption of the interspinal ligament, anterior and posterior longitudinal ligaments from C2 to C3, and cord contusion from C2 to C7, which was not apparent on CT. The fracture was also identified. (C) This is a lateral film after halo stabilization, and the cervical spine fracture is clearly seen in this film, highlighting the importance of screening cervical spine films in children, because most bony injuries are identified.

and specificity (98.5%, CI, 91.8%–99.7%) with a 100% NPV, allowing the safe discontinuation of cervical spine precautions without adverse neurologic outcomes. MRI has a sensitivity of 100%, specificity of 97%, and NPV of 75% and, when compared with CT, has a superior sensitivity for the detection of soft tissue injuries.[65] **Fig. 3**A is an example of the importance of a through neurologic examination for identification of soft tissue injuries, regardless of CT findings. The initial cervical spine CT scan on this 3-year-old who was involved in an MVC was normal. The patient, however, had right-sided paresis and an MRI was obtained (see **Fig. 3**B) that revealed a C1–C2 cord contusion and ligamentous injury, and the patient was placed in halo traction the following day.

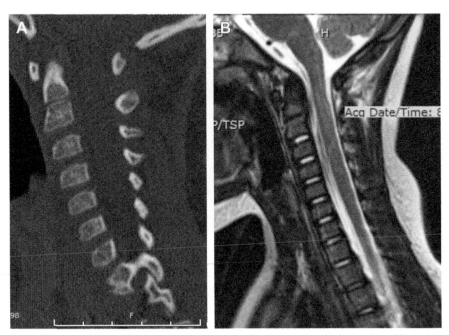

Fig. 3. (*A*) Normal cervical spine CT in a 3-year-old after a motor vehicle accident. (*B*) An MRI was obtained in this patient due to right-sided neurologic findings and revealed a C1–C2 cord contusion and ligamentous injury, underscoring the point that CT scans can be normal and miss the ligamentous injuries that are most common in young pediatric trauma patients. All patients with neurologic findings should undergo MRI.

MRI has a defined role in the clearance of CSI intubated or obtunded children. Frank and colleagues[95] found a decrease in time to cervical spine clearance and a reduction in the duration of ICU and hospital stay with the use of MRI. In any child who is likely to remain intubated or obtunded, an MRI within the first 72 hours is the best way to ensure no clinically significant CSI, even in the presence of normal plain radiographs.[72,96] If the cervical spine is unlikely to be cleared within 72 hours, and the child will undergo brain MRI for trauma, obtaining a cervical spine MRI at that time may also be useful.[61] All children with neurologic symptoms should undergo urgent MRI examination to rule out injuries that would warrant intervention.[64,75]

In 2000, Boston Children's Hospital instituted a cervical spine clearance algorithm for both conscious (**Fig. 4**) and the unconscious pediatric patients (**Fig. 5**) with possible CSI. Over a 10-year study period, the algorithm sensitivity was 94.4% and the NPV was 99.9%. There was only one missed injury that was a stable CSI found in a patient who remained in a collar at hospital discharge. These algorithms, or one similar, can be used in the evaluation children with suspected CSI while minimizing the risk of ionizing radiation (Arbuthnot M, Mooney, DP. Cervical spine clearance in pediatric trauma: a single institution's experience, submitted for publication).

MANAGEMENT

Table 5 outlines common CSIs in pediatric patients.[67] The management of injuries is beyond the scope of this article, but urgent consultation with a spine specialist and traumatologist is required in the setting of diagnosed CSI.

CLINICAL OUTCOMES

Traumatic spinal cord injury in children is a rare event. As discussed previously, the anatomic differences in the cervical spine result in a different pattern of injury in children and there is some evidence that children have a better neurosurgical recovery compared with adults.[97]

The mortality rate associated with spinal cord injury varies from 4% to 41%, and, of survivors, as many as 67% have neurologic deficits.[68] TBI is the most common concomitant injury.[98] Shin and colleagues[99] reviewed a decade of pediatric CSI from the Kids' Inpatient Database and found a 22.05% rate of TBI and determined the mortality rate was 11.07% in children with TBI and 3.14% in non-TBI patients.

In a large retrospective review by Leonard and colleagues,[66] children less than 2 years old had the poorest outcomes with the highest incidence of permanent neurologic damage and death. Patients with atlanto-occipital dislocations or C1–C2 dislocations were the most devastated, and children with axial injuries were 5 times more likely to die than those with subaxial injuries.[66]

Finally, there is insufficient evidence to recommend the use of steroids in CSI.[100] Steroid administration has been associated with worse clinical outcomes, and steroid administration is not recommended in children with spinal cord injuries.[66]

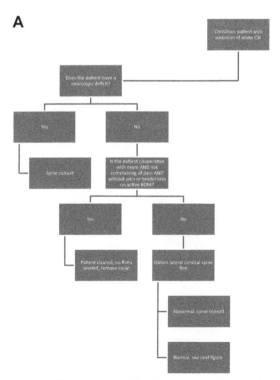

Fig. 4. (A, B) Cervical spine clearance algorithm for the conscious patient with concern for CSI. ROM, range of motion.

B

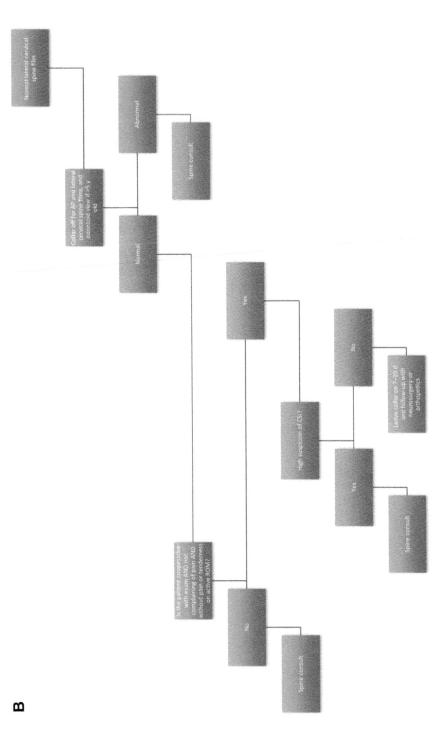

Fig. 4. (continued)

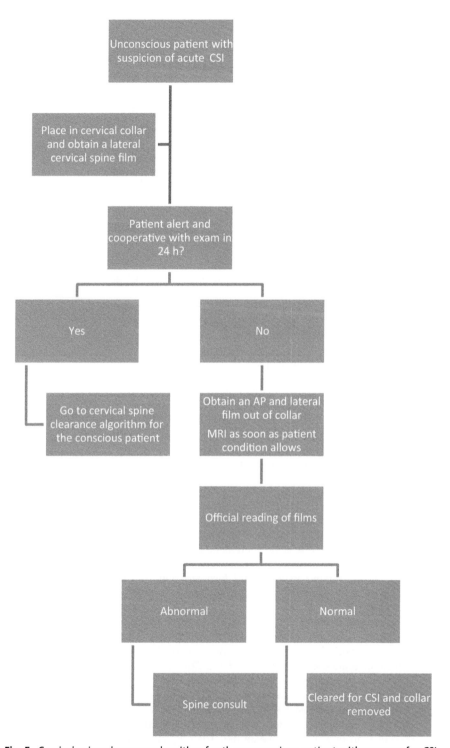

Fig. 5. Cervical spine clearance algorithm for the unconscious patient with concern for CSI.

Table 5
Cervical spine injuries in pediatric patients

Injury	Description
SCIWORA	• SCIWORA is likely related to transient deformation of the spinal column without bony fracture. • Requires MRI to evaluate
Atlanto-occipital injuries	• Associated with deceleration injuries, can be fatal. Atlanto-occipital dislocation is 2.5× more common in children than in adults. • Crucial to evaluate the craniocervical junction on imaging
Jefferson fracture	• Fracture of the ring of C1, due to axial loading injury • Stable when transverse ligament is still intact
Atlantoaxial injuries	• C1–C2 injuries can be due to ligamentous disruption, rotary subluxation, or odontoid separation • Can result in excess cervical rotation and spinal cord injury
Hangman fracture	• Hyperextension injury that results in fractures through the pars interarticularis of C2 and is associated with anterior subluxation of C2 on C3 • Important not to confuse with the normal variant of subluxation in children
Subaxial injuries	C3–C7 injuries are more common in older children and associated with MVC and sport-related injuries
Posterior ligamentous injuries	Diagnosed with MRI and often require operative intervention (posterior fusion)
Wedge compression fractures	• Associated with axial loading and flexion injuries resulting in loss of vertebral height • Usually stable fractures that heal easily
Facet dislocations	• Can be associated with facet fractures • Are unstable when bilateral and often associated with spinal cord syndromes

Data from Lustrin ES, Karakas SP, Ortiz AO, et al. Pediatric cervical spine: normal anatomy, variants, and trauma. Radiographics 2003;23(3):539–56.

SUMMARY

- Children younger than 8 are more likely to have ligamentous injuries located to the upper spine. After the age of 8, the pediatric spine starts to resemble the adult spine and there is an increased incidence of fractures and multilevel injuries.
- MVC, sports-related injuries, and falls are common mechanisms of injury. NAT should be in the differential diagnosis in children less than 2 years old with CSI.
- All unconscious patients and conscious patients who present after a significant mechanism of action or significant trauma to the head should be assumed to have a CSI and placed in proper cervical immobilization.
- Clinical clearance is possible in many children, although in older children it is easier due to improved ability to communicate. All children should undergo a complete neurologic examination.
- Plain radiographs (lateral ± AP) are the screening tool of choice in children who cannot be clinically cleared. The odontoid view can be reserved for children greater than or equal to 9 years old. There is little acute role for the oblique, flexion, or extension views.

- CT is associated with an increased malignancy risk and should not be used as a screening tool for pediatric CSI. It is good at evaluating fractures but cannot diagnose soft tissue or ligamentous injury and, as such, cannot be used solely to clear the cervical spine.
- In children less than 8 years old, an MRI may be the modality of choice to clear the cervical spine if it cannot be cleared clinically. Furthermore, an MRI should be obtained in all patients with neurologic symptoms. In patients who are expected to remain obtunded or intubated for greater than 24 to 48 hours, an MRI within the first 72 hours can be used to clinically clear the spine.
- Outcomes in spinal cord injury are related to age and type of injury. Generally, children have better neurologic outcomes compared with adults. Corticosteroids are currently not recommended in the treatment of pediatric spinal cord injury.
- A cervical spine clearance algorithm may assist in safe cervical spine clearance with a low missed injury rate.

REFERENCES

1. Mena JH, Sanchez AI, Rubiano AM, et al. Effect of the modified glasgow coma scale score criteria for mild traumatic brain injury on mortality prediction: comparing classic and modified glasgow coma scale score model scores of 13. J Trauma 2011;71(5):1185–93.
2. Salottolo K, Levy AS, Slone DS, et al. The effect of age on glasgow coma scale score in patients with traumatic brain injury. JAMA Surg 2014;149(7):727–34.
3. Emami P, Czorlich P, Fritzsche FS, et al. Impact of glasgow coma scale score and pupil parameters on mortality rate and outcome in pediatric and adult severe traumatic brain injury: a retrospective, multicenter cohort study. J Neurosurg 2016;1–8.
4. Bishop NB. Traumatic brain injury: a primer for primary care physicians. Curr Probl Pediatr Adolesc Health Care 2006;36(9):318–31.
5. Traumatic Brain Injury in the United States: Assessing outcomes in children. Available at: http://www.cdc.gov/traumaticbraininjury/assessing_outcomes_in_children.html. Accessed April 23, 2016.
6. Faul MXL, Wald MM, Coronado VG. Traumatic brain injury in the United States. Available at: http://www.cdc.gov/traumaticbraininjury/pdf/blue_book.pdf. Accessed April 23, 2016.
7. Percent Distributions of TBI-related Emergency Department Visits by Age Group and Injury Mechanism — United States cghwcgtdde. Available at: http://www.cdc.gov/traumaticbraininjury/data/dist_ed.html. Accessed April 29, 2016.
8. Rates of TBI-related Emergency Department Visits by Age Group — United States cghwcgtdrebhAA. Available at: http://www.cdc.gov/traumaticbraininjury/data/rates_ed_byage.html. Accessed April 29, 2016.
9. Keenan HT, Runyan DK, Marshall SW, et al. A population-based study of inflicted traumatic brain injury in young children. JAMA 2003;290(5):621–6.
10. Parks SE, Kegler SR, Annest JL, et al. Characteristics of fatal abusive head trauma among children in the USA: 2003-2007: an application of the CDC operational case definition to national vital statistics data. Inj Prev 2012;18(3):193–9.
11. Kim JJ, Gean AD. Imaging for the diagnosis and management of traumatic brain injury. Neurotherapeutics 2011;8(1):39–53.
12. Bodanapally UK, Sours C, Zhuo J, et al. Imaging of traumatic brain injury. Radiol Clin North Am 2015;53(4):695–715, viii.

13. Mokri B. The Monro-Kellie hypothesis: applications in CSF volume depletion. Neurology 2001;56(12):1746–8.
14. Jantzen J. Prevention and treatment of intracranial hypertension. Best Pract Res Clin Anaesthesiol 2007;21(4):517–38.
15. Schaller B, Graf R. Different compartments of intracranial pressure and its relationship to cerebral blood flow. J Trauma 2005;59(6):1521–31.
16. Pigula FA, Wald SL, Shackford SR, et al. The effect of hypotension and hypoxia on children with severe head injuries. J Pediatr Surg 1993;28(3):310–6.
17. Chambers IR, Kirkham FJ. What is the optimal cerebral perfusion pressure in children suffering from traumatic coma? Neurosurg Focus 2003;15(6):E3.
18. Ling GSF, Neal CJ. Maintaining cerebral perfusion pressure is a worthy clinical goal. Neurocrit Care 2005;2(1):75–81.
19. Allen BB, Chiu YL, Gerber LM, et al. Age-specific cerebral perfusion pressure thresholds and survival in children and adolescents with severe traumatic brain injury*. Pediatr Crit Care Med 2014;15(1):62–70.
20. White H, Venkatesh B. Cerebral perfusion pressure in neurotrauma: a review. Anesth Analg 2008;107(3):979–88.
21. National Clinical Guideline Centre (UK). Head Injury: Triage A, Investigation and Early Management of Head Injury in Children, Young People and Adults. London: National Institute for Health and Care Excellence (UK); 2014.
22. Levi L, Guilburd JN, Linn S, et al. The association between skull fracture, intracranial pathology and outcome in pediatric head injury. Br J Neurosurg 1991; 5(6):617–25.
23. Stein SC, Young GS, Talucci RC, et al. Delayed brain injury after head trauma: significance of coagulopathy. Neurosurgery 1992;30(2):160–5.
24. Davis RL, Mullen N, Makela M, et al. Cranial computed tomography scans in children after minimal head injury with loss of consciousness. Ann Emerg Med 1994;24(4):640–5.
25. Simon B, Letourneau P, Vitorino E, et al. Pediatric minor head trauma: indications for computed tomographic scanning revisited. J Trauma 2001;51(2):231–7 [discussion: 237–8].
26. Halley MK, Silva PD, Foley J, et al. Loss of consciousness: when to perform computed tomography? Pediatr Crit Care Med 2004;5(3):230–3.
27. Fundarò C, Caldarelli M, Monaco S, et al. Brain CT scan for pediatric minor accidental head injury. An Italian experience and review of literature. Childs Nerv Syst 2012;28(7):1063–8.
28. Lee LK, Monroe D, Bachman MC, et al. Isolated loss of consciousness in children with minor blunt head trauma. JAMA Pediatr 2014;168(9):837–43.
29. Ryan ME, Palasis S, Saigal G, et al. ACR appropriateness criteria head trauma–child. J Am Coll Radiol 2014;11:939–47.
30. Brown CVR, Weng J, Oh D, et al. Does routine serial computed tomography of the head influence management of traumatic brain injury? A prospective evaluation. J Trauma 2004;57(5):939–43.
31. Sifri ZC, Homnick AT, Vaynman A, et al. A prospective evaluation of the value of repeat cranial computed tomography in patients with minimal head injury and an intracranial bleed. J Trauma 2006;61(4):862–7.
32. Brown CVR, Zada G, Salim A, et al. Indications for routine repeat head computed tomography (CT) stratified by severity of traumatic brain injury. J Trauma 2007;62(6):1339–45.
33. Dias MS, Lillis KA, Calvo C, et al. Management of accidental minor head injuries in children: a prospective outcomes study. J Neurosurg Pediatr 2004;101(2):38–43.

34. Isokuortti H, Luoto TM, Kataja A, et al. Necessity of monitoring after negative head CT in acute head injury. Injury 2014;45(9):1340–4.
35. Holsti M, Kadish HA, Sill BL, et al. Pediatric closed head injuries treated in an observation unit. Pediatr Emerg Care 2005;21(10):639–44.
36. Powell EC, Atabaki SM, Wootton-Gorges S, et al. Isolated linear skull fractures in children with blunt head trauma. Pediatrics 2015;135(4):e851–7.
37. Blackwood BP, Bean JF, Sadecki-Lund C, et al. Observation for isolated traumatic skull fractures in the pediatric population: unnecessary and costly. J Pediatr Surg 2016;51(4):654–8.
38. Arrey EN, Kerr ML, Fletcher S, et al. Linear nondisplaced skull fractures in children: who should be observed or admitted? J Neurosurg Pediatr 2015;16(6): 703–8.
39. Addioui A, Saint-Vil D, Crevier L, et al. Management of skull fractures in children less than 1 year of age. J Pediatr Surg 2016;51(7):1146–50.
40. Hartwell JL, Spalding MC, Fletcher B, et al. You cannot go home: routine concussion evaluation is not enough. Am Surg 2015;81(4):395–403.
41. Berry C, Ley EJ, Bukur M, et al. Redefining hypotension in traumatic brain injury. Injury 2012;43(11):1833–7.
42. Brenner M, Stein DM, Hu PF, et al. Traditional systolic blood pressure targets underestimate hypotension-induced secondary brain injury. J Trauma Acute Care Surg 2012;72(5):1135–9.
43. Stevens RD, Shoykhet M, Cadena R. Emergency neurological life support: intracranial hypertension and herniation. Neurocrit Care 2015;23(Suppl 2):S76–82.
44. Mtaweh H, Bell MJ. Management of pediatric traumatic brain injury. Curr Treat Options Neurol 2015;17(5):348.
45. Kochanek PM, Carney N, Adelson PD, et al. Guidelines for the acute medical management of severe traumatic brain injury in infants, children, and adolescents–second edition. Pediatr Crit Care Med 2012;13(Suppl 1):S1–82.
46. Miller Ferguson N, Shein SL, Kochanek PM, et al. Intracranial hypertension and cerebral hypoperfusion in children with severe traumatic brain injury: thresholds and burden in accidental and abusive insults. Pediatr Crit Care Med 2016;17(5):444–50.
47. Pelletier EB, Émond M, Lauzier F, et al. Hyperosmolar therapy in severe traumatic brain injury: a Survey of Emergency Physicians from a Large Canadian Province. PLoS One 2014;9(4):e95778.
48. Brophy GM, Human T, Shutter L. Emergency neurological life support: pharmacotherapy. Neurocrit Care 2015;23(Suppl 2):S48–68.
49. Kamel H, Navi BB, Nakagawa K, et al. Hypertonic saline versus mannitol for the treatment of elevated intracranial pressure: a meta-analysis of randomized clinical trials. Crit Care Med 2011;39(3):554–9.
50. Shein SL, Ferguson NM, Kochanek PM, et al. Effectiveness of pharmacological therapies for intracranial hypertension in children with severe traumatic brain injury—results from an automated data collection system time-synched to drug administration. Pediatr Crit Care Med 2016;17(3):236–45.
51. Burgess S, Abu-Laban RB, Slavik RS, et al. A systematic review of randomized controlled trials comparing hypertonic sodium solutions and mannitol for traumatic brain injury: implications for emergency department management. Ann Pharmacother 2016;50(4):291–300.
52. Alderson P, Roberts I. Corticosteroids for acute traumatic brain injury. Cochrane Database Syst Rev 2005;(1):CD000196.
53. Babikian T, Asarnow R. Neurocognitive outcomes and recovery after pediatric TBI: meta-analytic review of the literature. Neuropsychology 2009;23(3):283–96.

54. Rivara FP, Vavilala MS, Durbin D, et al. Persistence of disability 24 to 36 months after pediatric traumatic brain injury: a cohort study. J Neurotrauma 2012;29(15): 2499–504.

55. Zonfrillo MR, Durbin DR, Koepsell TD, et al. Prevalence of and risk factors for poor functioning after isolated mild traumatic brain injury in children. J Neurotrauma 2014;31(8):722–7.

56. Ryan NP, van Bijnen L, Catroppa C, et al. Longitudinal outcome and recovery of social problems after pediatric traumatic brain injury (TBI): contribution of brain insult and family environment. Int J Dev Neurosci 2016;49:23–30.

57. Max JE, Wilde EA, Bigler ED, et al. Psychiatric disorders after pediatric traumatic brain injury: a prospective, longitudinal, controlled Study. J Neuropsychiatry Clin Neurosci 2012;24(4):427–36.

58. Deans KJ, Minneci PC, Lowell W, et al. Increased morbidity and mortality of traumatic brain injury in victims of nonaccidental trauma. J Trauma Acute Care Surg 2013;75(1):157–60.

59. Fulkerson DH, White IK, Rees JM, et al. Analysis of long-term (median 10.5 years) outcomes in children presenting with traumatic brain injury and an initial Glasgow Coma Scale score of 3 or 4. J Neurosurg Pediatr 2015;16(4):410–9.

60. Platzer P, Jaindl M, Thalhammer G, et al. Cervical spine injuries in pediatric patients. J Trauma 2007;62(2):389–96 [discussion: 394–6].

61. Booth TN. Cervical spine evaluation in pediatric trauma. AJR Am J Roentgenol 2012;198(5):W417–25.

62. Rosati SF, Maarouf R, Wolfe L, et al. Implementation of pediatric cervical spine clearance guidelines at a combined trauma center: twelve-month impact. J Trauma Acute Care Surg 2015;78(6):1117–21.

63. Hale DF, Fitzpatrick CM, Doski JJ, et al. Absence of clinical findings reliably excludes unstable cervical spine injuries in children 5 years or younger. J Trauma Acute Care Surg 2015;78(5):943–8.

64. Chung S, Mikrogianakis A, Wales PW, et al. Trauma association of Canada Pediatric Subcommittee National Pediatric Cervical Spine Evaluation Pathway: consensus guidelines. J Trauma 2011;70(4):873–84.

65. Henry M, Riesenburger RI, Kryzanski J, et al. A retrospective comparison of CT and MRI in detecting pediatric cervical spine injury. Childs Nerv Syst 2013; 29(8):1333–8.

66. Leonard JR, Jaffe DM, Kuppermann N, et al. Cervical spine injury patterns in children. Pediatrics 2014;133(5):e1179–88.

67. Lustrin ES, Karakas SP, Ortiz AO, et al. Pediatric cervical spine: normal anatomy, variants, and trauma. Radiographics 2003;23(3):539–60.

68. Easter JS, Barkin R, Rosen CL, et al. Cervical spine injuries in children, part I: mechanism of injury, clinical presentation, and imaging. J Emerg Med 2011; 41(2):142–50.

69. Patel JC, Tepas JJ 3rd, Mollitt DL, et al. Pediatric cervical spine injuries: defining the disease. J Pediatr Surg 2001;36(2):373–6.

70. Tat ST, Mejia MJ, Freishtat RJ. Imaging, clearance, and controversies in pediatric cervical spine trauma. Pediatr Emerg Care 2014;30(12):911–5 [quiz: 916–8].

71. Knox JB, Schneider JE, Cage JM, et al. Spine trauma in very young children: a retrospective study of 206 patients presenting to a level 1 pediatric trauma center. J Pediatr Orthop 2014;34(7):698–702.

72. Slack SE, Clancy MJ. Clearing the cervical spine of paediatric trauma patients. Emerg Med J 2004;21(2):189–93.

73. Basu S. Spinal injuries in children. Front Neurol 2012;3:96.

74. Robson KA. Os odontoideum: rare cervical lesion. West J Emerg Med 2011; 12(4):520–2.
75. Schoneberg C, Schweiger B, Hussmann B, et al. Diagnosis of cervical spine injuries in children: a systematic review. Eur J Trauma Emerg Surg 2013;39(6): 653–65.
76. Kreykes NS, Letton RW Jr. Current issues in the diagnosis of pediatric cervical spine injury. Semin Pediatr Surg 2010;19(4):257–64.
77. Knox J, Schneider J, Wimberly RL, et al. Characteristics of spinal injuries secondary to nonaccidental trauma. J Pediatr Orthop 2014;34(4):376–81.
78. Rozzelle CJ, Aarabi B, Dhall SS, et al. Management of pediatric cervical spine and spinal cord injuries. Neurosurgery 2013;72(Suppl 2):205–26.
79. Leonard JC, Kuppermann N, Olsen C, et al. Factors associated with cervical spine injury in children after blunt trauma. Ann Emerg Med 2011;58(2):145–55.
80. Hoffman JR, Mower WR, Wolfson AB, et al. Validity of a set of clinical criteria to rule out injury to the cervical spine in patients with blunt trauma. National Emergency X-Radiography Utilization Study Group. N Engl J Med 2000;343(2):94–9.
81. Stiell IG, Wells GA, Vandemheen KL, et al. The Canadian C-spine rule for radiography in alert and stable trauma patients. JAMA 2001;286(15):1841–8.
82. Stiell IG, Clement CM, McKnight RD, et al. The Canadian C-spine rule versus the NEXUS low-risk criteria in patients with trauma. N Engl J Med 2003;349(26): 2510–8.
83. Viccellio P, Simon H, Pressman BD, et al. A prospective multicenter study of cervical spine injury in children. Pediatrics 2001;108(2):E20.
84. Ehrlich PF, Wee C, Drongowski R, et al. Canadian C-spine rule and the national emergency X-radiography utilization low-risk criteria for C-spine radiography in young trauma patients. J Pediatr Surg 2009;44(5):987–91.
85. Lee SL, Sena M, Greenholz SK, et al. A multidisciplinary approach to the development of a cervical spine clearance protocol: process, rationale, and initial results. J Pediatr Surg 2003;38(3):358–62 [discussion: 358–62].
86. Pieretti-Vanmarcke R, Velmahos GC, Nance ML, et al. Clinical clearance of the cervical spine in blunt trauma patients younger than 3 years: a multi-center study of the american association for the surgery of trauma. J Trauma 2009; 67(3):543–9 [discussion: 549–50].
87. Nigrovic LE, Rogers AJ, Adelgais KM, et al. Utility of plain radiographs in detecting traumatic injuries of the cervical spine in children. Pediatr Emerg Care 2012; 28(5):426–32.
88. Bennett TD, Bratton SL, Riva-Cambrin J, et al. Cervical spine imaging in hospitalized children with traumatic brain injury. Pediatr Emerg Care 2015;31(4): 243–9.
89. Mazrani W, McHugh K, Marsden PJ. The radiation burden of radiological investigations. Arch Dis Child 2007;92(12):1127–31.
90. Garton HJ, Hammer MR. Detection of pediatric cervical spine injury. Neurosurgery 2008;62(3):700–8 [discussion: 700–8].
91. Hernandez JA, Chupik C, Swischuk LE. Cervical spine trauma in children under 5 years: productivity of CT. Emerg Radiol 2004;10(4):176–8.
92. Jimenez RR, Deguzman MA, Shiran S, et al. CT versus plain radiographs for evaluation of c-spine injury in young children: do benefits outweigh risks? Pediatr Radiol 2008;38(6):635–44.
93. Mahajan P, Jaffe DM, Olsen CS, et al. Spinal cord injury without radiologic abnormality in children imaged with magnetic resonance imaging. J Trauma Acute Care Surg 2013;75(5):843–7.

94. Muchow RD, Resnick DK, Abdel MP, et al. Magnetic resonance imaging (MRI) in the clearance of the cervical spine in blunt trauma: a meta-analysis. J Trauma 2008;64(1):179–89.
95. Frank JB, Lim CK, Flynn JM, et al. The efficacy of magnetic resonance imaging in pediatric cervical spine clearance. Spine 2002;27(11):1176–9.
96. Keiper MD, Zimmerman RA, Bilaniuk LT. MRI in the assessment of the supportive soft tissues of the cervical spine in acute trauma in children. Neuroradiology 1998;40(6):359–63.
97. Parent S, Mac-Thiong JM, Roy-Beaudry M, et al. Spinal cord injury in the pediatric population: a systematic review of the literature. J Neurotrauma 2011;28(8): 1515–24.
98. Cirak B, Ziegfeld S, Knight VM, et al. Spinal injuries in children. J Pediatr Surg 2004;39(4):607–12.
99. Shin JI, Lee NJ, Cho SK. Pediatric cervical spine and spinal cord injury: a national database study. Spine 2016;41(4):283–92.
100. Easter JS, Barkin R, Rosen CL, et al. Cervical spine injuries in children, part II: management and special considerations. J Emerg Med 2011;41(3):252–6.

Abdominal Trauma Evaluation for the Pediatric Surgeon

Sabrina Drexel, MD[a], Kenneth Azarow, MD[a],
Mubeen A. Jafri, MD[a,b],*

KEYWORDS

- Pediatric trauma • Abdominal evaluation • Pediatric surgeon
- Nonoperative management solid organ injury • Abdominal injury

KEY POINTS

- The evaluation of abdominal trauma in children should be guided by the Advanced Trauma Life Support algorithms accounting for the unique anatomy and physiology of pediatric patients.
- In children with mild trauma who are clinically stable, physical examination, laboratory results, and imaging avoiding ionizing radiation should be used; computed tomography imaging is reserved for more severe injury.
- Nonoperative management of many injuries, including solid organ trauma, has become the standard of care for children, although hemodynamically unstable patients must receive expeditious intervention.

INTRODUCTION

Trauma is the leading cause of childhood mortality. More than 20 million children are injured each year, and unintentional injury is the leading cause of death for children in all age groups over 1 year of age. Abdominal trauma is the third leading cause of death in this population, after head and thoracic injuries. It is the most common cause of death owing to unrecognized injury.[1] The evaluation of the injured child with a focus on abdominal trauma is a significant portion of the practice of pediatric surgery. Pediatric trauma differs from adult trauma by mechanisms, injury patterns, anatomy, and long-term effects on growth and development. A focus on clinical examination and, when appropriate, reduction in ionizing radiation, are important considerations. We

Disclosure: None of the authors have anything to disclose, with no commercial or financial conflicts.
[a] OHSU Doernbecher Children's Hospital, Division of Pediatric Surgery, 3181 SW Sam Jackson Park Road, Portland, OR, 97239, USA; [b] Randall Children's Hospital at Legacy Emanuel, 501 N. Graham St, Suite 300, Portland, OR 97227, USA
* Corresponding author. 501 North Graham Street, Suite 300, Portland, OR 97227.
E-mail address: jafri@ohsu.edu

focus this discussion on a systematic evaluation of injured children, centering on abdominal injuries, and highlighting areas where significant differences exist with an adult workup.

BACKGROUND

Intraabdominal injury (IAI) can result from blunt or penetrating mechanisms. Blunt injuries are much more common than penetrating injuries (85% vs 15%). Among children with blunt abdominal trauma, 5% to 10% sustain IAI. Despite improvements in emergency diagnostics and evaluation, controversy still exists regarding the optimal assessment and management of pediatric trauma patients with IAI.

Certain mechanisms of injury are more common in the pediatric population. Infants and young children are likely to sustain injuries from motor vehicle collisions (MVC), drowning, suffocation, burns, falls, and abuse. School-aged children are susceptible to MVC, pedestrian injuries, bicycle injuries, and firearm injuries. Adolescents are at risk from MVC, firearm injuries, falls, and intentional injuries.[2]

Unfortunately, socioeconomic and ethnic disparities related to pediatric trauma exist and vary by age and mechanism. African Americans and Native Americans are at higher risk of fatal injuries than other ethnic groups.[3] Their care and outcomes also differ along these same ethnic lines. Algorithms and guidelines that aim to standardize care may work to reduce some of these disparities.

PRESENTATION AND DIAGNOSIS

Children are more susceptible to blunt injury than adults. A smaller body size allows for a greater distribution of injury; therefore, children often suffer multiple traumatic injuries in several regions. Additionally, pediatric internal organs are more likely to be injured owing to a smaller torso, larger and more mobile viscera, and decreased amount of intraabdominal fat.[4]

There are several common mechanisms leading to blunt abdominal trauma in children. The leading cause is MVC, accounting for more than 50% of pediatric abdominal trauma. Physical examination findings from blunt trauma include ecchymosis, abrasions, lacerations, abdominal tenderness, or abdominal distention. The liver and spleen are the most common solid organs injured. The most concerning and often subtle finding results from abrasions or ecchymosis from restraining belts, the "seat belt sign." When these belt marks are not over the bony pelvis, significant injury may result. The injuries can result from either the lap portion of the belt being too high or the shoulder portion being too low (**Fig. 1**). Patients with a seat belt sign are at greater risk for intraabdominal injury, particularly hollow viscus injury.[5] These injuries are also associated with Chance fractures, flexion–distraction injuries of the spine at the area of the lap belt, owing to limited mobility of the spine from the compressing seat belt. Chance fractures occur in about 5% of restrained children involved in an MVC.[6] The belts may also injure solid organs including the liver, spleen, or pancreas. We have seen several associated aortic injuries in our patient population resulting from the similar compression that causes spine fractures. These injuries can be very difficult to address in young children and should not be overlooked.

Other causes of abdominal trauma include sport injuries, bicycle and all-terrain vehicle injuries, pedestrian injuries, falls, and child abuse. Sports-related injuries are more commonly associated with isolated organ injury as a result of impact to the abdomen, in particular the spleen, kidney, and gastrointestinal tract. Although

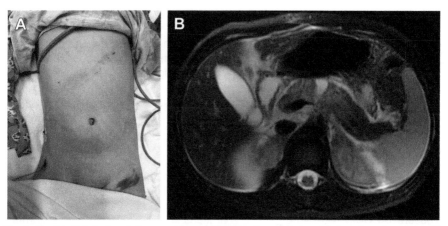

Fig. 1. Seat belt injuries. A 3-year-old restrained back seat passenger in a booster seat with lap and shoulder restraints presented with upper and pelvic bruising from the restraining belts. The lower abrasions over the anterior superior iliac spines demonstrate appropriate positioning and did not contribute to injury. The shoulder belt was too low over the upper abdomen, resulting in a pancreatic transection. (*A*) Clinical photo. (*B*) MRI demonstrating pancreatic laceration.

abdominal injury secondary to child abuse only occurs in about 5% of total child abuse cases, it is the second most common cause of death from abuse.

Penetrating trauma represents about 15% of abdominal trauma. The overwhelming majority of penetrating abdominal injuries are secondary to gunshots and stabbings.[7] More than 90% of gunshots occur in children 12 years or older.[8] Other causes of penetrating traumas include stab wounds and impalements. Trajectories of knives and projectiles may require whole body survey to evaluate for multiple wounds and guide clinical decision making (**Fig. 2**). The most commonly injured structures secondary

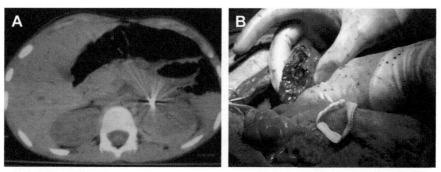

Fig. 2. Gunshot wound to the abdomen. An 8-year-old with a gunshot wound to the flank. Owing to an unclear trajectory and hemodynamic stability of the child, a computed tomography (CT) scan was undertaken, demonstrating tract of bullet into the left kidney with active extravasation of contrast. At laparotomy, an isolated renal injury was demonstrated and treated with partial nephrectomy. (*A*) CT demonstrating tract of projectile into left kidney. (*B*) Operative image demonstrating a well-perfused kidney with a laceration amenable to partial nephrectomy.

to penetrating trauma in this location are the gastrointestinal tract, liver, abdominal vasculature, kidney, and spleen.[9]

Other types of injuries include disasters, combat, and blast-type injuries. These injuries often combine blunt and penetrating mechanisms owing to the force of explosions and air-borne high-velocity projectiles. Explosions cause polytrauma to multiple organ systems including significant burn injuries, requiring multidisciplinary management for adequate resuscitation, evaluation, and treatment of these significantly injured patients.

INITIAL EVALUATION AND STABILIZATION

The initial management of abdominal trauma is similar in the pediatric and adult populations. The core principles of the Advanced Trauma Life Support[10] algorithm apply, with the primary survey evaluating airway, breathing, circulation, disability, and exposure (ABCDE). Any emergent interventions that are needed are performed during the primary survey, such as establishing an airway, decompression of tension pneumothorax, or recognition of life-threatening hemorrhage. In addition, control of exsanguinating hemorrhage has been show to be the most efficacious maneuver performed in prehospital resuscitation of children with relation to improved mortality.[11]

The airway is assessed by asking the patient verbal patients questions or assessing for phonation in nonverbal patients. Indications for intubation include: inability to ventilate by bag–valve–mask ventilation, Glasgow Coma Scale score of less than 8, hypoxemia, hypoventilation, decompensated shock patient not responsive to fluid resuscitation, or loss of protective airway reflexes. Intubation of a child requires consideration of age, size, and mechanism of injury. In general, cuffed endotracheal tubes have been shown to be safe in infants and young children. However, uncuffed tubes are generally used in children less than 8 years old unless there is need for a cuffed tube. For children ages 1 to 10 years, the following formulas estimate the proper size of endotracheal tube:

Uncuffed endotracheal tube size (mm internal diameter) = (age in years + 16)/4

Cuffed endotracheal tube size (mm internal diameter) = (age in years + 12)/4

Breathing is assessed by chest rise, respiratory rate, and auscultated breath sounds. Tachypnea may be a sign of impending respiratory collapse. Pulse oximetry is an excellent adjunct to assess oxygenation and should be used in the trauma bay on all patients. Capnography is a vital adjunct in confirming endotracheal tube position.

Circulation is assessed by physical examination findings including pulse, skin color, and capillary refill. Children have an extraordinary capacity for vasoconstriction, so a normal blood pressure does not rule out hemorrhagic shock. Minimum acceptable systolic blood pressures based on age are:

60 mm Hg in term neonates (0–28 days)
70 mm Hg in infants (1–12 months)
70 mm Hg + (2 × age in years) in children 1 to 10 years of age
90 mm Hg in children 10 years of age or older

In a hypovolemic patient, a bolus infusion of 20 mL/kg of isotonic crystalloid should be initiated promptly. In a patient with obvious hemorrhage, we advocate blood products as the initial resuscitative measure with prompt surgical control of bleeding.

Disability is then assessed via neurologic examination and a Glasgow Coma Scale score is given to the patient. Finally, the primary survey includes exposure, which involves removing all clothing to adequately proceed with the secondary survey. Hypothermia can occur rapidly in children owing to increased surface area relative to weight in children compared with adults. Warming measures should be in place from the onset of evaluation.

The secondary survey is then conducted to identify any traumatic injuries not identified on primary survey along with a more detailed history. A head-to-toe inspection is performed, focusing on pupillary size and reactivity; palpation of cranium and cervical spine; palpation of the mid face for stability; palpation of the chest and abdomen for crepitus or tenderness; inspection of each extremity for deformity, strength, and sensation; inspection and palpation of the cervical, thoracic, and lumbar spine for tenderness or deformity; and examination of the perineum for injury or open fracture often with a rectal examination for sphincter tone. An AMPLE history may be taken, which includes allergies, medications, past medical history, last meal, and events and details explaining the injury.

EVALUATION OF ABDOMINAL TRAUMA

Once a patient is appropriately stabilized with a secure airway and controlled breathing, a focus on abdominal trauma is appropriate. In a patient with profound instability or peritonitis, this evaluation may require emergent laparotomy as the initial diagnostic and therapeutic measure. We advocate a policy of direct transport to the operating room for the initial evaluation of all patients deemed unstable during the course of transport. This is a resource-intense practice and may not be appropriate for all centers. In our center, the computed tomography (CT) scanner is adjacent to the trauma operating rooms allowing transport to and from the operating room after stabilization, if appropriate (**Fig. 3**). If imaging is not warranted by mechanism or patient stability,

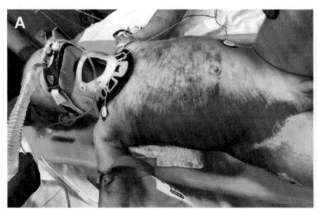
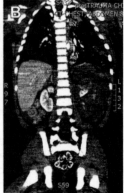

Fig. 3. Unstable trauma patient direct operating room transport. An 18-month-old sustained a crush injury from a motor vehicle collision with severe right-sided injuries, including a grade 4 spleen injury and completely devascularized left kidney with active extravasation. The patient was stable on initial evaluation at transferring facility, but during transport became hemodynamically unstable and was transported directly to the operating room for further evaluation. Laparotomy demonstrated a nonsalvagable spleen and left renal injuries. (*A*) External signs of significant trauma. (*B*) Computed tomography scan obtained during period of stability demonstrating severe spleen and left renal injury.

surgical intervention is not delayed. The hemodynamically stable patient allows for a more measured approach to the evaluation of abdominal injuries that, in addition to physical examination, includes laboratory studies, imaging, and diagnostic tests.

Laboratory Studies

Laboratory studies are an important aspect of the trauma evaluation. Often, blood is drawn and sent during the primary and secondary survey. However, there is no single value that can reliably predict IAI. For the stable patient without signs or symptoms of IAI, a hemoglobin, hematocrit, urinalysis, and liver function tests are typically sufficient. For patients with suspected intraabdominal injury, a complete blood count, lipase, blood gas, and type and screen are added. For the unstable patient, a coagulation panel, complete metabolic panel, and type and cross of blood are included, although none of these results should delay intervention.[12]

The usefulness of elevated transaminases to predict clinically significant liver injury is debatable. A study of blunt abdominal trauma revealed a correlation between AST and ALT levels and the severity of injury. However, about 50% of patients with elevated transaminases did not have any IAI on CT scan.[13] In nonaccidental trauma, elevated AST or ALT greater than 80 IU/L correlated with IAI, even in children with minimal physical examination findings.[14] The general usefulness of laboratory testing is limited, although anemia is an obvious predictor of hemorrhage, and significant acidosis with elevated lactate or base deficit may have prognostic value. Our practice is to use abnormal laboratory findings to increase the suspicion for injury and subsequent need for imaging, particularly in nonverbal or obtunded patients.

Imaging

Multiple imaging modalities exist for the trauma patient. Plain films of the chest and pelvis are often obtained in the trauma bay. The chest radiograph is often the only imaging that is needed in an unstable patient to confirm adequate placement of the endotracheal tube, as well as excluded pathology that should be immediately addressed (tension pneumothorax, significant hemothorax). Plain films of the abdomen are of limited usefulness in the trauma patient outside of identifying projectile trajectory/retention and identify grossly unstable fractures. Plain imaging of the cervical spine has some usefulness in clearance from injury in the stable, communicative patient without neck tenderness.

CT imaging is often the modality of choice for most trauma patients, given it is easily accessible, noninvasive, and accurate. The adoption of the use of CT imaging in stable patients has decreased significantly the rate of nontherapeutic laparotomies in the traumatically injured child. Indications for CT imaging include abdominal tenderness, seat belt sign, elevated transaminases, gross hematuria, downtrending hematocrit, inability to get an accurate examination with suspicious mechanism, or positive Focal Assessment with Sonography in Trauma (FAST) examination. However, unstable patients should not undergo CT scanning. These patients must first be adequately resuscitated or undergo laparotomy/thoracotomy if unable to resuscitate. Alternate imaging may be obtained via the modalities described elsewhere in this paper. The overuse of CT in stable, minimally injured children is another important area of concern that provides a stark contrast to adult trauma protocols.[15–17]

The FAST examination has been validated in the pediatric population.[18] The FAST examination includes ultrasonography of the pouch of Morrison in the right upper quadrant, pouch of Douglas around the bladder, the splenorenal plane in the left upper quadrant, and a subxiphoid view to look for pericardial fluid around the heart. This bedside examination has a high specificity rate to rule in free abdominal fluid, but low sensitivity, signifying its poor ability to rule out significant IAI. The use of FAST increases with clinician suspicion of abdominal injury, and patients who undergo FAST have a lesser chance of receiving an abdominal CT scan if clinician suspicion for IAI is low.[19]

Diagnostic peritoneal lavage (DPL) was once a mainstay of trauma evaluations. However, it is an invasive test, and with the advent of newer assessment tests such as FAST or CT scanning, it has largely been replaced by these faster and often more reliable noninvasive diagnostic tests. There may still be a role for DPL in an unstable patient who cannot undergo CT imaging where they may be multiple sites for blood loss. It may also be used for occult bowel injury where abdominal free fluid was attributed to solid organ injury. Finally, DPL may be considered in a patient undergoing emergent decompressive craniotomy before adequate evaluation of the abdomen owing to impending herniation. Our practice is to use diagnostic laparoscopy in this circumstance with DPL used rarely.

Diagnostic laparoscopy is an excellent modality for further investigation in the hemodynamically stable patient. Unlike bedside tests such as FAST or DPL, laparoscopy can readily localize injury and reduce the rate of negative laparotomy. Our use of diagnostic laparoscopy has increased steadily. We use it as a tool for evaluation in suspected diaphragmatic injuries, suspected bowel injury, and in cases of penetrating injury to evaluate for violation of the peritoneum. In the stable patient, we have expanded the role of laparoscopy beyond diagnostic realms and routinely use minimally invasive techniques for the repair of injuries including the diaphragm, pancreas, bowel, and colon.

Diagnostic cystoscopy is another adjunct that can be extremely useful. It can be used to diagnose bladder injuries as well as treat any ureteral injury with stent placement. It can be used with fluoroscopy to evaluate and treat injuries of the lower gastrointestinal tract as well. Evaluation of the ureters is best accomplished with intravenous contrast CT scan with delayed imaging. Suspected injuries can be further evaluated using retrograde fluoroscopic imaging at time of cystoscopy in both blunt and penetrating trauma.

The evaluation of penetrating trauma to the abdomen remains the same as blunt injury. However, in the unstable patient with penetrating trauma, expedient resuscitation with blood products and operative intervention should be used. In the stable patient, many of the modalities including imaging to determine projectile/stab tract may be used.

For the stable patient with penetrating trauma, FAST is a useful modality to assess for free peritoneal fluid. If the FAST is positive, the patient has a greater likelihood of needing operative exploration. CT scanning is the preferred imaging to definitely identify injuries. In patients with superficial wounds who are stable, local wound exploration is another option. If the injury penetrates the fascia, it requires further workup. If the injury does not penetrate the fascia, the wound can be irrigated and closed at the bedside without further imaging. Owing to anxiety in children, we rarely used the emergency department for wound exploration, usually conducting these in the operating room and often using diagnostic laparoscopy as a more definitive evaluation if suspicion is high.

Finally, angiography plays both a diagnostic and therapeutic role in the evaluation of abdominal trauma. Bleeding in locations that are difficult to access or can result in exsanguinating hemorrhage when approached in an open operative manner can be diagnosed expediently and addressed with embolization. The most common sites in children include troublesome pelvic bleeding, as well as significant liver and spleen injuries. We have found, however, that its usefulness in pediatric liver and spleen injuries is more limited. Often children who have an arterial "blush" signifying active extravasation of contrast and thus hemorrhage from liver and spleen injuries can be managed without embolization if clinically stable according to solid organ injury protocols described elsewhere in this paper. A majority of these injuries will tamponade and cease bleeding without intervention. The usefulness of angiography in the diagnosis of most other vascular injuries has been largely replaced with enhanced CT angiography protocols, but its therapeutic role continues to increase.

SPECIFIC INJURIES
Liver and Spleen

The liver and spleen are the 2 most commonly injured solid organs in blunt abdominal trauma, with an injury incidence of about 33% each. Many liver and spleen injuries can now be successfully managed nonoperatively. Indeed, isolated blunt liver and spleen injuries are managed nonoperatively more than 90% of the time. The classification of severity of injury remains an important aspect of nonoperative management. Liver and spleen injury scales as according to the American Association for the Surgery of Trauma are displayed in **Table 1**.[20] Please see David M. Notrica and Maria E. Linnaus's article, "Nonoperative Management of Blunt Solid Organ Injury in Pediatric Surgery," in this issue on solid organ injury for more detail regarding pediatric solid organ injuries.

Stomach and Small Bowel

Hollow viscus injury is much less common than solid organ injury in blunt trauma, occurring less than 10% of the time. The viscera are susceptible to injury via crush, compression, or shearing forces at points of fixation such as the ligament of Treitz or ileocecal region. Blunt bowel injuries may not be immediately apparent on initial CT imaging. CT findings to suggest bowel injury include free fluid without solid organ injury, bowel wall thickening or enhancement, extraluminal air, mesenteric stranding,

Table 1 Classification of spleen and liver injuries in trauma		
Grade	Type	Description
I	Hematoma	Subcapsular, <10% surface area
	Laceration	Capsular tear, <1 cm depth
II	Hematoma	Subcapsular, 10%–50% surface area, intraparenchymal <5 cm (Spleen), <10 cm (liver) diameter
	Laceration	Capsular tear, 1-3 cm depth, does not involve trabecular vessel (spleen), <10 cm length (liver)
III	Hematoma	Subcapsular, >50% surface area, intraparenchymal >5 cm
	Laceration	(spleen), >10 cm (liver) diameter
		>3 cm depth, involves trabecular vessel (spleen)
IV	Laceration	Spleen: Segmental or hilar vessels producing >25% devascularization Liver: 25%–75% hepatic lobe or >3 Couinaud's segments
V	Laceration	Spleen: Completely shattered or hilar injury resulting in devascularization
		Liver: >75% of hepatic lobe or >3 Couinaud's segments
	Vascular	Juxtahepatic venous injuries, retrohepatic vena cava/central major hepatic veins
VI	Vascular	Complete hepatic avulsion

From Tinkoff G, Esposito TJ, Reed J, et al. American Association for the Surgery of Trauma organ injury scale I: spleen, liver, and kidney, validation based on the national trauma data bank. J Am Coll Surg. 2008;207(5):648; with permission.

or bowel wall discontinuity. In children with these findings, it is challenging to decide if or when to intervene. Although a delay in surgical management could lead to adverse events, a study of 214 patients with bowel injury owing to trauma did not show any difference in complications or duration of hospital stay based on time to intervention.[21] Injuries to the stomach and small bowel can typically be repaired during the initial operation. Stomach injuries typically occur on the greater curvature and debridement with primary repair is sufficient. Small bowel injuries can be resected with primary anastomosis, even in the setting of contamination, if the patient is hemodynamically stable. We routinely observe these patients with serial abdominal examinations before intervention.

Genitourinary

Owing to the retroperitoneal position of the kidneys, signs of renal injury are often more occult. Patients often have dull back pain, ecchymosis in the costovertebral region, or hematuria. Renal ultrasound and CT examinations are useful modalities to assess degree of renal injury. However, CT scanning is preferred for the evaluation of hematuria in the trauma patient because the evaluation of the bladder and associated injuries to intraperitoneal structures can also be accomplished simultaneously. The American Association for the Surgery of Trauma has a similar grading scale for kidney injuries. Injuries to the ureters have also been classified by the American Association for the Surgery of Trauma, but with a slightly distinct schema. The injuries are graded with increasing severity as simple hematomas, transection (≤50% or >50%), or based on amount of devascularization (<2 or >2 cm) in the setting of complete transection.

Pancreas

Pancreas injuries occur around 3% to 12% in children with blunt abdominal trauma. Treatment of pancreatic injuries remains controversial, because individual centers have small sample sizes and thereby treatment is largely based on surgeon preference. One case series concluded that distal injuries should be treated with distal pancreatectomy, proximal injuries with observation, and pseudocysts with observation or cyst gastrostomy.[22] Endoscopic retrograde cholangiopancreatography is also an excellent modality to diagnose and treat pancreatic duct injuries via stent placement. Other studies show excellent results with nonoperative management in almost all cases of pancreatic injury.[23] Later data showed increased complication rates and dependency on total parenteral nutrition in the nonoperative management of high-grade pancreatic injuries.[24] Several ongoing studies are investigating the role of the nonoperative management of blunt pancreatic injuries in the setting of major duct disruption.

Colon and Rectum

Similar to the stomach and small bowel, the colon is susceptible to similar forces in trauma. Shearing can occur at the rectosigmoid junction, causing contamination of the abdominal cavity. However, repair in colon injuries is usually delayed compared with small bowel injuries. Often, colon injuries are not immediately apparent owing to a retroperitoneal position of some injuries, resulting in fecal contamination. Classically, an end-colostomy with Hartmann's pouch was the recommended intervention in this setting. In the pediatric population, most injuries can be handled with primary repair in the hemodynamically stable patient without significant fecal contamination. Diversion is more often the exception rather than the rule.

Diaphragm

Patients in MVC wearing seat belts are at increased risk of diaphragmatic herniation. Sudden compressive force to the abdomen results in increased intraabdominal pressure, resulting in rupture of the diaphragm. Patients often have concurrent seatbelt signs and are at risk for small bowel injury or Chance fractures. These injuries are not always obvious on CT imaging, depending on the degree of abdominal content herniation. One study in the adult literature reported CT imaging alone was only 80% sensitive in finding diaphragmatic injuries.[25] Treatment requires surgical repair but not emergently depending on concomitant injuries. Stabilization of the associated pulmonary contusion and evaluation/treatment of liver/splenic injury takes priority. In our center, laparoscopy/thoracoscopy is used to diagnose and occasionally repair suspected diaphragm injury, based on the appearance on imaging or location of penetrating injury (greater suspicion if injury spans from nipples to costal margin).

DECISION MAKING AND TREATMENT
Imaging Protocols

Pediatric Emergency Care Applied Research Network

The Pediatric Emergency Care Applied Research Network sought to develop a prediction tool to identify very low-risk patients for IAI needing acute intervention, and thereby defer CT scanning in the emergency department.[26] They prospectively studied more than 12,000 children at 20 emergency departments with blunt torso trauma; 46% received CT scans in the emergency department and 6.3% were diagnosed with IAI. They identified 7 variables of patient history and physical examination making IAI less likely in descending order: evidence of abdominal wall trauma or seatbelt sign, a Glasgow Coma Scale score of less than 14, abdominal tenderness, evidence of thoracic wall trauma, complaints of abdominal pain, decreased breath sounds, and vomiting. The study did not incorporate laboratory findings or FAST examination, because these modalities were variable across institutions. Children without any of these findings had a 0.1% risk for IAI undergoing acute intervention. This tool had a 98.9% negative predictive value if all 7 variables were negative, and CT imaging was deemed to be unnecessary. Children with 1 or more positive variables do not necessarily need CT imaging, but may need further evaluation with laboratory studies, FAST, further observation, or consideration of CT scan based on clinical suspicion for injury. The tool helps to risk stratify patients with blunt abdominal trauma and avoid CT imaging in children at low risk for IAI, although clinical judgment must still be applied in all cases.

Doernbecher/Randall children's evaluation algorithm

We have developed a clinical protocol for the evaluation of stable pediatric patients with abdominal trauma (**Fig. 4**).[26,27] The first and second decision points are based on the Pediatric Emergency Care Applied Research Network prediction rule. The use of laboratory studies and the FAST examination were also incorporated into this algorithm for the pediatric trauma patient. Although patient history, physical examination, laboratory studies, and the FAST examination have been validated individually as predictors of IAI, this comprehensive clinical algorithm is presently being validated and has shown promising results.

Solid Organ Injury Protocols

Over the past 30 years, there has been a large shift to nonoperative management in hemodynamically stable patients with traumatic solid organ injuries, with subsequent decreases in morbidity and mortality. However, there remains great variability in the

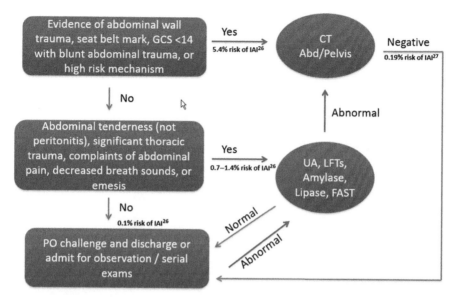

Fig. 4. Pediatric Abdominal Trauma Evaluation. Abd, abdomen; CT, computed tomography; FAST, Focal Assessment with Sonography in Trauma; GCS, Glasgow Coma Scale; IAI, intraabdominal injury requiring intervention; PO, oral; UA, urinalysis. (*Data from* Holmes JF, Lillis K, Monroe D, et al. Identifying children at very low risk of clinically important blunt abdominal injuries. Ann Emerg Med. 2013;62(2):107–16.e2; and Hom J. The risk of intra-abdominal injuries in pediatric patients with stable blunt abdominal trauma and negative abdominal computed tomography. Acad Emerg Med 2010;17(5):469–75.)

decision-making algorithms used by individual surgeons and institutions. Multiple solid organ injury protocols exist to aid in decision making and help to standardize care for these patients (see detailed description in David M. Notrica and Maria E. Linnaus's article, "Nonoperative Management of Blunt Solid Organ Injury in Pediatric Surgery," in this issue). The Oregon Health and Science University has created a protocol for managing liver and splenic injuries based on grade of injury and stability of the patient (**Fig. 5**).

American Pediatric Surgery Association Trauma Committee
In 2000, the American Pediatric Surgery Association Trauma Committee proposed guidelines for the management of stable patients with isolated blunt spleen or liver injuries, including standards for intensive care admission, duration of hospital stay, and interval imaging. These guidelines led to reductions in intensive care stay, hospital stay, follow-up imaging, and activity restriction.[28] The severity of injury was classified by CT grade, and all grade V patients were excluded. Five guidelines were proposed: intensive care unit admission for grade IV injury only, limited hospital stay, no predischarge or postdischarge imaging, and progressive activity restrictions. One center created clinical practice guidelines based on the American Pediatric Surgery Association recommendations and did not have any deaths or splenectomy for isolated blunt splenic trauma over the past 20 years.[29] They had reductions in duration of hospitalization, despite increases in splenic trauma severity. Despite these advances, the 2000 guidelines were still based on historical data and conservatively chosen to avoid any secondary injury as a patient was mobilized. Several studies within the past 5 to 10 years have demonstrated that more aggressive enhanced recovery pathways based on the patient's physiologic parameters can be adopted safely.[30,31]

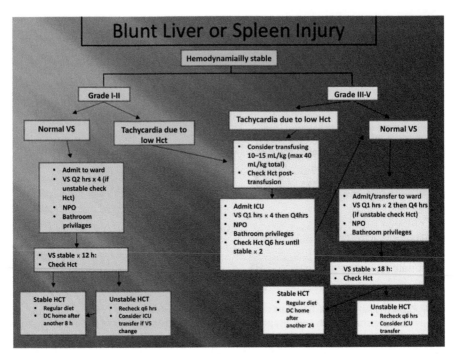

Fig. 5. Pediatric solid organ injury protocol. DC, discharge; Hct, hematocrit; ICU, intensive care unit; NPO, nil per os; VS, vital signs.

Doernbecher/Randall children's solid organ injury protocol

An abbreviated solid organ injury protocol with decreased hospital stay, abbreviated bed rest, and decreased phlebotomy is presently being studied at our institutions and has demonstrated clinical success with no increase in morbidity.

CONTROVERSIAL TOPICS

Focal Assessment with Sonography in Trauma Examination

The use of the FAST examination remains a point of debate in the pediatric population.[32] The FAST aims to detect intraperitoneal fluid, whether from hemorrhage, succus, bile, or urine. Although multiple studies have shown a high specificity for the FAST examination, its sensitivity remains variable. One study revealed more than one-third of low-grade liver and spleen injuries did not have any free fluid on ultrasonography.[33] Another study proposed the use of FAST in conjunction with transaminases. A negative FAST with transaminases of less than 100 IU/L was sufficient to rule out IAI and avoid CT scanning.[34] We use FAST in all injured children, although we have noted that its accuracy is less predictable in younger children.

Multiple scoring systems using ultrasonography have been proposed to effectively rule out IAI. The Blunt Abdominal Trauma in Children (BATiC) score uses physical examination findings and laboratory values in conjunction with Doppler ultrasound imaging.[35] The BATiC score includes 10 clinical parameters to predict IAI with the following scoring system: abnormal abdominal Doppler ultrasound examination (4 points), abdominal pain (2 points), peritoneal irritation (2 points), hemodynamic instability (2 points), AST greater than 60 IU/L (2 points), ALT greater than 25 IU/L (2 points), white blood cell count greater than 9.5 g/L (1 point), lactate dehydrogenase greater than 330

IU/L (1 point), lipase greater than 30 IU/L (1 point), and creatinine greater than 50 µg/L (1 point). A BATiC score of less than or equal to 7 have has a negative predictive value of 97%, which would obviate the need for CT imaging or hospital admission. However, a formal Doppler ultrasound examination and multiple laboratory values take time to obtain, potentially limiting the practicality of this scoring system.

Contrast-enhanced ultrasound imaging has also been studied to enhance the detection of IAI. There is evidence to suggest contrast-enhanced ultrasound imaging is more accurate than conventional ultrasonography in children in detecting solid organ injuries.[36] Wider use and clinical experience with this modality is necessary before its routine use can be advocated. MRI presently does not have a large role in the acute evaluation of abdominal trauma, but newer "quick" protocols may have usefulness in the future. We do use MRI/MR cholangiopancreatography in the evaluation of the pancreaticobiliary tree in patients with suspected bile duct and pancreatic duct injuries after their initial evaluation (usually with CT scanning).

All of these studies seek to find alternatives to CT imaging in the pediatric population. There is utility in applying these scoring systems to patients; however, the ultimate decision to obtain CT imaging remains with the practicing clinician in the appropriate clinical situation.

Negative Workup

Traditionally, children with normal physical examinations and CT imaging were admitted to the hospital for serial abdominal examinations to avoid missing a delayed bowel injury. An observational study of 1085 children with normal CT imaging revealed that 737 (68%) were still admitted to the hospital. Although 2 patients were subsequently found to have IAI, neither required intervention.[37] Another study reviewed data from almost 2600 patients with negative abdominal CT scans and found the incidence of IAI was 0.19%. Two patients required laparotomy, one for bowel perforation and one for mesenteric hematoma with serosa tear.[27] The overall negative predictive value of abdominal CT was 99.8%, making it an extremely reliable test to rule out IAI. Routine admission after abdominal trauma in the setting of normal initial CT imaging may not be necessary. We use discharge from the emergency department in the appropriate setting or a short period of observation in the emergency department before discharge if any suspicion remains. This has been an effective and reliable means to decrease the need for admission in the child with minor injuries and negative imaging.

Adult Versus Pediatric Trauma Centers

Differences in the evaluation and management of pediatric trauma patients have been documented between adult and pediatric centers. The use of whole body CT imaging in trauma varies based on location. Pediatric patients managed at adult trauma centers were 1.8 times more likely to receive whole body CT imaging with the associated increased risk of radiation without a difference in clinical outcomes.[38] It is crucial for adult trauma practitioners to be aware of the increased risk of malignancy in children and the current Pediatric Emergency Care Applied Research Network and other clinical guidelines for the use of CT imaging in children.

We have demonstrated in our own center that a focus on reduction in ionizing radiation through a focused cervical spine imaging protocol reduced use of CT imaging for other sites. This unintended benefit was the result of decreasing imaging in children with lower injury severity scores. This likely is owing to a greater focus on serial examinations in stable patients and a more measured approach to the evaluation of children with minor injuries. The overall reduction in radiation exposure and subsequent risk of malignancy was substantial.[39] This has led to guidelines for imaging all areas, including the head, chest, cervical spine, and abdomen.

Additionally, mass dissemination of imaging and solid organ injury protocols needs to occur. It has been shown that children treated outside of a pediatric trauma center have a higher rate of surgical exploration for blunt spleen injuries compared with children at dedicated trauma facilities. One study showed the risk-adjusted odds ratio for laparotomy at a nonpediatric facility to be as high as 6.2.[40] Dissemination of imaging and solid organ injury protocols is paramount to create practice changes in the management of traumatic solid organ injuries in children. However, the ability to manage these injuries relies on the surgeon's comfort with pediatric guidelines and experience with nonoperative management.

SUMMARY

The field of trauma is ever evolving and pediatric trauma is no exception. With the advent of newer technologies, clinical guidelines, and minimally invasive and percutaneous interventions, the world of trauma care is dramatically different today than just a few years ago. The field of pediatric trauma continues to build on research done in the adult world, but also needs to be tailored for the pediatric patient. Multiple imaging and treatment protocols exist for clinicians to follow; yet each pediatric trauma patient remains unique owing to the mechanism of injury, personal history, and access to care. The main challenge for any clinician caring for the pediatric abdominal trauma patient remains to align these individual characteristics with the most current and safest approach to management of traumatic injuries.

REFERENCES

1. National Vital Statistics System, National Center for Health Statistics (CDC). 10 Leading causes of death by age group, Unites States—2014. Available at: http://www.cdc.gov/injury/wisqars/pdf/leading_causes_of_death_by_age_group_2014-a.pdf. Accessed February 1, 2016.
2. Centers for Disease Control and Prevention (CDC). Vital signs: unintentional injury deaths among persons aged 0-19 years - United States, 2000-2009. MMWR Morb Mortal Wkly Rep 2012;61:270–6.
3. Bernard SJ, Paulozzi LJ, Wallace DL, Centers for Disease Control and Prevention (CDC). Fatal injuries among children by race and ethnicity–United States, 1999-2002. MMWR Surveill Summ 2007;56:1.
4. Avarello JT, Cantor RM. Pediatric major trauma: an approach to evaluation and management. Emerg Med Clin North Am 2007;25:803–36.
5. Borgialli DA, Ellison AM, Ehrlich P, et al, Pediatric Emergency Care Applied Research Network (PECARN). Association between the seat belt sign and intra-abdominal injuries in children with blunt torso trauma in motor vehicle collisions. Acad Emerg Med 2014;21(11):1240–8.
6. Sturm PF. Lumbar compression fractures secondary to lap-belt use in children. J Pediatr Orthop 1995;15:521–3.
7. Cotton BA, Nance ML. Penetrating trauma in children. Semin Pediatr Surg 2004;13:87.
8. Srinivasan S, Mannix R, Lee LK. Epidemiology of paediatric firearm injuries in the USA, 2001-2010. Arch Dis Child 2014;99:331.
9. Amick LF. Penetrating trauma in the pediatric patient. Clin Pediatr Emerg Med 2001;Col2(1):63–70.

10. American College of Surgeons Committee on Trauma. Advanced trauma life support. 10th edition. American College of Surgeons; 2010.

11. Sokol KK, Black GE, Azarow KS, et al. Prehospital interventions in severely injured pediatric patients: Rethinking the ABCs. J Trauma Acute Care Surg 2015;79(6):983–9.

12. Capraro AJ, Mooney D, Waltzman ML. The use of routine laboratory studies as screening tools in pediatric abdominal trauma. Pediatr Emerg Care 2006;22(7):480–4.

13. Karam O, La Scala G, Le Coultre C, et al. Liver function tests in children with blunt abdominal traumas. Eur J Pediatr Surg 2007;17:313–6.

14. Lindberg D, Makoroff K, Harper N, et al. Utility of hepatic transaminases to recognize abuse in children. Pediatrics 2009;124:509–16.

15. Brenner DJ, Hall EJ. Computed tomography—an increasing source of radiation exposure. N Engl J Med 2007;357:2277–84.

16. Mueller DL, Hatab M, Al-Senan R, et al. Pediatric radiation exposure during the initial evaluation for blunt trauma. J Trauma 2011;70(3):724–31.

17. Feng ST, Law MW, Huang B, et al. Radiation dose and cancer risk from pediatric CT examinations on 64-slice CT: a phantom study. Eur J Radiol 2010;76(2):e19–23.

18. Partrick DA, Bensard DD, Moore EE, et al. Ultrasound is an effective triage tool to evaluate blunt abdominal trauma in the pediatric population. J Trauma 1998;45:57–63.

19. Menaker J, Blumberg S, Wisner DH, et al, Intra-abdominal Injury Study Group of the Pediatric Emergency Care Applied Research Network (PECARN). Use of the focused assessment with sonography for trauma (FAST) examination and its impact on abdominal computed tomography use in hemodynamically stable children with blunt torso trauma. J Trauma Acute Care Surg 2014;77(3):427–32.

20. Tinkoff G, Esposito TJ, Reed J, et al. American Association for the Surgery of Trauma organ injury scale I: spleen, liver, and kidney, validation based on the national trauma data bank. J Am Coll Surg 2008;207(5):646–55.

21. Letton RW, Worrell V. Delay in diagnosis and treatment of blunt intestinal injury does not adversely affect prognosis in the pediatric trauma patient. J Pediatr Surg 2010;45:161–5.

22. Canty TG Sr, Weinman D. Management of major pancreatic duct injuries in children. J Trauma 2001;50(6):1001–7.

23. de Blaauw I, Winkelhorst JT, Rieu PN, et al. Pancreatic injury in children: good outcome of nonoperative treatment. J Pediatr Surg 2008;43(9):1640–3.

24. Beres AL, Wales PW, Christison-Lagay ER, et al. Non-operative management of high-grade pancreatic trauma: is it worth the wait? J Pediatr Surg 2013;48(5):1060–4.

25. Mihos P, Potaris K, Gakidis J, et al. Traumatic rupture of the diaphragm: experience with 65 patients. Injury 2003;34:169–72.

26. Holmes JF, Lillis K, Monroe D, et al, Pediatric Emergency Care Applied Research Network (PECARN). Identifying children at very low risk of clinically important blunt abdominal injuries. Ann Emerg Med 2013;62(2):107–16.

27. Hom J. The risk of intra-abdominal injuries in pediatric patients with stable blunt abdominal trauma and negative abdominal computed tomography. Acad Emerg Med 2010;17:469–75.

28. Stylianos S. APSA Trauma Committee. Evidence-based guidelines for resource utilization in children with isolated spleen or liver injury. J Pediatr Surg 2000;35:164–9.

29. Bairdain S, Litman HJ, Troy M, et al. Twenty-years of splenic preservation at a level 1 pediatric trauma center. J Pediatr Surg 2015;50(5):864–8.

30. Notrica DM, Eubanks JW, Tuggle DW, et al. Nonoperative management of blunt liver and spleen injury in children: Evaluation of the ATOMAC guideline using GRADE. J Trauma Acute Care Surg 2015;79(4):683–93.
31. St. Peter SD, Aguayo P, Juang D, et al. Follow up of prospective validation of an abbreviated bedrest protocol in the management of blunt spleen and liver injuries in children. J Pediatr Surg 2013;48(12):2437–41.
32. Holmes JF, Gladman A, Chang CH. Performance of abdominal ultrasonography in pediatric blunt trauma patients: a meta-analysis. J Pediatr Surg 2007;42:1588–94.
33. Bixby SD, Callahan MJ, Taylor GA. Imaging in pediatric blunt abdominal trauma. Semin Roentgenol 2008;43:72–82.
34. Sola JE, Cheung MC, Yang R, et al. Pediatric FAST and elevated liver transaminases: an effective screening tool in blunt abdominal trauma. J Surg Res 2009;157:103–7.
35. Karam O, Sanchez O, Chardot C, et al. Blunt abdominal trauma in children: a score to predict the absence of organ injury. J Pediatr 2009;154:912–7.
36. Valentino M, Ansaloni L, Catena F, et al. Contrast-enhanced ultrasonography in blunt abdominal trauma: considerations after 5 years of experience. Radiol Med 2009;114:1080–93.
37. Awasthi S, Mao A, Wooton-Gorges SL, et al. Is hospital admission and observation required after a normal abdominal computed tomography scan in children with blunt abdominal trauma? Acad Emerg Med 2008;15:895–9.
38. Pandit V, Michailidou M, Rhee P, et al. The use of whole body computed tomography scans in pediatric trauma patients: Are there differences among adults and pediatric centers? J Pediatr Surg 2015;51(4):649–53.
39. Connolly CR, Yonge JD, Eastes LE, et al. Performance improvement and patient safety program guided quality improvement initiatives can significantly reduce CT imaging in pediatric trauma patients. J Trauma Acute Care Surg 2016;81(2):278–84.
40. Davis DH, Localio AR, Stafford PW, et al. Trends in operative management of pediatric splenic injury in a regional trauma system. Pediatrics 2005;115(1):89–94.

The Role of Minimally Invasive Surgery in Pediatric Trauma

Erik G. Pearson, MD[a], Matthew S. Clifton, MD[b],*

KEYWORDS

• Minimally invasive surgery • Trauma • Laparoscopy • Thoracoscopy

KEY POINTS

• Laparoscopy and thoracoscopy possess high levels of diagnostic accuracy with low associated missed injury rates.
• Minimally invasive surgery (MIS) is used in pediatric trauma patients who are hemodynamically stable.
• MIS offers diagnostic and therapeutic capabilities in pediatric trauma patients.
• MIS confers a lower postoperative morbidity profile than traditional open approaches.

The role of minimally invasive surgery (MIS) in the management of blunt and penetrating injuries to the chest and abdomen has evolved over the last 3 decades. In 1972, Gans and Berci first demonstrated the diagnostic capacity of laparoscopy in 16 children and shortly after Carnevale and associates published a broad experience with laparoscopy in trauma patients.[1,2] Subsequently, several groups published case series demonstrating both the safety and efficacy of laparoscopy in trauma, and perhaps more importantly its effect on reducing nontherapeutic laparotomy rates by up to 60% in both blunt and penetrating injury.[3–5] Although early technical limitations precluded the full diagnostic and therapeutic potential of MIS, this was quickly overcome. MIS is now routinely used as a therapeutic strategy encompassing the full spectrum of traumatic injuries, including repair of lung, diaphragm, bowel, pancreas, and solid organ injuries.[6–10]

Disclosures: The authors do not have any commercial or financial conflicts of interest that interfere with the production of this article.
[a] Department of Surgery, Emory University School of Medicine, 1405 Clifton Road Northeast, Atlanta, GA 30322, USA; [b] Department of Surgery, Children's Healthcare of Atlanta, Emory University School of Medicine, 1405 Clifton Road Northeast, Atlanta, GA 30322, USA
* Corresponding author.
E-mail address: mclifto@emory.edu

The current gold standard therapeutic intervention for an unstable patient with blunt or penetrating abdominal injury remains exploration through a midline laparotomy; similarly, a sternotomy or thoracotomy may be required in the unstable patient with a thoracic injury. It is important to note, however, that negative open exploration carries with it a significant mortality of up to 5% and an 18% incidence of morbidity. Most notably, this includes the risk of future adhesive intestinal obstruction and potential for abdominal wall hernia.[11] Across pediatric and adult case series, diagnostic and therapeutic laparoscopy has demonstrated significant benefit for the treatment of traumatic injuries. In hemodynamically stable patients requiring exploration, MIS offers a safe diagnostic or therapeutic alternative with several advantages, including less pain, shorter recovery time and hospital stay, and decreased financial burden, as well as decreased morbidity and mortality through avoidance of unnecessary procedures.[12,13] In an examination of the National Trauma Data Bank, Zafar and colleagues[14] evaluated 916 patients at 467 trauma centers undergoing therapeutic laparoscopic interventions for blunt and penetrating trauma, including diaphragm repair, bowel repair or resection, and splenectomy. The authors found that patients treated with therapeutic laparoscopy had a significantly shorter hospital stay with no increased risk of mortality or morbidity compared with patients undergoing laparotomy. In addition, the accuracy of MIS in diagnosing traumatic injury approaches 100%, with several studies documenting zero missed injuries in pediatric trauma patients.[12,15,16] Further, maintaining the intestines within the peritoneal cavity prevents tissue desiccation and minimizes fluid and temperature shifts.[8] Across pediatric and adult case series, diagnostic and therapeutic laparoscopy has demonstrated significant benefit for the treatment of traumatic injury to the abdomen and thorax.

Children suffer higher rates of solid organ injury than adults from both blunt and penetrating trauma because they have proportionally larger solid organs, less subcutaneous fat, and less protective muscle.[17] Blunt abdominal trauma related to motor vehicle collision is the most common cause of unrecognized fatal injury in children, and approximately one third of children with major trauma will suffer intraperitoneal injuries.[18] The Advanced Trauma Life Support system outlines the initial evaluation and management of children with traumatic injuries and follows the same sequence as that in an adult: primary survey, resuscitation, secondary survey, and definitive care. The management of children with solid organ injury after blunt abdominal trauma has evolved significantly since Upadhyay and Simpson[19] in 1968 first suggested the nonoperative management of splenic trauma in children. Hemodynamically unstable children with free fluid identified on ultrasound examination proceed immediately to exploratory laparotomy, whereas hemodynamically stable children with free fluid on ultrasound examination undergo computed tomography. This strategy has demonstrated accuracy in identifying greater than 95% of intraabdominal injuries.[20] Diagnostic peritoneal lavage in the pediatric population has become relatively obsolete owing to the diagnostic accuracy of high-resolution computed tomography and Focused Abdominal Sonography for Trauma examinations. Currently, children who suffer blunt abdominal trauma with solid organ injury involving liver and/or spleen are now managed according to the ATOMAC guideline used at many pediatric trauma centers.[21] The ATOMAC protocol for the management of blunt liver or spleen injury guides the surgeon along a nonoperative management pathway until the child develops recurrent hypotension, bleeding, or fails to have a sustained response to blood transfusion. When surgery is indicated, MIS offers diagnostic and therapeutic equivalency to open surgery in the hemodynamically stable child.

LAPAROSCOPY FOR THE DIAGNOSIS AND TREATMENT OF ACUTE TRAUMATIC INJURY

In a recent analysis of the use of MIS for trauma, Alemayehu and colleagues[15] characterized the practice patterns at 6 pediatric trauma centers across the United States. The retrospective study included 200 patients, each receiving laparoscopy (94%), thoracoscopy (4%), or both (2%). The most common mechanism of injury was all terrain vehicle or motor vehicle collision (37%) followed by stab wounds (17%), bicycle crashes (14%), gunshot wounds (12%), and falls (11%). The most common indications for laparoscopy included penetrating injury (32%), peritonitis (16%), and free fluid with abdominal pain (14%). Of the 192 children undergoing laparoscopy for abdominal trauma, 120 operations (63%) were completed without conversion, including 77 diagnostic and 43 therapeutic procedures. The conversion rate to laparotomy was 37%. Most of the repairs performed after conversions were related to intestinal injury. As a diagnostic tool, laparoscopy provided insufficient information to exclude an injury in only 6 (3%) of the 192 procedures. Additionally, using MIS as an extension of the diagnostic evaluation for trauma resulted in zero missed injuries, a testament to its efficacy.[22,23] In a sense, diagnostic laparoscopy has become an extension of the secondary survey.

As a therapeutic tool, the most common operations performed included bowel resection or repair of enterotomies, distal pancreatectomy, splenectomy, or repair of traumatic hernias. If a bowel resection or complex repair of an enterotomy was required, 73% of these cases were converted to laparotomy. Repair of hollow viscera is more difficult laparoscopically, but it has been reported in several studies as a safe option.[7,24,25] The success of this approach depends on the expertise of the surgeon. Even when conversion is necessary, the incision is typically much smaller than that for a primary trauma laparotomy, because other potential sites of injury have been explored and excluded. In a metaanalysis of 51 studies evaluating the use of laparoscopy in penetrating abdominal trauma as both a diagnostic and therapeutic modality, 51.8% of patients were spared a nontherapeutic laparotomy, with most studies reporting 100% sensitivity for the detection of injury.

A separate study from an American College of Surgeons–designated level 1 pediatric trauma center reviewed 20 years of experience using MIS in the management of trauma patients.[12] The authors found that, in addition to its diagnostic capabilities, MIS therapeutic interventions are possible in up to 65% of cases without conversion to an open procedure. Furthermore, 19% of negative laparoscopies did not require any further intervention, thus avoiding the morbidity of a negative laparotomy. In a 13-year analysis of 16,321 trauma admissions with 119 patients requiring abdominal exploration for blunt and penetrating injury, Tharakan and colleagues[16] retrospectively reviewed 38 hemodynamically stable children who underwent diagnostic and therapeutic laparoscopy. In 13 children (34%), laparoscopic exploration ruled out injuries and avoided the need for a negative laparotomy. In 9 children (24%), laparoscopy identified an injury for which no surgical intervention was necessary and in another 9 children (24%) an injury was repaired laparoscopically. The authors identified 7 children (6%) who required conversion to laparotomy and concluded that in the hemodynamically stable patient with a concerning examination and inconclusive imaging, laparoscopy is a sensitive diagnostic modality that provides the opportunity for therapeutic intervention with substantially less morbidity than open exploration.

Diagnostic laparoscopy is an established surgical approach in penetrating abdominal trauma with sensitivity, specificity, and accuracy of up to 100%.[26] The screening, diagnostic, and therapeutic potential of MIS in the management of penetrating injuries to the abdomen was well-documented in a recent retrospective analysis by Koto and colleagues.[27] In a series of 114 patients including 81 stab injuries and 33 gunshot wounds, hemodynamically stable patients or hemodynamically unstable patients who responded to initial resuscitation were managed with MIS with only a 7% conversion rate. Of the patients converted to an open procedure, extensive bleeding was the most common surgical indication. Liver injury not requiring repair was the most common finding during nontherapeutic diagnostic laparoscopy and the most common therapeutic procedure was diaphragm repair. The use of laparoscopy for the repair of diaphragm injuries can be done entirely intracorporeally or via a laparoscopic assisted technique.[24] Bowel injuries were either managed laparoscopically with intracorporeal suturing of the enterotomy or by a laparoscopic-assisted technique with a small, focused incision. Current guidelines recommend the use of laparoscopy only in hemodynamically stable patients; however, other studies have demonstrated the safety of diagnostic laparoscopy in adults in both the hemodynamic responder and nonresponder to resuscitation.[7,26–28]

The hemodynamic changes induced during laparoscopy are well-described. Pneumoperitoneum reduces lung volumes and cardiac index with systemic hypercapnia, increased cardiac filling pressures and increased systemic vascular resistance.[29] These physiologic changes may lead to greater hemodynamic instability in the underresuscitated or unstable trauma patient. Cherkasov and colleagues[28] reviewed 1332 adult patients with abdominal trauma with varying degrees of hemodynamic instability (51%, 25%, and 16% of patients were in mild, moderate, and severe shock, respectively). Diagnostic and therapeutic laparoscopy was taken to completion in 89% of patients irrespective of hemodynamic status. Gasless laparoscopy has been proposed as an alternative to the use of pneumoperitoneum as a tactic to avoid hemodynamic instability as well as the other complications of pneumoperitoneum, including hypercapnia, acidosis, gas embolism, pneumothorax, and deep venous thrombosis.[30] In a review of 15 adult patients sustaining intraabdominal trauma, gasless laparoscopy was used successfully to manage both blunt and penetrating injury with no effect of hemodynamic status. In our hospital, we continue to manage hemodynamically unstable pediatric trauma patients with open exploration by midline laparotomy and believe this remains the safest strategy for the critically injured child.

Children selected for an MIS approach to traumatic abdominal injury should not have an absolute contraindication to laparoscopy such as hemodynamic instability (**Box 1**). Relative contraindications such as peritonitis, evisceration, or multiorgan injury should be weighed carefully. Other relative contraindications to consider include an inability to tolerate abdominal insufflation, increased intracranial pressure, uncorrected coagulopathy, or congestive heart failure. These factors must be reviewed by the anesthesia and trauma team in the multiply injured patient before an MIS approach is undertaken. Clear indications for diagnostic and/or therapeutic laparoscopy include penetrating injuries to the anterior abdominal wall, thoracoabdominal trauma, suspected hollow viscus injury, and presentation suggestive of a diaphragm injury. Children with blunt trauma and a worsening abdominal examination with free fluid on ultrasound examination or inadequate imaging may be candidates for laparoscopy. A common pediatric scenario demonstrating the usefulness of laparoscopy is a child with a Chance fracture and worsening abdominal examination after a motor vehicle collision. Bowel injury is present in a significant number of these children and this injury pattern occurs with enough frequency to warrant a standardized minimally invasive approach.

Box 1
Indications and contraindications for minimally invasive surgery in pediatric blunt and penetrating trauma

Indications

Penetrating injury abdominal wall

Suspected diaphragm injury

Thoracoabdominal trauma

Suspected hollow viscus injury

Worsening abdominal examination

Contraindications

Absolute
  Hemodynamic instability

Relative
  Increased intracranial pressure
  Congestive heart failure
  Uncorrected coagulopathy
  Peritonitis
  Evisceration
  Multiple organ injury

TREATMENT ALGORITHM FOR THE USE OF MINIMALLY INVASIVE SURGERY IN BLUNT AND PENETRATING TRAUMA

Many algorithms have been developed for the triage of patients for MIS in blunt and penetrating abdominal trauma.[23,27] In a retrospective review of 7127 trauma admissions with 113 children requiring surgical exploration, 32 patients with initial diagnostic laparoscopy were reviewed in detail and a clinical decision making tree was created.[23] Hemodynamically stable children with blunt abdominal trauma and a concerning abdominal examination, elevated liver function tests, or a positive Focused Abdominal Sonography for Trauma examination should undergo a computed tomography scan (**Fig. 1**). If injuries are limited to solid organs, a nonoperative management pathway should be chosen. Children with clear evidence of hollow viscus or diaphragm injury should undergo laparoscopy for either diagnostic or therapeutic purposes. The child without solid organ injury who has free fluid and an equivocal examination may be managed with serial abdominal examinations or upfront laparoscopy.[23] Hemodynamically stable children with anterior abdominal stab wounds or tangential gun shot injuries with questionable fascial penetration are excellent candidates for diagnostic laparoscopy (**Fig. 2**). If at any point the child is unstable hemodynamically, exploratory laparotomy is the procedure of choice.

TECHNICAL CONSIDERATIONS IN TRAUMA LAPAROSCOPY

After the decision has been made to proceed with surgical intervention, the patient is taken directly to the operating room with cross-matched blood available and induced with general anesthesia. After surgical preparation with chlorhexidine gluconate solution, access to the peritoneum is achieved via the umbilicus using either a Veress needle or Hassan technique. The initial approach begins with CO_2 insufflation of the abdomen to 9 to 12 mm Hg with a flow of 0.5 to 2 mL/min. A 4- or 5-mm port is placed at the umbilicus. Additional port placement is tailored to the nature of the injury.

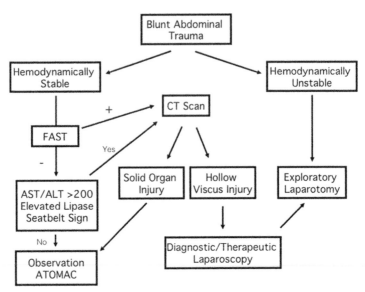

Fig. 1. Management algorithm for blunt abdominal trauma. CT, computed tomography; FAST, Focused Abdominal Sonography for Trauma.

Common configurations include a 5-mm port in the right and left mid abdomen, or 2 additional 5-mm ports placed in the left flank. The latter triangulates the approach for running the entirety of the small bowel, although in some cases a 5-mm port in the right lower quadrant is necessary for additional exposure. If an injury clearly penetrates the peritoneum, this wound may be used to establish laparoscopic access. Once ports are safely established, the peritoneal cavity is evaluated with a 30°

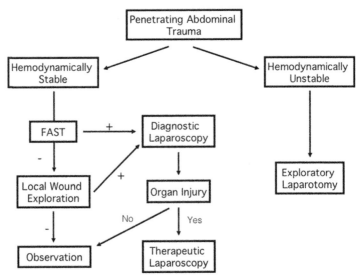

Fig. 2. Management algorithm for penetrating abdominal trauma. FAST, Focused Abdominal Sonography for Trauma.

telescope for the presence of blood, bile, or enteric contents. A systematic evaluation of the peritoneal cavity and its contents has been shown to be reproducible, reduce the incidence of missed injury, and increase the safety and efficacy of laparoscopy in trauma patients.[31] The rate of missed injuries can be decreased significantly by following 3 strategies[1]: systematic and careful inspection,[2] changing the patient's position to optimize evaluation,[3] and using atraumatic graspers to handle the bowel. Intraabdominal contents are evaluated systematically beginning with the liver, spleen, stomach, diaphragm, pancreas, and abdominal wall in the reverse Trendelenburg position. The patient is then positioned in the level supine position and using atraumatic graspers, the transverse colon is elevated superiorly. The small bowel and its mesentery should be examined in segments beginning at the ligament of Treitz, proceeding distally until the ileocecal valve is reached. By crossing the graspers, the reverse side of the bowel is brought into view, because a detailed inspection of all surfaces of the intestine and its mesentery is necessary to avoid missed injuries.[32] The large intestine is then examined, followed by the rectum and pelvic contents with the patient in the Trendelenburg position.

Once an injury is discovered, the surgeon must judge whether the repair can safely be completed laparoscopically. Simple gastric, small bowel, and colon perforations (<50% of bowel wall circumference) are repaired with 3-0/4-0 absorbable sutures sewn intracorporeally.[8] If more complex injuries exist requiring bowel resection, a "minilaparotomy" of greater than 4 cm is extended from the nearest trocar or umbilicus and an extracorporeal resection with stapled or hand sewn anastomosis can be performed (after the entire abdomen has been fully explored for additional injuries). Using these techniques, Streck and colleagues[8] retrospectively evaluated 50 hemodynamically stable children explored for suspected bowel injury. The authors noted that children sustaining penetrating trauma were operated on shortly after arrival (4.2 hours), whereas patients with isolated bowel injuries after blunt abdominal trauma had a delay in diagnosis and treatment (16 hours after arrival). The decision to operate was made based on a worsening abdominal examination or the presence of pneumoperitoneum or a progression of free air or fluid on serial radiographs. In this study, laparoscopic repair was completed in 6 children and an additional 6 children found to have complex intestinal injury underwent laparoscopic-assisted bowel resection. No patient undergoing laparoscopic exploration and repair experienced an early (missed injury, wound infection, bleeding) or late (need for reoperation) complication. In addition to bowel injury, myriad other therapeutic procedures have been documented as safe and efficacious in the hands of an experienced surgeon with advanced laparoscopic skills.

Although laparoscopy is safe and efficacious, it can be associated with significant risks, including access-related complications, equipment failure, inadequate visualization of injuries, insufflation-related injuries, intraoperative injuries, and postoperative complications.[33] The physiologic consequences of CO_2 insufflation have been described and include impaired venous return, pneumomediastinum, venous gas embolism, and subcutaneous emphysema. These changes may have an effect on preload, causing bradycardia and hypotension. Access-related complications include injury to the abdominal wall or intraabdominal vessels as well as solid and hollow organs with associated sequelae. Hemorrhagic complications during laparoscopy occur during 0.3% of cases with an associated mortality of 15%. Omental injuries occur in as many as 1.6% of laparoscopic cases, although most do not require repair. Visceral injuries occur in up to 0.5% of cases. Importantly, up to one-half of visceral injuries caused by iatrogenic laparoscopic intervention go undiagnosed during surgery, leading to significant morbidity or mortality.[33] These injuries may be attributed to trocar insertion, direct mechanical instrument injury, and thermal injury from electrocautery.

Other potential complications include bladder puncture by trocar insertion, port site hernias, and inadequate visualization or missed injuries.

MINIMALLY INVASIVE SURGERY AND THORACIC TRAUMA

The resuscitation and clinical management of the child with thoracic and thoracoabdominal trauma remains a clinical challenge and treatment algorithms are poorly defined in the pediatric population. In the adult population, thoracoscopy has been used at an increasing rate over the last decade for both diagnosis and treatment of trauma to the chest cavity. Authors have demonstrated reduced rates of postoperative complications, bleeding, drainage, and a shortened hospitalization when comparing thoracoscopy to open thoracotomy.[34] In a recent metaanalysis of 26 studies of adult chest trauma, the authors found that video-assisted thoracoscopic surgery is an effective and better treatment for improving preoperative outcomes of hemodynamically stable patients with reduced postoperative complications. The range of thoracoscopic interventions that have been successful include, but are not limited to, hemostasis of bleeding vessels, decortication and evacuation of hemothorax, repair of lung laceration or pulmonary wedge resection, repair of diaphragm injury, control of air leak, removal of foreign bodies, and widening of pericardial lacerations. Contraindications to thoracoscopic management of chest trauma include obliterated pleural spaces, inability to tolerate single lung ventilation, hemodynamic instability, circulatory shock, and life-threatening thoracic injury.[34]

The management of thoracic trauma by video-assisted thoracoscopic surgery has not been studied exhaustively in the pediatric literature and data are limited to small case series and reports. In a single institutional review of a 20-year experience using MIS for trauma, the authors reported just 2 children with diagnostic thoracoscopy after trauma with successful thoracoscopic repair of a diaphragmatic repair in 1 child and conversion to open thoracotomy for repair in the other patient.[12] In a much larger study including 6 pediatric trauma centers, Alemayehu and colleagues[15] reviewed 13 patients that underwent video-assisted thoracoscopic surgery repair for penetrating injury, failed chest tube management, or a large hemothorax. In this cohort, the rate of conversion was only 11%. Interventions included evacuation of hemothorax, repair of diaphragmatic injury, and wedge resection for lung injury. Perioperative thoracic complications included complex hemothorax, pleural effusion, and empyema. Thoracoabdominal trauma presents a particular challenge to the trauma surgeon, who must decide which cavity to explore, especially if occult injuries may be present and not identified on imaging. In a recent review of 30 adult patients with thoracoabdominal stab wounds who underwent thoracoscopy to identify a possible diaphragmatic injury, 17% of patients were found to have injuries and the accuracy of thoracoscopy reached 100%.[35]

In the multiply injured child, the minimally invasive treatment paradigm is expanding into the realm of vascular surgery as well. Although still in its development phase, the advent of resuscitative endovascular balloon occlusion of the aorta and other wire-based or catheter-based interventions make it conceptually possible that in the near future children with severe thoracic and abdominal injuries will be treated using techniques that are entirely minimally invasive.

SUMMARY

MIS in the management of blunt and penetrating pediatric trauma is finding its place in the armamentarium of the pediatric trauma surgeon. Several studies have demonstrated the safety and efficacy of laparoscopy and thoracoscopy with diagnostic accuracy approaching 100% and a missed injury rate of 0% to 1%. Although some studies have shown safety in the management of patients who are hemodynamically unstable or who are transient responders to initial trauma resuscitation, the currently available data advocate limiting the use of MIS to blunt or penetrating injuries in the hemodynamically stable child. In the pediatric trauma population, MIS offers both diagnostic and therapeutic potential, as well as reduced postoperative pain, a decreased rate of postoperative complications, shortened hospital stay, and potentially reduced cost.

REFERENCES

1. Carnevale N, Baron N, Delany HM. Peritoneoscopy as an aid in the diagnosis of abdominal trauma: a preliminary report. J Trauma 1977;17:634–41.
2. Gans SL, Berci G. Peritoneoscopy in infants and children. J Pediatr Surg 1973;8: 399–405.
3. Chen MK, Schropp KP, Lobe TE. The use of minimal access surgery in pediatric trauma: a preliminary report. J Laparoendosc Surg 1995;5:295–301.
4. Brandt CP, Priebe PP, Jacobs DG. Potential of laparoscopy to reduce non-therapeutic trauma laparotomies. Am Surg 1994;60:416–20.
5. Livingston DH, Tortella BJ, Blackwood J, et al. The role of laparoscopy in abdominal trauma. J Trauma 1992;33:471–5.
6. Berg RJ, Karamanos E, Inaba K, et al. The persistent diagnostic challenge of thoracoabdominal stab wounds. J Trauma Acute Care Surg 2014;76:418–23.
7. Lin HF, Wu JM, Tu CC, et al. Value of diagnostic and therapeutic laparoscopy for abdominal stab wounds: reply. World J Surg 2013;37:2721–2.
8. Streck CJ, Lobe TE, Pietsch JB, et al. Laparoscopic repair of traumatic bowel injury in children. J Pediatr Surg 2006;41:1864–9.
9. Koehler RH, Smith RS, Fry WR. Successful laparoscopic splenorrhaphy using absorbable mesh for grade III splenic injury: report of a case. Surg Laparosc Endosc 1994;4:311–5.
10. Sosa JL, Arrillaga A, Sleeman D, et al. Missed diaphragmatic injuries that were diagnosed and treated thoracoscopically. J Trauma 1994;37:515.
11. Ross SE, Dragon GM, O'Malley KF, et al. Morbidity of negative coeliotomy in trauma. Injury 1995;26:393–4.
12. Stringel G, Xu ML, Lopez J. Minimally invasive surgery in pediatric trauma: one institution's 20-Year Experience. JSLS 2016;20(1):1–5.
13. Sosa JL, Arrillaga A, Puente I, et al. Laparoscopy in 121 consecutive patients with abdominal gunshot wounds. J Trauma 1995;39:501–4 [discussion: 504].
14. Zafar SN, Onwugbufor MT, Hughes K, et al. Laparoscopic surgery for trauma: the realm of therapeutic management. Am J Surg 2015;209:627–32.
15. Alemayehu H, Clifton M, Santore M, et al. Minimally invasive surgery for pediatric trauma-a multicenter review. J Laparoendosc Adv Surg Tech A 2015;25:243–7.
16. Tharakan SJ, Kim AG, Collins JL, et al. Laparoscopy in Pediatric Abdominal Trauma: A 13-year Experience. Eur J Pediatr Surg 2015. [Epub ahead of print].
17. Avarello JT, Cantor RM. Pediatric major trauma: an approach to evaluation and management. Emerg Med Clin North Am 2007;25:803–36, x.
18. McFadyen JG, Ramaiah R, Bhananker SM. Initial assessment and management of pediatric trauma patients. Int J Crit Illn Inj Sci 2012;2:121–7.
19. Upadhyaya P, Simpson JS. Splenic trauma in children. Surg Gynecol Obstet 1968;126:781–90.
20. Uranüs S, Pfeifer J. Nonoperative treatment of blunt splenic injury. World J Surg 2001;25:1405–7.

21. Notrica DM, Eubanks JW, Tuggle DW, et al. Nonoperative management of blunt liver and spleen injury in children: evaluation of the ATOMAC guideline using GRADE. J Trauma Acute Care Surg 2015;79:683–93.
22. Marwan A, Harmon CM, Georgeson KE, et al. Use of laparoscopy in the management of pediatric abdominal trauma. J Trauma 2010;69:761–4.
23. Feliz A, Shultz B, McKenna C, et al. Diagnostic and therapeutic laparoscopy in pediatric abdominal trauma. J Pediatr Surg 2006;41:72–7.
24. Shaw JM, Navsaria PH, Nicol AJ. Laparoscopy-assisted repair of diaphragm injuries. World J Surg 2003;27:671–4.
25. Fabiani P, Iannelli A, Mazza D, et al. Diagnostic and therapeutic laparoscopy for stab wounds of the anterior abdomen. J Laparoendosc Adv Surg Tech A 2003;13:309–12.
26. O'Malley E, Boyle E, O'Callaghan A, et al. Role of laparoscopy in penetrating abdominal trauma: a systematic review. World J Surg 2013;37:113–22.
27. Koto MZ, Matsevych OY, Motilall SR. The role of laparoscopy in penetrating abdominal trauma: our initial experience. J Laparoendosc Adv Surg Tech A 2015;25:730–6.
28. Cherkasov M, Sitnikov V, Sarkisyan B, et al. Laparoscopy versus laparotomy in management of abdominal trauma. Surg Endosc 2008;22:228–31.
29. Carey JE, Koo R, Miller R, et al. Laparoscopy and thoracoscopy in evaluation of abdominal trauma. Am Surg 1995;61:92–5.
30. Liao CH, Kuo IM, Fu CY, et al. Gasless laparoscopic assisted surgery for abdominal trauma. Injury 2014;45:850–4.
31. Choi GS. Systematized laparoscopic surgery in abdominal trauma. J Korean Surg Soc 1998;54:492–500.
32. Lim KH, Chung BS, Kim JY, et al. Laparoscopic surgery in abdominal trauma: a single center review of a 7-year experience. World J Emerg Surg 2015;10:16.
33. Kindel T, Latchana N, Swaroop M, et al. Laparoscopy in trauma: An overview of complications and related topics. Int J Crit Illn Inj Sci 2015;5:196–205.
34. Wu N, Wu L, Qiu C, et al. A comparison of video-assisted thoracoscopic surgery with open thoracotomy for the management of chest trauma: a systematic review and meta-analysis. World J Surg 2015;39:940–52.
35. Bagheri R, Tavassoli A, Sadrizadeh A, et al. The role of thoracoscopy for the diagnosis of hidden diaphragmatic injuries in penetrating thoracoabdominal trauma. Interact Cardiovasc Thorac Surg 2009;9:195–7 [discussion: 197].

Pediatric Airway and Esophageal Foreign Bodies

Elizabeth A. Berdan, MD, MS[a], Thomas T. Sato, MD[b],*

KEYWORDS

- Aerodigestive foreign bodies • Bronchoscopy • Button battery
- Esophageal bougienage

KEY POINTS

- Common airway foreign bodies include peanuts, seeds, and vegetable matter.
- Many children with airway foreign bodies initially have normal chest radiographs.
- Suspicion of an airway foreign body mandates bronchoscopy.
- The most commonly retained esophageal foreign bodies are coins.
- Lithium button battery ingestion must be distinguished from coins. Button batteries require emergent diagnosis and removal to prevent life-threatening injury.

INTRODUCTION

Aerodigestive foreign bodies (FBs) in children are commonly encountered clinical problems with the potential for life-threatening complications. FB aspiration into the tracheobronchial tree or ingestion with esophageal retention requires prompt surgical diagnosis and management. The identification of a foreign object lodged in the trachea or esophagus can be difficult owing to a delay in presentation and nonspecific symptoms. This article focuses on the clinical presentation, treatment approach, and risks associated with pediatric aerodigestive FBs.

Gustav Killian performed the first bronchoscopic removal of a FB in a farmer in 1897. Decades later, Chevalier Jackson developed the lighted bronchoscope and several specialized instruments for removal of FBs.[1] Contemporary management of airway or esophageal FBs is characterized by evaluation and stabilization of the physiologic status of the child with the performance of appropriate diagnostic and therapeutic procedures designed to achieve safe, successful removal. These procedures mandate

Disclosure: The authors have no financial disclosures to report.
[a] Children's Hospital of Wisconsin, Medical College of Wisconsin, Milwaukee, WI, USA;
[b] Division of Pediatric Surgery, Children's Hospital of Wisconsin, Medical College of Wisconsin, Children's Corporate Center, Suite C320, 999 North 92nd Street, Milwaukee, WI 53226, USA
* Corresponding author.
E-mail address: ttsato@chw.org

coordinated efforts between the primary care provider, emergency room, pediatric surgeon, anesthesiologist, and the operating room team.[2]

AIRWAY FOREIGN BODIES: CLINICAL PRESENTATION

Aspiration is common for infants and children, and, in particular, between 1 and 4 years of age.[2–5] Many FBs are either partially or completely expelled by coughing and spitting reflexes. Frequently inhaled FBs include organic materials such as nuts, seeds, vegetable matter, or dried fruits, and inorganic material such as toy pieces and pins.[6] Most aspirated objects lodge in the bronchial tree, with the right main stem bronchus being the most common location because of its straighter trajectory relative to the trachea.[2,5,7] The diagnostic difficulty is increased by the observation that the FB is visible on radiograph in only 10% to 20% of cases.[4,5] Clinically, this is made more complex by an initially normal chest radiograph appearance in many infants and children who have aspirated a FB.[8] A positive history or even a plausible history of witnessed aspiration of a FB should prompt evaluation and management for definitive diagnosis, because a delay in diagnosis increases the rate and severity of complications.[9]

FB aspiration typically presents with at least 1 symptom of coughing, choking, stridor, and/or wheezing at the time of aspiration.[7,10,11] On physical examination, the character of persistent stridor may reflect the anatomic location of partial airway obstruction. High-pitched inspiratory stridor is usually a result of supraglottic obstruction or physiologic collapse. Biphasic stridor indicates an obstruction in the glottis or subglottic region. Expiratory stridor is generally characteristic of tracheal or bronchial obstruction. The presence of decreased breath sounds and wheezing is highly correlated with an aspirated FB.[4] The aspiration or ingestion event is often not witnessed, making the clinical history less clear in infants and preverbal children.

A high index of suspicion should be maintained for any infant, child, or adolescent who has a history consistent with aspiration. The degree of respiratory distress determines the urgency of intervention. Tachypnea, nasal flaring, retractions, or cyanosis requires immediate intervention, and acute respiratory distress necessitates emergent establishment of a secure airway. In a physiologically normal child, the urgency of intervention may change precipitously based on the location of the FB. Delay in diagnosis is common, and many children do not present acutely following FB aspiration. Subacute or chronic airway FB in the bronchi may cause chronic pulmonary infection, bronchiectasis, asthma, lung collapse, or lung abscess.[5,12]

AIRWAY ASPIRATION: DIAGNOSTIC AND THERAPEUTIC PROCEDURES

Simulation courses can provide the foundation for trainees to become familiar with the assembly and utility of a ventilating bronchoscope, as well as how to address laryngospasm and other potential intraoperative issues. Most importantly, a simulated setting is an excellent way to provide experience to trainees and the team in the technical and communication aspects of the procedure.[13]

Radiographic findings of an aspirated FB include asymmetric air trapping with hyperinflation; unilateral atelectasis; and, later, pneumonia with distal chronic parenchymal infection.[8,11] In children older than 3 years of age, inspiratory and expiratory radiographs may be attempted. Bilateral decubitus radiographs may also be helpful. The sensitivity and specificity of chest radiography in identifying an aspirated FB are 61% and 77%, respectively.[9] For this reason, children with characteristic history and symptoms of FB aspiration should undergo prompt bronchoscopy regardless of radiographic findings.[7,8]

Extraction of airway FB is performed under general anesthesia. The team should have the necessary equipment, personnel, and experience before attempting airway FB removal in an infant or child; this includes resources, infrastructure, and experience with complicated pediatric airway management. Preoperative communication between the pediatric anesthesiologist, surgeon, and operating room team are essential to establish a plan of action. Spontaneous respiration is generally safer than an apneic technique with positive pressure ventilation to prevent distal displacement of the FB in the airway.

Rigid bronchoscopy is the mostly commonly used technique for airway FB removal.[14] The ability to control the airway, the excellent telescopic visualization, various sizes of bronchoscopes, and the array of available extraction instruments make rigid bronchoscopy the technique of choice; however, this does not allow for evaluation of the most distal peripheral airways. Flexible bronchoscopy may be used for objects in the smaller, peripheral airways. The limiting factor for flexible bronchoscopy is the 2-mm instrument channel, which requires specialized extraction equipment that is not readily available.[15]

For airway FB removal, appropriate instruments should be assembled and the child well oxygenated before induction of anesthesia. Once a suitable plane of anesthesia is achieved, direct laryngoscopy is performed with insertion of the bronchoscope into the airway with the child in supine position. Contemporary ventilating bronchoscopes allow for adequate gas exchange during the procedure. A systematic approach to the inspection of the trachea and bronchi is essential. The FB is identified and suction performed as needed to aspirate secretions. The FB is typically removed with optical forceps; rarely, impacted debris in the distal bronchi can be carefully extracted into the trachea with a Fogarty catheter and subsequently removed with forceps. Following successful extraction, bronchoscopy should be repeated to evaluate for retained FB or secretions, and an endotracheal tube placed for emergence from anesthesia. Complicated FBs include pins, teeth, and thin flexible material that can occlude the airway. Should symptomatic tracheal occlusion occur during attempts to extract an airway FB, the FB can be temporarily pushed into the right or left bronchus, allowing for single lung ventilation for further attempts at removal. Passage of catheters for distal airway ventilation; tracheostomy instruments; and, in rare cases, cardiopulmonary bypass should be available resources for complicated airway management.

ESOPHAGEAL FOREIGN BODIES: CLINICAL PRESENTATION

Symptoms of FB ingestion vary with the age of the patient and the location and size of the FB. Infants may show nonspecific symptoms such as drooling, gagging, or poor feeding. Larger objects in the esophagus may rarely cause obstruction of the airway if lodged proximal to the upper esophageal sphincter. Some children present immediately following witnessed ingestion of a coin or other FB; other children are found to have an incidental retained FB from a chest radiograph taken for other symptoms. Older children may report odynophagia, dysphagia, and chest pain. The physical examination includes airway and oropharyngeal evaluation, palpation of the neck and upper thorax to assess for crepitus, and auscultation of the lungs. Symptomatic patients with retained esophageal FB who are unable to swallow or in acute respiratory distress require prompt evaluation based on physiologic status. For most infants and children, symptoms and physical signs of a retained esophageal FB are not dramatic.

ESOPHAGEAL FOREIGN BODIES: DIAGNOSTIC AND THERAPEUTIC PROCEDURES

Essential diagnostic procedures for a retained esophageal FB include frontal and lateral radiograph imaging for radiopaque items such as coins and metal FBs. The images should include the neck and chest. If a retained esophageal object is suspected by history, examination, or symptoms, and plain radiographs of the neck are normal, an esophagram may be helpful, particularly for food impaction. The most commonly retained object in the esophagus in infants and children is a coin. Some esophageal coins spontaneously pass within 24 hours. Persistent esophageal coins may be removed by rigid endoscopy. Alternatively, esophageal coin removal using a balloon catheter passed into the esophagus under fluoroscopy may be used.[16,17] The balloon of the catheter is passed distal to the coin, inflated with contrast, and the coin is brought into the oropharynx under fluoroscopic guidance. In addition, the authors have reported our experience using bougienage for the management of uncomplicated esophageal coins in children.[18]

If the retained esophageal FB is a suspected button battery, it must be emergently removed given the potential for clinically significant esophageal injury within 2 hours.[19] Button batteries, and in particular the 3-V, 20-mm lithium button batteries that are approximately the size of a United States penny, are particularly dangerous and can lead to rapid, serious injury and death. Once in contact with a wet mucosal surface, the electrical current from the battery generates hydroxide alkaline injury that can rapidly proceed to full-thickness oropharyngeal or esophageal injury, which can lead to esophageal perforation with mediastinal infection, tracheoesophageal fistula, or erosion into major vascular structures with life-threatening hemorrhage. Batteries have a distinctive radiographic appearance, and the combination of frontal and lateral radiograph imaging is useful.[20] An anterior radiographic battery image may show a double-density shadow, or halo, caused by the bilaminar structure of the battery. A lateral view may also show the step-off at the junction of the cathode and anode. Once diagnosed or suspected, retained esophageal batteries require emergent removal via rigid or flexible esophagoscopy. Asymptomatic gastric batteries may be allowed to pass spontaneously, but passage should be documented with follow-up radiographs. Symptomatic patients with gastric batteries require urgent retrieval of the battery. Retrieval of gastric button batteries is also recommended if a magnet was also ingested, if the battery is greater than or equal to 15 mm in diameter, the child is younger than 6 years, or the battery remains in the stomach for greater than or equal to 4 days.[21]

Rigid esophagoscopy is performed under general anesthesia with placement of an endotracheal tube to reduce the risk of aspiration. Positioning the table lateral to the anesthesiology team and securing the endotracheal tube to the left side of the child's mouth is helpful. Plain films or esophagram images with preoperative localization of the foreign object should be available in the operating room. The child is placed supine; placing the neck in slight extension with a towel roll under the shoulders may be useful. The esophagoscope is directed posteriorly and through the upper esophagus under direct visualization. The object may be removed with either optical forceps or, with older esophagoscopes, with forceps placed through the viewing channel. In general, objects larger than the esophagoscope diameter require removal of the forceps, FB, and esophagoscope together. Repeat esophagoscopy should be performed to assess for any esophageal mucosal injury, and, if found, the depth of injury should be documented.

If the FB is accurately identified as a coin retained in the esophagus, the coin may be removed by rigid or flexible esophagoscopy under general anesthesia, fluoroscopically guided balloon retrieval, or pushed into the stomach using esophageal bougienage. All of these techniques in the management of retained esophageal coins are similar in safety and efficacy; balloon retrieval and bougienage do not require anesthesia, making these more cost-effective approaches.[17] The authors have used esophageal bougienage for the management of acute, uncomplicated esophageal coins for several decades. The rationale for bougienage of esophageal coins is to push the coin from the esophagus into the stomach, with subsequent passage of the coin through the gastrointestinal tract. **Box 1** lists our current criteria for esophageal bougienage.[18]

Box 1
Clinical criteria for bougienage of an esophageal coin

Single coin

Present with 24 hour of ingestion

No esophageal abnormalities or surgeries

Coin located inferior to the clavicles and cephalad the diaphragm on plain film

No respiratory distress

No prior foreign body ingestions

Adapted from Heinzerling NP, Christensen MA, Swedler R, et al. Safe and effective management of esophageal coins in children with bougienage. Surgery 2015;158(4):1066; with permission.

CLINICAL OUTCOMES

The complication rate of rigid endoscopy for either airway or esophageal FB is low (0.2%–5%) and mortality is rare (<0.1%).[2,15,16,22,23] Postoperative complications increase for children who present with a delay in diagnosis greater than 24 hours, whereas the morbidity of diagnostic rigid bronchoscopy is almost zero in children without a tracheobronchial FB.[6] Airway FBs that are not diagnosed and promptly removed may lead to pneumonia and continued obstructive pulmonary parenchymal infection and injury. The impact of delayed diagnosis is reflected in the significant mortality associated with childhood airway FBs. A retrospective, administrative database review identified 2771 children admitted to the hospital during 2003 for an FB causing airway obstruction, with 94 deaths (3.4%) while in the hospital.[6] Known complications include extraction failure, retained fragments, laryngeal edema or bronchospasm requiring tracheotomy or reintubation, tracheal or bronchial laceration, pneumothorax, pneumomediastinum, respiratory infection, airway or esophageal injury, cardiac arrest, and hypoxic brain damage.

Consideration should be given to performing esophagoscopy in children who undergo bronchoscopy for suspected aspiration with a negative bronchoscopic examination. The trachea is compressible in young children and an esophageal FB may cause obstruction of the trachea as well.[23] Complications related to endoscopic removal of esophageal FB are generally related to the type of FB and duration of time the FB is retained in the esophagus. The risk of erosion of metallic and plastic esophageal FBs into the mediastinum and great vessels increases with duration of retention, and life-threatening hemorrhage requiring emergent intervention has been reported from our institution.[24] For partial-thickness or full-thickness esophageal injury from a retained FB, follow up esophagram at 4 to 6 weeks following extraction may be useful to evaluate for esophageal narrowing secondary to inflammatory stricture.

SUMMARY

Aerodigestive tract FBs are common in infants and children. The most commonly retrieved airway FBs in young children are food products, particularly peanuts and seeds; in older children, pins, toy pieces, pen caps, and nonfood objects are commonly found. Airway FBs require prompt diagnosis and management given the complications associated with diagnostic delay. Rigid bronchoscopy under general anesthesia is the most widely accepted diagnostic and therapeutic intervention. For esophageal FBs, retained button batteries must be removed emergently. For retained food or coins, rigid esophagoscopy is commonly used. For a selected population with retained esophageal coins, experience with balloon catheter retrieval or esophageal bougienage suggests these methods as safe, efficient, and cost-effective methodologies.

REFERENCES

1. Clerf LH. Chevalier Jackson. Arch Otolaryngol 1966;83(3):292–6.
2. Fidkowski CW, Zheng H, Firth PG. The anesthetic considerations of tracheobronchial foreign bodies in children: a literature review of 12,979 cases. Anesth Analg 2010;111(4):1016–25.
3. Cevik M, Gókdemir MT, Boleken ME, et al. The characteristics and outcomes of foreign body ingestion and aspiration in children due to lodged foreign body in the aerodigestive tract. Pediatr Emerg Care 2013;29(1):53–7.
4. Sink JR, Kitsko DJ, Georg MW, et al. Predictors of foreign body aspiration in children. Otolaryngol Head Neck Surg 2016;155(3):501–7.
5. Lakhkar BB, Kini P, Shenoy V, et al. Foreign body aspiration: Manipal experience. Indian Pediatr 2000;37(2):193–5.
6. Shah RK, Patel A, Lander L, et al. Management of foreign bodies obstructing the airway in children. Arch Otolaryngol Head Neck Surg 2010;136(4):373–9.
7. Black RE, Johnson DG, Matlak ME. Bronchoscopic removal of aspirated foreign bodies in children. J Pediatr Surg 1994;29(5):682–4.
8. Zerella JT, Dimler M, McGill LC, et al. Foreign body aspiration in children: value of radiography and complications of bronchoscopy. J Pediatr Surg 1998;33(11):1651–4.
9. Foltran F, Ballali S, Passali FM, et al. Foreign bodies in the airways: a meta-analysis of published papers. Int J Pediatr Otorhinolaryngol 2012;76(Suppl 1):S12–9.
10. Rodríguez H, Passali GC, Gregori D, et al. Management of foreign bodies in the airway and oesophagus. Int J Pediatr Otorhinolaryngol 2012;76(Suppl 1):S84–91.
11. Even L, Heno N, Talmon Y, et al. Diagnostic evaluation of foreign body aspiration in children: a prospective study. J Pediatr Surg 2005;40(7):1122–7.
12. Mu L, He P, Sun D. The causes and complications of late diagnosis of foreign body aspiration in children. Report of 210 cases. Arch Otolaryngol Head Neck Surg 1991;117(8):876–9.
13. Deutsch ES. High-fidelity patient simulation mannequins to facilitate aerodigestive endoscopy training. Arch Otolaryngol Head Neck Surg 2008;134(6):625–9.
14. Hsu WC, Sheen TS, Lin CD, et al. Clinical experiences of removing foreign bodies in the airway and esophagus with a rigid endoscope: a series of 3217 cases from 1970 to 1996. Otolaryngol Head Neck Surg 2000;122(3):450–4.
15. Endoh M, Oizumi H, Kanauchi N, et al. Removal of foreign bodies from the respiratory tract of young children: treatment outcomes using newly developed foreign-body grasping forceps. J Pediatr Surg 2016;51(8):1375–9.
16. Harned RK 2nd, Strain JD, Hay TC, et al. Esophageal foreign bodies: safety and efficacy of Foley catheter extraction of coins. AJR Am J Roentgenol 1997;168(2):443–6.
17. Conners GP. A literature-based comparison of three methods of pediatric esophageal coin removal. Pediatr Emerg Care 1997;13(2):154–7.
18. Heinzerling NP, Christensen MA, Swedler R, et al. Safe and effective management of esophageal coins in children with bougienage. Surgery 2015;158(4):1065–70.
19. Yardeni D, Yardeni H, Coran AG, et al. Severe esophageal damage due to button battery ingestion: can it be prevented? Pediatr Surg Int 2004;20(7):496–501.

20. Guelfguat M, Kaplinskiy V, Reddy SH, et al. Clinical guidelines for imaging and reporting ingested foreign bodies. Am J Roentgenol 2014;203(1):37–53.
21. Litovitz T, Whitaker N, Clark L, et al. Emerging battery-ingestion hazard: clinical implications. Pediatrics 2010;125(6):1168–77.
22. Tomaske M, Gerber AC, Weiss M. Anesthesia and periinterventional morbidity of rigid bronchoscopy for tracheobronchial foreign body diagnosis and removal. Paediatr Anaesth 2006;16(2):123–9.
23. Yalçin S, Karnak I, Ciftci AO, et al. Foreign body ingestion in children: an analysis of pediatric surgical practice. Pediatr Surg Int 2007;23(8):755–61.
24. Stuth EA, Stucke AG, Cohen RD, et al. Successful resuscitation of a child after exsanguination due to aortoesophageal fistula from undiagnosed foreign body. Anesthesiology 2001;95(4):1025–6.

Pediatric Appendicitis

Rebecca M. Rentea, MD[a], Shawn D. St. Peter, MD[b],*

KEYWORDS

- Appendicitis • Surgery • Appendectomy • Children • Nonoperative management
- Abdominal pain • Right lower quadrant

KEY POINTS

- Appendicitis is less likely to present in a classic manner than commonly thought.
- Appendicitis can be managed nonoperatively in selected children.
- For children with perforated appendicitis, a laparoscopic appendectomy should be performed.
- The long-term risk of recurrence of appendicitis is unknown.

INTRODUCTION

Appendicitis is the most common surgical emergency in children.[1] The lifetime risk of developing appendicitis is 7% to 8%, with a peak incidence in the teenage years.[2] It is estimated that 86 cases of appendicitis per 100,000 people occur annually, with an estimated 70,000 pediatric appendectomies performed in the United States each year with a mean cost of $9000.[3,4] In the recent decade appendicitis has become more protocolized with greater efforts to minimize antibiotic durations and radiation exposure as well as to begin to study the nonoperative management of appendicitis. Much variation still exists, however, in the diagnosis and management of appendicitis. This article serves to highlight and update some of the controversies and recent literature regarding pediatric appendicitis.

Diagnosis

The peak incidence of appendicitis occurs in the second decade of life with the median age between 10 and 11 years. The male/female ratio is 1.4:1. There is a seasonal variation with increased presentation of appendicitis in the summer months with perforated appendicitis occurring more frequently in the fall and winter.[5]

Funding/Grant Support: None.
Disclosures: The authors have no disclosures or conflicts of interest.
[a] Department of Surgery, Children's Mercy Hospital, 2401 Gillham Road, Kansas City, MO 64108, USA; [b] Pediatric Surgical Fellowship and Scholars Programs, Department of Surgery, Children's Mercy Hospital, 2401 Gillham Road, Kansas City, MO 64108, USA
* Corresponding author.
E-mail address: sspeter@cmh.edu

SYMPTOMS

The symptoms of appendicitis have been classically described as the gradual onset of dull periumbilical pain migrating to the right lower quadrant over the course of a day. Additional and variable symptoms include nausea, vomiting, anorexia, fever, and, less frequently, diarrhea. Classically, it is thought that perforation occurs within 24 to 36 hours from the onset of symptoms of pain. The pain, which was localized, improves and then becomes generalized. This description of symptoms, however, occurs in less than 50% of children.[6] Many other classic symptoms also variably present in children without appendicitis, including nausea, right lower quadrant guarding, or migrating pain.[7] Certain findings have been shown to increase or decrease the likelihood of appendicitis, including the midabdominal pain migrating to the right lower quadrant (likelihood ration [LR] 1.9–3.1) and the presence of fever (LR 3.4), which, if not present, lowers the likelihood of appendicitis by two-thirds.[6] The overlap in symptoms makes the diagnosis a clinical challenge, which is amplified in young children who do not understand or articulate the early symptoms.[8] Children less than 3 years of age present with perforated appendicitis more than 80% of the time compared with 20% of those aged 10 to 17 years.[6]

SIGNS

Physical examination findings include tenderness palpation and guarding in the right lower quadrant and rebound tenderness. Rovsing sign (left lower quadrant palpation resulting in referred pain to the right lower quadrat), obturator sign (internal rotation of the right lower extremity), and psoas sign (pain while lying on the left side and extending the right hip) are nonspecific physical examination findings of appendicitis. Only rebound tenderness has correlated with an increased likelihood of appendicitis (LR 2.3–3.9), whereas lack of tenderness in the right lower quadrant reduces the likelihood of appendicitis by half.[7,9]

LABORATORY STUDIES

Although no single laboratory value has a high sensitivity and specificity for appendicitis, white blood cell (WBC) count, absolute neutrophil count (ANC), and C-reactive protein (CRP) are most often used to aid diagnose appendicitis. The use of these laboratory tests alone is not helpful or predictive. WBC, ANC, and CRP all have wide ranges in specificity and sensitivity for predicting appendicitis.[9–14] An elevated WBC count does not predict appendicitis, as appendicitis may be present in children with a normal WBC count.[12] However, an increased WBC (>10–12,000 cells per cubic millimeter) increases the odds of appendicitis. In children less than 4 years of age, a normal WBC count has a negative predictive value of 95.6%, whereas the negative predictive value in those 4 to 12 years old is 89.5%. The negative predictive value of a low or normal WBC count among adolescents is 92%.[9] A left shift or increase in the number of immature forms of neutrophils also has a strong association with appendicitis, because only 3.7% of pediatric patients without a left shift have appendicitis. Although CRP is nonspecific as an isolated laboratory value, a higher mean level may predict complicated or perforated appendicitis or those children more likely to form an abscess.[12,15,16]

SCORING

The Alvarado score and the Pediatric Appendicitis Score (PAS) are the 2 systems that have been extensively evaluated for their ability to predict appendicitis based on symptoms, physical examination findings, and laboratory values (**Tables 1** and **2**).[17,18] The

Table 1 Alvarado score	
Migration of pain	1
Anorexia	1
Nausea/vomiting	1
Right lower quadrant tenderness	2
Rebound pain	1
Increase in temperature (>37.3°C)	1
Leukocytosis (>10,000/mL)	2
Polymorphonuclear neutrophilia (>75%)	1
Total	10

From Alvarado A. A practical score for the early diagnosis of acute appendicitis. Ann Emerg Med 1986;15(5):558.

Alvarado score is composed of 8 components with a total score of 10 (migration of pain, anorexia, nausea/vomiting, right lower quadrant tenderness, rebound pain, increased temperature >37°C, leukocytosis >10,000/mL, polymorphonuclear neutrophilia >75%).[17] The PAS score is composed of 8 components with a total score of 10 (migration of pain, anorexia, nausea/vomiting, right lower quadrant tenderness, coughing/hopping/percussion tenderness in right lower quadrant, increase in temperature, leukocytes >10,000/mL, polymophoyclear neutrophila >75%).[18] Both systems have been divided into low, medium, and high range scores to aid in management and give a likelihood of appendicitis. Intermediate scores, or those with Alvarado scores of 5 to 8 or PAS scores of 4 to 7, typically precipitate further imaging. Both scoring systems initially demonstrated sensitivity, specificity, and negative and positive predictive values in the high 90s.[17,18] However, large validation studies have only found sensitivity and specificity in the 70s and 80s.[19–23] In specific groups of children, such as adolescent girls, the scoring ranges and cutoff values further decrease, underscoring the need for further investigation of the scoring systems performance in specific subpopulations.[24] When the PAS score was compared with the Alvarado score in 311 patients, the investigators concluded that both scoring systems can be of assistance in the diagnosis of acute appendicitis but that neither has adequate predictive values to be definitive.[22]

Table 2 Pediatric Appendicitis Score	
Migration of pain	1
Anorexia	1
Nausea/vomiting	1
Right lower quadrant tenderness	2
Cough/hopping/percussion tenderness in right lower quadrant	2
Increase in temperature	1
Leukocytes >10,000/mL	1
Polymorphonuclear neutrophilia >75%	1
Total	10

From Samuel M. Pediatric appendicitis score. J Pediatr Surg 2002;37(6):878.

CLINICAL PATHWAYS

Clinical pathways consist of multidisciplinary management tools based on evidence-based practice for a specific group of patients in order to decrease unnecessary variation and improve outcomes while reducing fragmentation and cost.[25] Additional qualities of a pathway are standardization, efficiency, and reproducibility. Pathways have been able to reduce hospital costs and time spent in the hospital for patients with acute and perforated appendicitis.[26] Many investigators noted that utilization of clinical pathways decreased the use of radiation exposure demonstrated by decreased utilization of computed tomography (CT) scans and the ability to discharge patients with low probability of having appendicitis.[27–30]

DIFFERENTIAL DIAGNOSIS

The differential diagnosis for right lower quadrant abdominal pain is exhaustive. The authors of a previous review on appendicitis, the authors characterize 5 general categories: inflammatory, infectious, vascular, congenital, and genitourinary conditions. Inflammatory mimickers of appendicitis include mesenteric adenitis (primary or secondary), inflammatory bowel disease, intussusception, omental infarction, epiploic appendagitis, and cecal diverticulitis. Infectious causes include viral infections, bacterial infections, and parasitic infections. Among vascular causes, Henoch-Schönlein purpura can initially present as severe abdominal pain. Congenital causes include Meckel diverticulum, Meckel diverticulitis, and duplication cysts. Genitourinary causes include pyelonephritis, nephrolithiasis, ovarian torsion, ovarian tumors, hemorrhagic ovarian cysts, pelvic inflammatory disease, and infected urachal remnants. Constipation cannot be forgotten when evaluating pediatric patients because it is often a culprit in abdominal pain.[31]

Imaging

Imaging provides an adjunct to the diagnosis of appendicitis. Ideal imaging is rapid, inexpensive, and reproducible and has high sensitivity and specificity. In settings where operative care for children with appendicitis is not available, resources for appropriate pediatric imaging and interpretation of radiographic findings may also be lacking.[32] These children should avoid diagnostic imaging and be transferred to an appropriate pediatric facility. In an era of increased reliance on imaging, clinical judgment remains paramount, as it has been documented that a pediatric surgeon can differentiate appendicitis from other abdominal disorders with 92% accuracy.[33]

ULTRASOUND

In centers with experience and high utilization of ultrasound (US), US has been adopted as an adjunct in the diagnosis of appendicitis. Advantages are its lack of sedation, contrast agents, and radiation and low cost.[34–36] Sensitivity and specificity for US is 88% and 94%.[37] Disadvantages of US include the following: operator experience is required; there may be a lack of regular availability during off hours; and visualizing the appendix can be difficult in obese individuals or those with low clinical suspicion.[37–41] Increased sensitivity and specificity using US can be obtained by changing parameters of thickness of the appendix (>7 vs 6 mm), having dedicated sonographers, using US with greater frequency, and increased duration of abdominal pain (>48 vs <12 hours).[42–45] Studies have also demonstrated that surgeon-performed US with clinical evaluation may yield similar accuracy as radiologist-performed US.[46]

COMPUTED TOMOGRAPHY

CT scans combine the advantages of many other imaging modalities, including rapid acquisition time and a lack of operator dependency.[42] The sensitivity of CT scan for appendicitis is 97%, specificity of 99%, positive predictive value of 98%, negative predictive value of 98%, and accuracy 96%. Intravenous (IV) contrast enhances the CT scan sensitivity and specificity,[35,47,48] whereas contrast administered enterally (oral or rectal) in observational studies does not further improve test performance over IV contrast CT alone.[49,50] The accuracy of CT scan for perforation is around 72%, with a sensitivity of 62% and specificity of 82%.[51] Nonvisualization of the appendix on CT scan has been shown to have a high negative predictive value (98.7%).[52] The advantages of CT scan come at the cost of ionizing radiation. One CT scan of the abdomen in a 5-year-old child increases the lifetime risk of radiation-induced cancer to 26.1 per 100,000 in women and 20.1 per 100,000 in men.[53] In order to lower overall radiation dose, one study evaluated decreasing the radiation dose by 50% and another examined targeted CT imaging; both demonstrated high sensitivity and specificity.[37,54] It has been shown that a dedicated pediatric facility has much lower doses of radiation when using CT to diagnoses appendicitis compared with adult centers without pediatric-specific protocols.[55]

MRI

MRI has a high diagnostic accuracy for appendicitis and does not expose the child to ionizing radiation. The obvious disadvantages, though, have limited its utility, including lack of availability at many hospitals, lengthy acquisition time, high cost compared with CT and US, and often requires sedation or anesthesia.[56–59] Overall sensitivity and specificity are 96.8% and 97.4%, with a negative appendectomy rate of 3.1%.[58] Future research is required to define its role and position in the workup of appendicitis.

TREATMENT
Antibiotics

Antibiotics are initiated once the diagnosis of appendicitis is made. Initially a triple-antibiotic regimen consisting of ampicillin, gentamicin, and clindamycin was used. With the changes in the adult antibiotic regimens, pediatric surgery has evolved as well. Both piperacillin/tazobactam and cefoxitin have been shown to be at least as efficacious as the triple-drug regimen and may also decrease length of stay (LOS) and pharmaceutical costs.[60] Other studies suggest that metronidazole must be added to a third-generation cephalosporin to cover anaerobic isolates.[61,62] The authors' center begins with a single dose of ceftriaxone sodium (Rocephin) and metronidazole (Flagyl). If children are perforated, they receive additional IV doses until they are ready for discharge, at which time a WBC count, if elevated, results in discharge with a 5-day oral antibiotic course.[63] A recent prospective observational study of 1975 adult and pediatric patients with acute and perforated appendicitis demonstrated there was no difference in either 3 or 5 days of antibiotic treatment on the development of infectious complications after laparoscopic appendectomy for complicated appendicitis.[64]

Nonoperative Management of Acute Appendicitis

Although appendectomy is generally a simple procedure, it requires general anesthesia and is an abdominal operation with inherent risks and potential complications. Complications related to surgery or anesthesia occur in more than 10% of children within 30 days of appendectomy.[65] Even with current imaging methods, 6.3% of children in Canada and 4.3% in the United States undergoing appendectomy are subsequently found to have a normal appendix.[66] Consequently, this could be considered an unnecessary operation.

The interest in nonoperative management of appendicitis has largely been revived by the research and management of several intra-abdominal infectious processes, including diverticulitis, abscess resulting from Crohn disease, and tubo-ovarian abscess, that are all now treated with antibiotics alone with surgery reserved for failures of medical management.[67,68] Nonoperative management of uncomplicated appendicitis has been studied in several international adult trials (**Table 3**).[69–75] Overall, these trials demonstrated successful nonoperative management of acute appendicitis in 70% to 85% of cases at the 1-year follow-up. A 2012 meta-analysis concluded that, although there were benefits to nonoperative treatment, including fewer complications, better pain control, and shorter sick leave, the combined failure and recurrence rates in nonoperative patients made this approach less effective overall.[76] Predictors of failure of nonoperative management in the literature were abdominal pain greater than 48 hours; presence of an appendicolith, phlegmon, or abscess on imaging; and elevated laboratory measures, specifically WBC greater than 18,000 and CRP greater than 4 mg/dL.[69–75]

There is a moderate amount of existing literature on the nonoperative management of pediatric appendicitis. This literature consists of a mix of retrospective and prospective cohort studies[77–85] and one pilot randomized controlled trial.[84] Previous studies in children revealed a success rate ranging from 75% to 80% with no increased rates of perforated appendicitis in patients initially managed nonoperatively. In a patient choice study from 2007 to 2013 with an average 4.3-year follow-up, 78 chose nonoperative management with a 99% success rate initially but a 29% recurrence at 1 year.[85] In a feasibility study, 24 patients aged 5 to 18 years with less than 48 hours of symptoms of acute appendicitis were compared with 50 controls.[80] At a mean follow-up of 14 months, 3 of the 24 failed on therapy and 2 of those 21 returned with recurrent appendicitis. Two patients elected to undergo an interval appendectomy despite absence of symptoms. The appendectomy-free rate at 1 year was, therefore, 71% with no patient developing perforation or other complications and having an overall cost savings of $1359 (from $4130 to $2771 per nonoperatively treated patient).[80] Minneci and colleagues[83] performed a prospective single-institution patient choice trial in which a total of 102 patients were enrolled (65 chose appendectomy, 37 families chose nonoperative management). The inclusion criteria were 7 to 18 years of age, less than 48 hours of abdominal pain, WBC less than 18,000 cells per microliter, and US or CT demonstrating an appendix less than 1.2 cm in diameter without appendicolith, abscess, or phlegmon. Patients in the operative arm received urgent laparoscopic appendectomy. Those patients in the nonoperative arm received a diet after 12 hours; if at 24 hours they had no clinical improvement, they underwent laparoscopic appendectomy. The success rate of nonoperative management was 89.2% with an incidence of complicated appendicitis of 2.7% in the nonoperative group and 12.3% in the surgery group (8 of 65 children). These investigators demonstrated that nonoperative patients reported higher quality-of-life scores at 30 days and fewer days off and overall lower costs associated with the hospitalization.[83]

The only randomized controlled trial performed to date was a recently performed pilot study in Sweden evaluating 24 nonoperative and 26 operative pediatric patients with a follow-up to 1 year. The investigators reported a 92% (24 of 26 patients) successful treatment with antibiotics.[84] Based off the results of a pilot randomized controlled trial,[84] there is currently an international, multicenter, randomized trial to

Table 3
Existing literature relating to nonoperative treatment of acute uncomplicated appendicitis in children

Study	Country of Origin	Study Design	No. of Children Receiving NOM	Comparative Study[a]	Criteria	No. Days IV Antibiotics in NOM	No. Days Hospital Stay	No. Children Requiring Appendectomy in NOM	Follow-up Interval (mo)
Kaneko et al,[81] 2004	Japan	Prospective cohort	22	No	3–15 y US classification	4.2	NR	6 (27.3%)	13
Abes et al,[77] 2007	Turkey	Retrospective cohort	16	No	5–13 y US	5.0	5.0	2 (13.3%)	12
Armstrong et al,[78] 2014	Canada	Nonrandomized retrospective cohort	12	Yes	<18 y US	1.5	1.5	3 (25%)	12
Koike et al,[82] 2014	Japan	Retrospective cohort	130	No	1–15 y Clinical diagnosis	6.7	6.7	24 (19.2%)	2–36
Gorter et al,[79] 2015	Holland	Nonrandomized prospective cohort	25	Yes	7–17 y Imaging	2–4	4.0	2 (8%)	1.5

(continued on next page)

Table 3
(continued)

Study	Country of Origin	Study Design	No. of Children Receiving NOM	Comparative Study[a]	Criteria	No. Days IV Antibiotics in NOM	No. Days Hospital Stay	No. Children Requiring Appendectomy in NOM	Follow-up Interval (mo)
Hartwich et al,[80] 2016	United States	Prospective parent preference-based feasibility trial	24	Yes	5–18 y Clinical diagnosis	1.0	2.0	7 (29%)	14
Minneci et al,[83] 2016	United States	Prospective parent preference-based trial	30	Yes	7–17 y US/CT	1.0	2.0	3 (10%)	1
Svensson et al,[136] 2015	Sweden	Pilot RCT	24	Yes	5–15 y Clinical diagnosis	2.0	2.0	9 (37%)	12
Steiner et al,[137] 2015	Israel	Nonrandomized prospective cohort	45	No	4–15 y US	3.3	3.8	7 (16.6%)	6–14
Tanaka et al,[85] 2015	Japan	Nonrandomized retrospective cohort	78	Yes	5–15 y US	6.0	6.6	22 (28.6%)	12

Abbreviations: NOM, nonoperative management; NR, not recorded; RCT, randomized controlled trial.
[a] Included a comparison group who underwent appendectomy.

evaluate the nonoperative management of acute pediatric appendicitis. Inclusion criteria are children aged 5 to 16 years, clinical and/or radiological diagnosis (US and/or CT scan) of acute nonperforated appendicitis, and written informed parental consent. Exclusion criteria include suspicion of perforated appendicitis, presentation with an appendix mass or phlegmon (on physical examination and/or imaging), nonoperative management (2 or more doses of IV antibiotic) initiated at an outside institution, previous episode of appendicitis or appendix mass/phlegmon treated nonoperatively, and current treatment of malignancy.

One of the greatest predictors of failure of nonoperative management seems to be the presence of an appendicolith on imaging studies.[84,85] A prospective nonrandomized trial comparing the nonoperative management of uncomplicated acute appendicitis with an appendicolith performed in children aged 7 to 17 years was halted early because the failure of nonoperative management was 60% (3 of 5 patients) at a median follow-up of 5 months.[86] Another interesting point in many of the patient/family choice–based nonoperative trials is that despite patient characteristics being similar up until treatment selection, parents may ultimately be able to recognize if their child would be successful at nonoperative management.

One of the more complex aspects of understanding this pediatric appendicitis is changing the previous misconceptions and perceptions of the diagnosis of appendicitis. A feasibility study performed highlighted the striking knowledge gap in the participant perception of appendicitis. One hundred subjects (caregivers and patients ≥15 years of age) were questioned before and after an education session about their understanding of appendicitis. Eighty-two percent of respondents thought it was *likely* or *very likely* that the appendix would rupture if the operation was at all delayed and that rupture of the appendix would rapidly lead to severe complications and death. These feelings increased when subjects knew at least one friend or relative who had a negative experience with appendicitis. The investigators concluded that appropriate education can correct anecdotally supported misconceptions. Adequate education may empower patients to make better-informed decisions about their medical care and may be important for future studies in alternative treatments for appendicitis in children.[87]

Surgical Options for Appendicitis

Appendicitis presents in a spectrum from acute to perforated with and without organized abscess. The goals of surgical care for appendicitis are to minimize complications and cost, alleviate patient anxiety, and improve quality of life.

Acute appendicitis

Traditional thinking was that emergent appendectomy should be performed at the time of diagnosis. When comparing emergent appendectomy (within 5 hours of admission) with urgent appendectomy (within 17 hours), no difference in gangrenous/perforated appendixes, operative length, readmission, postoperative complications, hospital stay, or charges have been noted.[88] Many centers now perform appendectomies in the morning for patients presenting at night, although it is recommended that patients begin antibiotics at the time of diagnosis.[31] A recent multicenter study including 1300 patients demonstrated that delay in appendectomy did not impact the incidence of surgical site infections.[89] A recent study in 230 children with appendicitis presenting with greater than 48 hours of symptoms had 4.9 times increased odds of perforation and 56% greater hospital LOS than those presenting within 0 to 23 hours. From diagnosis to appendectomy, those taken at 0 to 3 hours, 4 to 6 hours, or longer than 6 hours after diagnosis to the operating room (OR) had no statistically significant difference in hospital LOS or perforation rates and no clinically significant difference in OR times. The investigators were unable to demonstrate a difference in perforation rates based on emergency department LOS before surgery.[90] Thus, putting together the data that exist suggesting overnight appendectomies place stress on the family, surgeon, and hospital, midnight appendectomies are no longer justified.[91–93]

Perforated appendicitis

Perforation is defined as a hole in the appendix or a fecalith in the abdomen.[1] Approximately 30% of children with appendicitis present with perforated appendicitis.[94] The postoperative risk of an intra-abdominal abscess is approximately 20% for children with perforated appendicitis, and the risk for children with nonperforated appendicitis to develop an abscess is less than 0.8%.[1] There are still several controversies that exist in the management of children who present with perforated appendicitis. Three options exist: antibiotics only, antibiotics followed by an interval appendectomy, and an appendectomy at the time of presentation.

Children treated with antibiotics initially avoid a difficult operation while the peritonitis resolves. A wide range of recurrent appendicitis has been demonstrated in prospective studies, between 8% and 15%, with an unknown lifetime risk. It is estimated that the risk of appendicitis is 1% to 3% per year, which if true would argue for an appendectomy in children. Although infrequent, a small rate of pathologic findings in interval appendectomy specimens, including appendiceal neoplasms, has not resulted in a clear answer regarding the management of children with a history of perforated appendicitis and an appendicular mass.[95,96] Additionally, the lumen in most appendix specimens from interval appendectomy are found to be patent, with less than 16% being completely obliterated.[97,98]

Currently most surgeons surveyed would perform an interval appendectomy in a patient with previously perforated appendicitis.[99] The risk in the interval between treatment and presentation for elective operation is recurrent appendicitis, with an increased rate of recurrence among patients with appendicoliths or contamination beyond the right lower quadrant on imaging.[96,100–102] Additional problems with this management pathway are the difficulty in being able to predict perforation on a CT scan accurately (<80% accuracy to predict perforation by CT scan).[51] Treating a child with nonperforated appendicitis with a protracted course of antibiotics and interval appendectomy results in complications from antibiotic overuse and overtreatment.

Another point of controversy is when to perform interval appendectomy in a child with perforated appendicitis. Many studies have been performed; a meta-analysis evaluating early versus delayed appendectomy for perforated appendicitis concluded that patients who underwent a delayed operation were associated with significantly less overall complications, wound infections, intra-abdominal abscesses, bowel obstructions, and reoperations. No differences were found in the duration of first hospitalization, the overall duration of hospital stay, and the duration of IV antibiotics.[103] A randomized controlled trial compared appendectomy on presentation with initial antibiotic therapy and appendectomy 6 to 8 weeks later for children with presumptive perforated appendicitis with and without abscess. Early appendectomy, compared with interval appendectomy, significantly reduced the time away from normal activities (mean, 13.8 vs 19.4 days; $P<.001$). The overall adverse event rate was 30% for early appendectomy versus 55% for interval appendectomy (relative risk with interval appendectomy, 1.86; 95% confidence interval, 1.21–2.87; $P = .003$). Of the patients randomized to interval appendectomy, 23 (34%) had an appendectomy earlier than planned owing to failure to improve (n = 17), recurrent appendicitis (n = 5), or other reasons (n = 1). Importantly, children who had delayed appendectomy had higher costs and were more likely to receive a central line.[104] Children with a preoperative diagnosis of perforated appendicitis, thus, benefit from early laparoscopic appendectomy.

Patients who present with a well-defined abscess on imaging studies present another controversial group. Given the perceived technical demands of laparoscopic appendectomy and the expected postoperative morbidity in patients with a well-defined abscess, initial percutaneous drainage has become an attractive option.[105–108] Fifty-two patients with well-formed abscesses following perforated appendicitis were studied to evaluate outcomes following drainage of the abscess or drain placement. During the interval between initial presentation and interval appendectomy, 9 recurrent abscesses developed (17.3%) and 6 patients (11.5%) required another drainage procedure. The mean total charge to the patients was $40,414.02. There were 4 significant drain complications (ileal perforation, colon perforation, bladder perforation, and buttock/thigh necrotizing abscess).[105] A randomized trial comparing 40 patients with well-formed abscess to drainage with interval appendectomy versus early laparoscopic appendectomy at presentation demonstrated that, although operative time was slightly longer in those patients receiving initial appendectomy, overall quality-of-life assessments were improved.[105,109] Although the rare child may be doing clinically well at presentation, the authors recommend most children with abscesses receive early primary laparoscopic appendectomy.

OPERATIVE APPROACHES

In 1894, McBurney[110] first described the traditional appendectomy through a muscle-splitting incision in the right lower quadrant, 4 years before he wrote his article regarding the utility of rubber gloves in surgery.[110,111] Today, laparoscopic appendectomies have largely replaced the open approach, as greater than 91% of appendectomies are performed laparoscopically versus 22% in the late 1990s.[112] Several different operative approaches using various minimally invasive techniques have been described and summarized,[31] including a traditional 3-port appendectomy, transumbilical laparoscopic appendectomy (2 ports) whereby the appendix is ultimately delivered through the umbilicus, and single-incision laparoscopic appendectomy whereby instruments are placed through the same incision used for the camera port with an intracorporeal or extracorporeal appendix. Many trials have evaluated single-incision versus traditional 3-port appendectomy, and no differences have been found between the groups regarding outcomes.[113,114] Cosmetically, the initial excitement of a single incision fades at a longer interval follow-up between the two patient groups.[115]

Higher postoperative abscess rates were initially described following laparoscopic appendectomy compared with traditional open appendectomy.[116,117] Meta-analysis and multi-institutional reviews have found no differences in intra-abdominal abscess rates and continued low rates of wound infections at the port sites as well as less adhesive small bowel obstruction.[118–126]

IRRIGATION

Following operative intervention, the question of abdominal irrigation has been studied. No clear data existed from previous studies on the role of irrigation for peritoneal contamination in perforated appendicitis.[127] As late as 2004, more than 93% of North American surgeons reported using irrigation.[128] Two retrospective studies comparing laparoscopic irrigation with no irrigation during appendectomy demonstrated an increase in abscesses resulting from the use of irrigation.[129,130] A randomized trial of 220 patients comparing normal saline irrigation of greater than 500 mL to suction alone during laparoscopic appendectomy for perforated appendicitis in children demonstrated no differences in abscess rates or other clinical measures or hospital costs.[127]

INCIDENTAL APPENDECTOMIES

Incidental appendectomies (IAs), defined as the removal of the appendix accompanying another operation without evidence of acute appendicitis, are not routinely advocated except in specific situations, including any surgery that has a right lower quadrant incision, such as a Meckel diverticulectomy or intussusception reduction. A patient with an appendicolith evaluated for other issues is not an indication for appendectomy, as the risk of appendicitis is less than 5.8%.[131] Performing an appendectomy converts a procedure from clean to clean-contaminated. Most importantly, in a comprehensive review on IAs, the investigators concluded that the decision to perform a pediatric IA relies on informed consideration of the individual patient's comorbid conditions, the indications for the initial operation, the future utility of the appendix, and the risk of future appendiceal pathology.[132]

POSTOPERATIVE CARE

Postoperative care is best protocolized.[133] Children with acute appendicitis can be discharged a few hours following operative intervention.[134] Nonoperative management has yet to determine the optimal duration of admission, but 12 to 24 hours' duration seems to be sufficient. For children with perforated appendicitis, antibiotics are continued until fevers are no longer present and patients are tolerating a diet. Normalization of WBC is not required, and before discharge patients get a WBC and are sent home on additional oral antibiotics if the WBC count is elevated. If prolonged ileus and failure to progress results in a stay greater than 6 days, a CT scan is obtained to evaluate for intra-abdominal abscesses, which are then drained. Nasogastric tubes, abdominal drains, central lines, total parenteral nutrition, prolonged use of Foley catheters, and complex wound packing schema have been largely abandoned.[135]

SUMMARY

1. Appendicitis occurs most frequently between 10 and 11 years of age.
2. Classic symptoms include migrating pain to the right lower quadrant and fevers but are present in less than half of the children presenting with appendicitis.
3. Clinical judgment and judicious studies are the best methods when assessing for appendicitis. Scoring systems have been shown to be useful with the addition of selective imaging and laboratory tests.
4. US imaging continues to be the study of choice as CT increases radiation exposure.
5. Laparoscopic approaches now make up more than 90% of the operative approaches for appendicitis.
6. Nonoperative management for carefully selected children with acute appendicitis is possible.
7. Complex appendicitis with perforation is best managed with a minimally invasive operative technique in children without a well-defined abscess.

REFERENCES

1. St Peter SD, Sharp SW, Holcomb GW III, et al. An evidence-based definition for perforated appendicitis derived from a prospective randomized trial. J Pediatr Surg 2008;43(12):2242–5.

2. Addiss DG, Shaffer N, Fowler BS, et al. The epidemiology of appendicitis and appendectomy in the United States. Am J Epidemiol 1990;132(5):910–25.
3. Healthcare Cost and Utilization Project (HCUP). The SAGE encyclopedia of pharmacology and society. SAGE Publications. Available at: www. hcup.ahrq.gov. Accessed November 12, 2015.
4. Brennan GD. Pediatric appendicitis: pathophysiology and appropriate use of diagnostic imaging. CJEM 2006;8(6):425–32.
5. Deng Y, Chang DC, Zhang Y, et al. Seasonal and day of the week variations of perforated appendicitis in US children. Pediatr Surg Int 2010;26(7):691–6.
6. Pearl RH, Hale DA, Molloy M, et al. Pediatric appendectomy. J Pediatr Surg 1995;30(2):173–81.
7. Becker T, Kharbanda A, Bachur R. Atypical clinical features of pediatric appendicitis. Acad Emerg Med 2007;14(2):124–9.
8. Paulson EK, Kalady MF, Pappas TN. Suspected appendicitis. N Engl J Med 2003;348(3):236–42.
9. Wang LT, Prentiss KA, Simon JZ, et al. The use of white blood cell count and left shift in the diagnosis of appendicitis in children. Pediatr Emerg Care 2007;23(2): 69–76.
10. Beltrán MA, Almonacid J, Vicencio A, et al. Predictive value of white blood cell count and C-reactive protein in children with appendicitis. J Pediatr Surg 2007; 42(7):1208–14.
11. Benito J, Acedo Y, Medrano L, et al. Usefulness of new and traditional serum biomarkers in children with suspected appendicitis. Am J Emerg Med 2016; 34(5):871–6.
12. Grönroos P, Huhtinen H, Grönroos JM. Normal leukocyte count value do not effectively exclude acute appendicitis in children. Dis Colon Rectum 2009; 52(5):1028–9.
13. Mekhail P, Yanni F, Naguib N, et al. Appendicitis in paediatric age group: correlation between preoperative inflammatory markers and postoperative histological diagnosis. Afr J Paediatr Surg 2011;8(3):309.
14. Siddique K, Baruah P, Bhandari S, et al. Diagnostic accuracy of white cell count and C-reactive protein for assessing the severity of paediatric appendicitis. JRSM Short Rep 2011;2(7):59.
15. Chung J-L, Kong M-S, Lin S-L, et al. Diagnostic value of C-reactive protein in children with perforated appendicitis. Eur J Pediatr 1996;155(7):529–31.
16. Rodríguez-Sanjuán JC, Martín-Parra JI, Seco I, et al. C-reactive protein and leukocyte count in the diagnosis of acute appendicitis in children. Dis Colon Rectum 1999;42(10):1325–9.
17. Alvarado A. A practical score for the early diagnosis of acute appendicitis. Ann Emerg Med 1986;15(5):557–64.
18. Samuel M. Pediatric appendicitis score. J Pediatr Surg 2002;37(6):877–81.
19. Bhatt M, Joseph L, Ducharme FM, et al. Prospective validation of the pediatric appendicitis score in a Canadian pediatric emergency department. Acad Emerg Med 2009;16(7):591–6.
20. Goldman RD, Carter S, Stephens D, et al. Prospective validation of the pediatric appendicitis score. J Pediatr 2008;153(2):278–82.
21. Mandeville K, Pottker T, Bulloch B, et al. Using appendicitis scores in the pediatric ED. Am J Emerg Med 2011;29(9):972–7.
22. Pogorelić Z, Rak S, Mrklić I, et al. Prospective validation of Alvarado score and pediatric appendicitis score for the diagnosis of acute appendicitis in children. Pediatr Emerg Care 2015;31(3):164–8.

23. Schneider C, Kharbanda A, Bachur R. Evaluating appendicitis scoring systems using a prospective pediatric cohort. Ann Emerg Med 2007;49(6):778–84, 784.e1.

24. Scheller RL, Depinet HE, Ho ML, et al. Utility of pediatric appendicitis score in female adolescent patients. Acad Emerg Med 2016;23(5):610–5.

25. Panella M, Marchisio S, Di Stanislao F. Reducing clinical variations with clinical pathways: do pathways work? Int J Qual Health Care 2003;15(6):509–21.

26. Warner BW, Kulick RM, Stoops MM, et al. An evidenced-based clinical pathway for acute appendicitis decreases hospital duration and cost. J Pediatr Surg 1998;33(9):1371–5.

27. Anandalwar SP, Callahan MJ, Bachur RG, et al. Use of white blood cell count and polymorphonuclear leukocyte differential to improve the predictive value of ultrasound for suspected appendicitis in children. J Am Coll Surg 2015; 220(6):1010–7.

28. Fleischman RJ, Devine MK, Yagapen MA, et al. Evaluation of a novel pediatric appendicitis pathway using high- and low-risk scoring systems. Pediatr Emerg Care 2013;29(10):1060–5.

29. Garcia Pena BM, Taylor GA, Fishman SJ, et al. Costs and effectiveness of ultrasonography and limited computed tomography for diagnosing appendicitis in children. Pediatrics 2000;106(4):672–6.

30. Saucier A, Huang EY, Emeremni CA, et al. Prospective evaluation of a clinical pathway for suspected appendicitis. Pediatrics 2014;133(1):e88–95.

31. Pepper VK, Stanfill AB, Pearl RH. Diagnosis and management of pediatric appendicitis, intussusception, and Meckel diverticulum. Surg Clin North Am 2012;92(3):505–26, vii.

32. Klein MD. Referral to pediatric surgical specialists. Pediatrics 2014;133(2): 350–6.

33. Williams RF, Blakely ML, Fischer PE, et al. Diagnosing ruptured appendicitis preoperatively in pediatric patients. J Am Coll Surg 2009;208(5):819–25.

34. Binkovitz LA, Unsdorfer KML, Thapa P, et al. Pediatric appendiceal ultrasound: accuracy, determinacy and clinical outcomes. Pediatr Radiol 2015;45(13): 1934–44.

35. Peña BMG. Ultrasonography and limited computed tomography in the diagnosis and management of appendicitis in children. JAMA 1999;282(11):1041.

36. Rosen MP, Ding A, Blake MA, et al. ACR Appropriateness Criteria® right lower quadrant pain—suspected appendicitis. J Am Coll Radiol 2011;8(11):749–55.

37. Doria AS, Moineddin R, Kellenberger CJ, et al. US or CT for diagnosis of appendicitis in children and adults? A meta-analysis. Radiology 2006;241(1):83–94.

38. Burr A, Renaud EJ, Manno M, et al. Glowing in the dark: time of day as a determinant of radiographic imaging in the evaluation of abdominal pain in children. J Pediatr Surg 2011;46(1):188–91.

39. Butler M, Servaes S, Srinivasan A, et al. US depiction of the appendix: role of abdominal wall thickness and appendiceal location. Emerg Radiol 2011;18(6): 525–31.

40. Schuh S, Man C, Cheng A, et al. Predictors of non-diagnostic ultrasound scanning in children with suspected appendicitis. J Pediatr 2011;158(1):112–8.

41. Yiğiter M, Kantarcı M, Yalçin O, et al. Does obesity limit the sonographic diagnosis of appendicitis in children? J Clin Ultrasound 2010;39(4):187–90.

42. Bachur RG, Dayan PS, Bajaj L, et al. The effect of abdominal pain duration on the accuracy of diagnostic imaging for pediatric appendicitis. Ann Emerg Med 2012;60(5):582–90.e3.

43. Goldin AB, Khanna P, Thapa M, et al. Revised ultrasound criteria for appendicitis in children improve diagnostic accuracy. Pediatr Radiol 2011;41(8):993–9.
44. Mittal MK, Dayan PS, Macias CG, et al. Performance of ultrasound in the diagnosis of appendicitis in children in a multicenter cohort. Acad Emerg Med 2013; 20(7):697–702.
45. Trout AT, Sanchez R, Ladino-Torres MF, et al. A critical evaluation of US for the diagnosis of pediatric acute appendicitis in a real-life setting: how can we improve the diagnostic value of sonography? Pediatr Radiol 2012;42(7):813–23.
46. Burford JM, Dassinger MS, Smith SD. Surgeon-performed ultrasound as a diagnostic tool in appendicitis. J Pediatr Surg 2011;46(6):1115–20.
47. Callahan MJ, Kleinman PL, Strauss KJ, et al. Pediatric CT dose reduction for suspected appendicitis: a practice quality improvement project using artificial gaussian noise—part 1, computer simulations. Am J Roentgenol 2015;204(1): W86–94.
48. Sivit CJ, Applegate KE, Stallion A, et al. Imaging evaluation of suspected appendicitis in a pediatric population. Am J Roentgenol 2000;175(4):977–80.
49. Laituri CA, Fraser JD, Aguayo P, et al. The lack of efficacy for oral contrast in the diagnosis of appendicitis by computed tomography. J Surg Res 2011;170(1): 100–3.
50. Servaes S, Srinivasan A, Pena A, et al. CT diagnosis of appendicitis in children: comparison of orthogonal planes and assessment of contrast opacification of the appendix. Pediatr Emerg Care 2015;31(3):161–3.
51. Fraser JD, Aguayo P, Sharp SW, et al. Accuracy of computed tomography in predicting appendiceal perforation. J Pediatr Surg 2010;45(1):231–4 [discussion: 234].
52. Garcia K, Hernanz-Schulman M, Bennett DL, et al. Suspected appendicitis in children: diagnostic importance of normal abdominopelvic CT findings with non-visualized appendix 1. Radiology 2009;250(2):531–7.
53. Hall EJ. Lessons we have learned from our children: cancer risks from diagnostic radiology. Pediatr Radiol 2002;32(10):700–6.
54. Fefferman NR, Roche KJ, Pinkney LP, et al. Suspected appendicitis in children: focused CT technique for evaluation. Radiology 2001;220(3):691–5.
55. Sharp NE, Raghavan MU, Svetanoff WJ, et al. Radiation exposure - how do CT scans for appendicitis compare between a free standing children's hospital and non-dedicated pediatric facilities? J Pediatr Surg 2014;49(6):1016–9 [discussion: 1019].
56. Johnson AK, Filippi CG, Andrews T, et al. Ultrafast 3-T MRI in the evaluation of children with acute lower abdominal pain for the detection of appendicitis. Am J Roentgenol 2012;198(6):1424–30.
57. Koning JL, Naheedy JH, Kruk PG. Diagnostic performance of contrast-enhanced MR for acute appendicitis and alternative causes of abdominal pain in children. Pediatr Radiol 2014;44(8):948–55.
58. Kulaylat AN, Moore MM, Engbrecht BW, et al. An implemented MRI program to eliminate radiation from the evaluation of pediatric appendicitis. J Pediatr Surg 2015;50(8):1359–63.
59. Orth RC, Guillerman RP, Zhang W, et al. Prospective comparison of MR imaging and US for the diagnosis of pediatric appendicitis. Radiology 2014;272(1): 233–40.
60. Goldin AB, Sawin RS, Garrison MM, et al. Aminoglycoside-based triple-antibiotic therapy versus monotherapy for children with ruptured appendicitis. Pediatrics 2007;119(5):905–11.

61. Guillet-Caruba C, Cheikhelard A, Guillet M, et al. Bacteriologic epidemiology and empirical treatment of pediatric complicated appendicitis. Diagn Microbiol Infect Dis 2011;69(4):376–81.
62. St. Peter SD, Little DC, Calkins CM, et al. A simple and more cost-effective antibiotic regimen for perforated appendicitis. J Pediatr Surg 2006;41(5):1020–4.
63. Desai AA, Alemayehu H, Holcomb GW 3rd, et al. Safety of a new protocol decreasing antibiotic utilization after laparoscopic appendectomy for perforated appendicitis in children: a prospective observational study. J Pediatr Surg 2015; 50(6):912–4.
64. van Rossem CC, Schreinemacher MH, van Geloven AA, et al. Antibiotic duration after laparoscopic appendectomy for acute complicated appendicitis. JAMA Surg 2016;151(4):323–9.
65. Tiboni S, Bhangu A, Hall NJ. Outcome of appendicectomy in children performed in paediatric surgery units compared with general surgery units. Br J Surg 2014; 101(6):707–14.
66. Cheong LH, Emil S. Outcomes of pediatric appendicitis: an international comparison of the United States and Canada. JAMA Surg 2014;149(1):50–5.
67. Broderick-Villa G. Hospitalization for acute diverticulitis does not mandate routine elective colectomy. Arch Surg 2005;140(6):576.
68. Ricciardi R, Baxter NN, Read TE, et al. Is the decline in the surgical treatment for diverticulitis associated with an increase in complicated diverticulitis? Dis Colon Rectum 2009;52(9):1558–63.
69. Di SS, Sibilio A, Giorgini E, et al. The NOTA Study (Non Operative Treatment for Acute Appendicitis): prospective study on the efficacy and safety of antibiotics (amoxicillin and clavulanic acid) for treating patients with right lower quadrant abdominal pain and long-term follow-up of conservatively treated suspected appendicitis. Ann Surg 2014;260(1):109–17.
70. Hansson J, Körner U, Khorram-Manesh A, et al. Randomized clinical trial of antibiotic therapy versus appendicectomy as primary treatment of acute appendicitis in unselected patients. Br J Surg 2009;96(5):473–81.
71. Hansson J, Körner U, Ludwigs K, et al. Antibiotics as first-line therapy for acute appendicitis: evidence for a change in clinical practice. World J Surg 2012; 36(9):2028–36.
72. Salminen P, Paajanen H, Rautio T, et al. Antibiotic therapy vs appendectomy for treatment of uncomplicated acute appendicitis: the APPAC randomized clinical trial. JAMA 2015;313(23):2340–8.
73. Shindoh J, Niwa H, Kawai K, et al. Predictive factors for negative outcomes in initial non-operative management of suspected appendicitis. J Gastrointest Surg 2009;14(2):309–14.
74. Styrud J, Eriksson S, Nilsson I, et al. Appendectomy versus antibiotic treatment in acute appendicitis. A prospective multicenter randomized controlled trial. World J Surg 2006;30(6):1033–7.
75. Vons C, Barry C, Maitre S, et al. Amoxicillin plus clavulanic acid versus appendicectomy for treatment of acute uncomplicated appendicitis: an open-label, non-inferiority, randomised controlled trial. Lancet 2011;377(9777):1573–9.
76. Mason RJ, Moazzez A, Sohn H, et al. Meta-analysis of randomized trials comparing antibiotic therapy with appendectomy for acute uncomplicated (no abscess or phlegmon) appendicitis. Surg Infect (Larchmt) 2012;13(2):74–84.
77. Abeş M, Petik B, Kazıl S. Nonoperative treatment of acute appendicitis in children. J Pediatr Surg 2007;42(8):1439–42.

78. Armstrong J, Merritt N, Jones S, et al. Non-operative management of early, acute appendicitis in children: is it safe and effective? J Pediatr Surg 2014; 49(5):782–5.
79. Gorter RR, van der Lee JH, Cense HA, et al. Initial antibiotic treatment for acute simple appendicitis in children is safe: short-term results from a multicenter, prospective cohort study. Surgery 2015;157(5):916–23.
80. Hartwich J, Luks FI, Watson-Smith D, et al. Nonoperative treatment of acute appendicitis in children: a feasibility study. J Pediatr Surg 2016;51(1):111–6.
81. Kaneko K, Tsuda M. Ultrasound-based decision making in the treatment of acute appendicitis in children. J Pediatr Surg 2004;39(9):1316–20.
82. Koike Y, Uchida K, Matsushita K, et al. Intraluminal appendiceal fluid is a predictive factor for recurrent appendicitis after initial successful non-operative management of uncomplicated appendicitis in pediatric patients. J Pediatr Surg 2014;49(7):1116–21.
83. Minneci PC, Mahida JB, Lodwick DL, et al. Effectiveness of patient choice in nonoperative vs surgical management of pediatric uncomplicated acute appendicitis. JAMA Surg 2016;151(5):408–15.
84. Svensson JF, Patkova B, Almström M, et al. Nonoperative treatment with antibiotics versus surgery for acute nonperforated appendicitis in children. Ann Surg 2015;261(1):67–71.
85. Tanaka Y, Uchida H, Kawashima H, et al. Long-term outcomes of operative versus nonoperative treatment for uncomplicated appendicitis. J Pediatr Surg 2015;50(11):1893–7.
86. Mahida JB, Lodwick DL, Nacion KM, et al. High failure rate of nonoperative management of acute appendicitis with an appendicolith in children. J Pediatr Surg 2016;51(6):908–11.
87. Chau DB, Ciullo SS, Watson-Smith D, et al. Patient-centered outcomes research in appendicitis in children: bridging the knowledge gap. J Pediatr Surg 2016; 51(1):117–21.
88. Taylor M, Emil S, Nguyen N, et al. Emergent vs urgent appendectomy in children: a study of outcomes. J Pediatr Surg 2005;40(12):1912–5.
89. Boomer LA, Cooper JN, Anandalwar S, et al. Delaying appendectomy does not lead to higher rates of surgical site infections. Ann Surg 2016;264(1):164–8.
90. Mandeville K, Monuteaux M, Pottker T, et al. Effects of timing to diagnosis and appendectomy in pediatric appendicitis. Pediatr Emerg Care 2015;31(11): 753–8.
91. Stahlfeld K, Hower J, Homitsky S, et al. Is acute appendicitis a surgical emergency? Am Surg 2007;73(6):626–9 [discussion: 629–30].
92. Surana R, Quinn F, Puri P. Is it necessary to perform appendicectomy in the middle of the night in children? BMJ 1993;306(6886):1168.
93. Yardeni D, Hirschl RB, Drongowski RA, et al. Delayed versus immediate surgery in acute appendicitis: do we need to operate during the night? J Pediatr Surg 2004;39(3):464–9.
94. Barrett ML, Hines AL, Andrews RM. Trends in rates of perforated appendix, 2001-2010: statistical brief #159. Healthcare Cost and Utilization Project (HCUP) statistical briefs. Rockville (MD): Agency for Health Care Policy and Research (US); 2006.
95. Gahukamble DB, Gahukamble LD. Surgical and pathological basis for interval appendicectomy after resolution of appendicular mass in children. J Pediatr Surg 2000;35(3):424–7.

96. Puapong D, Lee SL, Haigh PI, et al. Routine interval appendectomy in children is not indicated. J Pediatr Surg 2007;42(9):1500–3.

97. Knott EM, Iqbal CW, Mortellaro VE, et al. Outcomes for interval appendectomy after non-operative management of perforated appendicitis: what are the operative risks and luminal patency rates? J Surg Res 2012;172(2):189.

98. Mazziotti MV, Marley EF, Winthrop AL, et al. Histopathologic analysis of interval appendectomy specimens: support for the role of interval appendectomy. J Pediatr Surg 1997;32(6):806–9.

99. Chen C, Botelho C, Cooper A, et al. Current practice patterns in the treatment of perforated appendicitis in children. J Am Coll Surg 2003;196(2):212–21.

100. Aprahamian CJ, Barnhart DC, Bledsoe SE, et al. Failure in the nonoperative management of pediatric ruptured appendicitis: predictors and consequences. J Pediatr Surg 2007;42(6):934–8.

101. Ein SH, Langer JC, Daneman A. Nonoperative management of pediatric ruptured appendix with inflammatory mass or abscess: presence of an appendicolith predicts recurrent appendicitis. J Pediatr Surg 2005;40(10):1612–5.

102. Levin T, Whyte C, Borzykowski R, et al. Nonoperative management of perforated appendicitis in children: can CT predict outcome? Pediatr Radiol 2006;37(3):251–5.

103. Simillis C, Symeonides P, Shorthouse AJ, et al. A meta-analysis comparing conservative treatment versus acute appendectomy for complicated appendicitis (abscess or phlegmon). Surgery 2010;147(6):818–29.

104. Blakely ML. Early vs interval appendectomy for children with perforated appendicitis. Arch Surg 2011;146(6):660.

105. Keckler SJ, Tsao K, Sharp SW, et al. Resource utilization and outcomes from percutaneous drainage and interval appendectomy for perforated appendicitis with abscess. J Pediatr Surg 2008;43(6):977–80.

106. Janik JS, Ein SH, Shandling B, et al. Nonsurgical management of appendiceal mass in late presenting children. J Pediatr Surg 1980;15(4):574–6.

107. Morrow SE, Newman KD. Current management of appendicitis. Semin Pediatr Surg 2007;16(1):34–40.

108. Owen A, Moore O, Marven S, et al. Interval laparoscopic appendectomy in children. J Laparoendosc Adv Surg Tech 2006;16(3):308–11.

109. St. Peter SD, Aguayo P, Fraser JD, et al. Initial laparoscopic appendectomy versus initial nonoperative management and interval appendectomy for perforated appendicitis with abscess: a prospective, randomized trial. J Pediatr Surg 2010;45(1):236–40.

110. McBurney C IV. The incision made in the abdominal wall in cases of appendicitis, with a description of a new method of operating. Ann Surg 1894;20(1):38–43.

111. McBurney C IV. The use of rubber gloves in operative surgery. Ann Surg 1898;28(1):108–19.

112. Jen HC, Shew SB. Laparoscopic versus open appendectomy in children: outcomes comparison based on a statewide analysis. J Surg Res 2010;161(1):13–7.

113. St. Peter SD, Adibe OO, Juang D, et al. Single incision versus standard 3-port laparoscopic appendectomy. Ann Surg 2011;254(4):586–90.

114. Zhang Z, Wang Y, Liu R, et al. Systematic review and meta-analysis of single-incision versus conventional laparoscopic appendectomy in children. J Pediatr Surg 2015;50(9):1600–9.

115. Gasior AC, Knott EM, Holcomb GW 3rd, et al. Patient and parental scar assessment after single incision versus standard 3-port laparoscopic appendectomy: long-term follow-up from a prospective randomized trial. J Pediatr Surg 2014; 49(1):120–2 [discussion: 122].
116. Gasior AC, St. Peter SD, Knott EM, et al. National trends in approach and outcomes with appendicitis in children. J Pediatr Surg 2012;47(12):2264–7.
117. Lintula H, Kokki H, Vanamo K, et al. Laparoscopy in children with complicated appendicitis. J Pediatr Surg 2002;37(9):1317–20.
118. Aziz O, Athanasiou T, Tekkis PP, et al. Laparoscopic versus open appendectomy in children. Ann Surg 2006;243(1):17–27.
119. Esposito C, Borzi P, Valla JS, et al. Laparoscopic versus open appendectomy in children: a retrospective comparative study of 2,332 cases. World J Surg 2007; 31(4):750–5.
120. Guller U, Hervey S, Purves H, et al. Laparoscopic versus open appendectomy. Ann Surg 2004;239(1):43–52.
121. Horwitz JR, Custer MD, May BH, et al. Should laparoscopic appendectomy be avoided for complicated appendicitis in children? J Pediatr Surg 1997;32(11): 1601–3.
122. Jaschinski T, Mosch C, Eikermann M, et al. Laparoscopic versus open appendectomy in patients with suspected appendicitis: a systematic review of meta-analyses of randomised controlled trials. BMC Gastroenterol 2015;15(1):48.
123. Katkhouda N, Mason RJ, Towfigh S. Laparoscopic versus open appendectomy: a prospective, randomized, double-blind study. Adv Surg 2006;40:1–19.
124. Menezes M, Das L, Alagtal M, et al. Laparoscopic appendectomy is recommended for the treatment of complicated appendicitis in children. Pediatr Surg Int 2008;24(3):303–5.
125. Paterson HM, Qadan M, de Luca SM, et al. Changing trends in surgery for acute appendicitis. Br J Surg 2008;95(3):363–8.
126. Yau KK, Siu WT, Tang CN, et al. Laparoscopic versus open appendectomy for complicated appendicitis. J Am Coll Surg 2007;205(1):60–5.
127. St Peter SD, Adibe OO, Iqbal CW, et al. Irrigation versus suction alone during laparoscopic appendectomy for perforated appendicitis. Ann Surg 2012; 256(4):581–5.
128. Muehlstedt SG, Pham TQ, Schmeling DJ. The management of pediatric appendicitis: a survey of North American pediatric surgeons. J Pediatr Surg 2004; 39(6):875–9.
129. Hartwich JE, Carter RF, Wolfe L, et al. The effects of irrigation on outcomes in cases of perforated appendicitis in children. J Surg Res 2013;180(2):222–5.
130. Moore CB, Smith RS, Herbertson R, et al. Does use of intraoperative irrigation with open or laparoscopic appendectomy reduce post-operative intra-abdominal abscess? Am Surg 2011;77(1):78–80.
131. Rollins MD, Andolsek W, Scaife ER, et al. Prophylactic appendectomy: unnecessary in children with incidental appendicoliths detected by computed tomographic scan. J Pediatr Surg 2010;45(12):2377–80.
132. Healy JM, Olgun LF, Hittelman AB, et al. Pediatric incidental appendectomy: a systematic review. Pediatr Surg Int 2016;32(4):321–35.
133. Willis ZI, Duggan EM, Bucher BT, et al. Effect of a clinical practice guideline for pediatric complicated appendicitis. JAMA Surg 2016;151(5):e160194.
134. Aguayo P, Alemayehu H, Desai AA, et al. Initial experience with same day discharge after laparoscopic appendectomy for non-perforated appendicitis. J Surg Res 2014;186(2):535.

135. Knott EM, Gasior AC, Ostlie DJ, et al. Decreased resource utilization since initiation of institutional clinical pathway for care of children with perforated appendicitis. J Pediatr Surg 2013;48(6):1395–8.
136. Svensson JF, Patkova B, Almstrom M, et al. Nonoperative treatment with antibiotics versus surgery for acute nonperforated appendicitis in children: a pilot randomized controlled trial. Ann Surg 2015;261(1):67–71.
137. Steiner Z, Buklan G, Stackievicz R, et al. A role for conservative antibiotic treatment in early appendicitis in children. J Pediatr Surg 2015;50(9):1566–8.

Vascular Access in the Pediatric Population

Joseph T. Church, MD[a], Marcus D. Jarboe, MD[b],*

KEYWORDS

- Vascular access • Central venous catheter • Ultrasound

KEY POINTS

- The selection of the appropriate central venous catheter requires knowledge of the indication for placement and the intended duration and frequency of use. Clear communication between the surgeon and the primary provider requesting the catheter is essential to performing the correct procedure.
- Seldinger or modified Seldinger technique is preferred for nearly all vascular access procedures. The authors recommend use of a 21-gauge (g) or 22-g access needle and thin (0.018-in) flexible-tip wire to establish access.
- Ultrasound guidance improves the safety and ease of most vascular access procedures. Transverse or in-line transducer orientations can be used depending on the anatomy and approach.
- Most central line–associated blood stream infections (CLABSIs) require catheter removal. Blood cultures should be negative for at least 48 hours before placing a new line except in rare circumstances.

INTRODUCTION

Vascular access procedures are a common and important part of pediatric surgical practice. Children require vascular access for numerous indications, including hydration, infusion of parental nutrition, administration of medications, and obtaining blood for laboratory analysis. Advances in vascular access have made many disease processes, such as intestinal atresia, short bowel syndrome, and various malignancies survivable.

Pediatric vascular access presents numerous challenges to the pediatric surgeon. In obtaining access, the pediatric surgeon must make several important preoperative

Disclosure Statement: The authors have no commercial or financial conflicts of interest or external funding sources.
[a] Department of Surgery, University of Michigan Health System, 2110 Taubman Center, 1500 East Medical Center Drive, Ann Arbor, MI 48109, USA; [b] Section of Pediatric Surgery, Department of Surgery, University of Michigan Health System, 1540 East Medical Center Drive, SPC 4211, Ann Arbor, MI 48109, USA
* Corresponding author.
E-mail address: marjarbo@med.umich.edu

http://dx.doi.org/10.1016/j.suc.2016.08.007
0039-6109/17/© 2016 Elsevier Inc. All rights reserved.
surgical.theclinics.com

decisions – what type of access to obtain, the size and number of lumens required, and where to place the catheter. Therefore, sound knowledge of the indications, contraindications, advantages, and disadvantages of different types of access is required to provide the best care for the patient. This article addresses these questions in decision making and presents the basic tenets of vascular access in children and how to manage this access postprocedurally. The majority of the article focuses on central venous access, but arterial access, peripheral venous access, and peripherally inserted central catheters (PICCs) are addressed as well.

SURGICAL TECHNIQUE
Preoperative Planning

Peripheral venous access
Peripheral venous access could be considered the mainstay of vascular access during hospital admission, because it is nearly ubiquitous in inpatients. Peripheral access is adequate for intravenous (IV) hydration, most medication administration, and often blood sampling. It is usually more technically straightforward and safer than central access and can be performed at the bedside without anesthesia, although topical analgesics are often helpful.

Peripheral access is often obtained by other skilled members of the patient care team, such as nurses and anesthesia staff. Peripheral venous access can be challenging, however, in children, and a pediatric surgeon may be called on if others are unsuccessful in obtaining access. Pediatric veins are small in caliber and often difficult to see and feel, especially in a patient who may be dehydrated. It is, therefore, helpful to be familiar with the anatomic locations amenable to peripheral IV insertions as well as the technology available to assist with access.

The anatomic options for peripheral IV insertion are summarized:

- Scalp: generally limited to neonates.
- External jugular vein: of adequate size and visibility but frequently difficult to access due to excessive mobility, difficult location, and ease of compression, even with the access needle
- Superficial veins of the arm and dorsal hand/wrist: good targets for peripheral venous access; however, the antecubital fossa must not be crossed with the catheter unless the arm is immobilized
- Greater saphenous vein: often a good target, especially anterior to the medial malleolus. This is best visualized with the foot held in plantar flexion. In an emergency when no other peripheral access can be acquired, the distal saphenous vein also represents a good target for peripheral cut-down. This is performed via a small transverse incision medial and superior to the medical malleolus, with suture ligature and direct venipuncture.[1]

Technology can be used to aid in peripheral venous access. Ultrasound offers good delineation of vascular anatomy (**Fig. 1**). It can distinguish arterial from venous structures based on compressibility and pulsatility and with use of color flow Doppler. Recent studies have demonstrated that ultrasound use in peripheral vascular access increases accuracy and decreases attempts required.[2,3] More recent technological advancements have included infrared-based vein finders. This modality improves vein visibility, thereby increasing accuracy and decreasing the pain associated with access.[4,5]

Central venous access
Central venous access is required for the administration of several medications and fluids, including many vasoactive medications; hyperosmolar fluid, including total

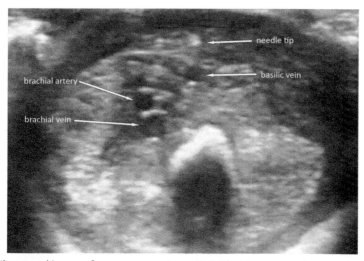

Fig. 1. Ultrasound image of upper arm anatomy. Note that in cross-section, vessels appear as anechoic circles. Arteries and veins can be differentiated by compressibility, pulsatility, and use of color flow Doppler. This particular image represented needle access to the basilic vein in a 460g premature neonate for PICC placement.

parenteral nutrition (TPN); and cytotoxic medications (most chemotherapy). Central access is also indicated any time venous access is required and peripheral access is unable to be obtained, which is a frequent challenge in the pediatric population. Central venous access can be approached in many different ways, however, depending on the medical therapy required. If a pediatric surgeon is not the primary provider using the catheter, clear communication between the primary provider and surgeon is essential to ensure the patient undergoes the correct procedure, with the correct catheter and number of lumens.

The types of central venous access are summarized in **Table 1**. The primary determinants in central venous catheter selection are intended duration and frequency of use. Central venous lines (CVLs) intended for long-term use, continuing after hospital discharge, are often tunneled under the skin to provide added stability. Cuffed CVLs, such as Broviac and Hickman catheters, exit the skin so they can be easily accessed, making them ideal for continuous use, such as for TPN. Ports, on the other hand, remain completely subcutaneous. This means needle puncture of the skin is required for use, but risks of infection and line damage are decreased. These ports are for long-term intermittent use, such as administration of chemotherapeutic drugs. Both these tunneled CVLs allow for more than 1 lumen if desired, depending on the intended medication administration plan.

Percutaneous, nontunneled CVLs are intended for acute use, generally during hospital admission. Similarly, acute hemodialysis lines allow for hemodialysis or plasmapheresis in the hospital setting in the absence of more durable access, such as an arteriovenous fistula or graft, but are not intended for long-term outpatient use. PICCs are more versatile. As the name implies, they are long, thin catheters inserted into a peripheral vein, with the tip in the central venous compartment. Their length and small diameter limit the flow they can tolerate, but they provide more stability and comfort than most percutaneous CVLs and, therefore, can be used in the outpatient setting for prolonged periods of time, such as during a weeks-long course of IV antibiotics.

Table 1
Types of central access

	Line	Duration of Use	Requires Operating Room?	Example Uses
Nontunneled	PICC	Intermediate to long term	No	Prolonged antibiotic administration (eg, after perforated appendicitis)
	Percutaneous CVL	Short term	No	Vasopressor or hyperosmolar fluid/medication administration as inpatient
	Acute hemodialysis line	Short term	No	Acute hemodialysis (no arteriovenous fistula/graft used)
Tunneled	Cuffed CVL	Long-term, regular use	No, but lower infection rate in operating rooms[6]	Prolonged/ outpatient parenteral nutrition
	Port	Long-term, intermittent use	Yes	Chemotherapy administration

Preoperatively, the surgeon must also decide where to place the CVL. Central access may be obtained via the external jugular or internal jugular (IJ) vein, facial vein, subclavian vein, saphenous vein or femoral vein, with the IJ, subclavian, and femoral the most common and well defined.[1] The advantages and disadvantages of each location are outlined in **Table 2**.

Table 2
Central venous line locations

Site	Advantages	Disadvantages
IJ vein	• Shortest distance to right atrium • Straightest route to right atrium • Decreased incidence of stenosis • Aided by use of ultrasound[7]	• Neck access, therefore potential discomfort • Line position may change with head movement (if placed high in neck)
Subclavian vein	• Short distance to right atrium • Relatively fixed position → comfort and line stability	• Ultrasound guidance precluded in subclavicular approach (must use landmarks unless approach from above clavicle) • Poor choice for dialysis access (higher stenosis incidence, difficulty with future AV fistula creation)
Femoral vein	• Relative ease of placement using landmarks • Aided by use of ultrasound[8]	Position in groin crease → limits comfort and mobility, decreases stability

Equipment

Access

Most venous access in children can be obtained with a 21-g or 22-g needle. Smaller needles preclude passage of all but the smallest guide wires and also risk bending on insertion. Larger needles present unnecessary risk of damage to nearby structure and the target vein itself. A 22-g needle allows passage of a 0.018-in coaxial wire. In the authors' practice, the 0.018-in Cope nitinol Mandril Wire Guide (Cook Medical, Bloomington, Indiana) is preferred. This wire has a flexible tip, which reduces risk of vascular damage from wire passage, but also a stiff shaft, which increases ease of dilator and catheter threading.

In general, J-wires or C-wires should be avoided in pediatric patients. Although the intention of these wires is to curl to form a blunt end while advancing the wire in adult patients, the radius of curvature is often too large for the size of a child's vein. This risks loss of access to the vascular lumen by the wire and needle.

Dilators and catheters

Once the target vein has been accessed by a 0.018-in wire, this can be exchanged for a larger, 0.035-in guide wire using a 3F to 4F dilator (3F dilator seated within a 4F dilator). These dilators are standardly included with the micropuncture vascular access kit. A 0.035-in wire allows for the passage of larger dilators. Depending on the catheter selected, the surgeon can then place the catheter directly over the wire (Seldinger technique) or place an introducer through which the catheter can be placed (modified Seldinger technique). In the very small vessels of the neonate, the catheters are made to go over smaller wires, such as 0.018-in and 0.010-in wires. In these cases, changing wire to 0.035 in is not helpful or necessary.

Ultrasound

Historically, central venous access was obtained using anatomic landmarks. The introduction of ultrasound guidance into the technique, however, has made the procedures safer and easier, particularly in children.[7,9,10] A high-frequency (7.5–20 MHz), linear array transducer is used because it gives best resolution without the need for significant tissue penetration.

It is important to clearly establish left-right orientation on ultrasound prior to attempting access (left side of the probe should be seen on the left side of the screen). Access is also aided by orienting the probe in such a way that the handle does not impede manipulation of the needle and wire. This is especially true of the hockey-stick probe, which has a handle that can be angled away from the working anatomy.

Fluoroscopy

Fluoroscopy is an essential tool for CVL placement in the operating room. It can be used to identify key landmarks before attempting access (eg, the carina in cases of IJ or subclavian access). It also guides wire advancement and dilator/peel-away sheath placement and ensures appropriate catheter position at the end of the procedure.

Preparation and Patient Positioning

Positioning

When ultrasound is used, the ultrasound machine should be placed across the table from the operating surgeon. The patient is placed supine on a radiolucent table for nearly all vascular access procedures in the operating room. The extremities are extended to optimize exposure if they contain the target vessel; otherwise, the arms are tucked. For jugular and subclavian access, the patient is placed in Trendelenburg position to distend target veins and prevent air embolism. A shoulder roll can be used to extend the neck and improve ease of access to the IJ; contrarily, the authors do not recommend use of a shoulder roll in subclavian access because it decreases the cross-sectional area of the subclavian vein.[11] Turning the head to the contralateral side is also helpful in IJ and subclavian access. Femoral vein exposure is aided by abduction and external rotation of the leg.

Sterile preparation
Standard skin preparation is used, in most cases consisting of chlorhexidine solution. Hats, masks, and sterile gloves and gowns are worn. If fluoroscopy is to be used, lead should be worn by all those in the operating room. Ultrasound requires a sterile probe cover, with nonsterile ultrasound gel directly on the transducer within the cover and sterile ultrasound gel available for use directly on the patient. Avoiding any air bubbles in the gel layer between the probe and the probe cover is extremely important because air causes shadowing and thus large areas of nonvisualization in the ultrasound field of view.

Procedural Approach

Cut-down technique
Historically, central venous access was obtained by surgical exposure of the target vessel. In this technique, a venotomy is performed, with or without proximal ligation of the vein, and the CVL placed. If the distal vein is not to be ligated, a lateral venotomy with a purse-string suture of 7-0 Prolene is used to secure the catheter. Anatomic targets of such cut-downs are the external jugular vein, facial vein, IJ vein just above the clavicle, and the proximal greater saphenous vein, with advancement of the catheter into the femoral vein. The greater saphenous vein still has some utility in critically ill infants requiring emergent access, but overall the cut-down technique has been largely replaced by percutaneous access.[1] Despite this, it remains an important technique that is indispensable in many circumstances.

Percutaneous technique – Seldinger and modified Seldinger
In 1953, Swedish radiologist Sven-Ivar Seldinger published a novel technique for vascular access involving a needle, a wire, and a catheter.[12] This technique, which now bears his name, has become the standard approach not only for vascular access but also for other percutaneous techniques, such as chest tube placement and biliary tract access.

The first step in Seldinger technique is access to the vascular lumen via needle venipuncture. As discussed previously, in children this can generally be performed with a 21-g or 22-g micropuncture needle. The bevel of the needle is oriented upwards. When using landmarks alone, a syringe is used and gentle suction applied so that successful luminal access is confirmed by the return of blood. When using ultrasound in the pediatric population, however, the authors recommend not using a syringe, because this hinders fine touch of the needle, and the suction applied by the syringe can cause vascular collapse and vasospasm. With the landmark technique, once blood is seen coming into the syringe, the syringe is taken off carefully without needle movement and a wire is advanced through the needle and into the lumen of the vessel.

When using ultrasound, needle tip entry into the vessel is visualized with the ultrasound. Once the needle tip is seen in the lumen of the vessel and the vessel wall is no longer tented (the needle has clearly pierced the wall as opposed to deforming it), the wire is advanced through the needle and into the vessel. For peripheral access, once the needle is noted to be in the lumen of the vessel, the needle is advanced some distances further (approximately 1 cm) down the barrel of the vessel lumen under ultrasound guidance. This prevents ejection of the needle and/or wire if the vessel spasms, a common phenomenon in children, especially newborns. It also ensures that the needle has not tented the vessel wall and ensures intraluminal location of the needle and/or catheter tip. This strategy has been shown to reduce the risk of extravasation during peripheral venous access.[13]

With the needle well into the vessel lumen, the wire is advanced. Care should be taken not to attempt to force the wire past any resistance. If resistance is met, ultrasound or fluoroscopy should be used to confirm proper wire placement and to guide advancement.

Once the wire is in place, maintaining control of its position becomes the surgeon's top priority. A small skin nick is made with an 11 blade adjacent to the wire, avoiding any skin bridge between the two. Dilators are passed over the wire to expand the tract to the necessary size. Preferably, serial dilation should be performed under fluoroscopy. Once the tract is appropriately dilated, the catheter is advanced over the wire. Proper position is confirmed with ultrasound and/or fluoroscopy, and the catheter is secured at the skin.

A modification to the Seldinger technique can be applied with silastic catheters, which are sometimes difficult to place bareback over a wire. In this situation, a combination introducer sheath and dilator is placed over the wire into the vein lumen. The wire and dilator are removed simultaneously, leaving the introducer in place. A finger is quickly placed over the opening of the introducer to prevent back-bleeding. The silastic catheter can then be advanced through the introducer into the vein lumen. Most introducers can then be split and peeled down their length to be removed around the catheter.

Anatomy

Prior to the widespread use of ultrasound, anatomic landmarks were the primary guides to central venous access. Although ultrasound has improved the accuracy, ease, and safety of these procedures, knowing the anatomic landmarks is still important to performing these procedures safely. The landmarks for the common sites of access are as follows:

- IJ vein: the right side provides a more direct route to the heart. The needle is inserted into the skin at just below the confluence of the sternal and clavicular heads of the sternocleidomastoid, directed inferiorly toward the ipsilateral nipple at a 30° angle to the skin.
- Subclavian vein: the skin is punctured just below the clavicle, approximately two-thirds of the distance from the manubrium to lateral clavicular head. The needle is directed medially toward just above the sternal notch, also at a 30° angle from the skin. Pushing down on the needle and taking a shallower approach may help avoid lung injury. Ultrasound is not as useful when using this subclavicular approach but does have utility if the subclavian vein is to be accessed from a supraclavicular approach. The subclavian vein can also be accessed with ultrasound guidance in larger patients near the deltopectoral groove.
- Femoral vein: the femoral artery is palpated just below the inguinal ligament approximately one-third of the way from the pubic tubercle to the anterior superior iliac spine (ASIS). The femoral vein lies just medial to this. The skin is punctured well below the inguinal ligament, with the needle directed toward the umbilicus at a 30° angle to the skin In neonates, the femoral vein tends to lie more posterior than medial to the femoral artery (**Fig. 2**A, B). In this situation, the needle can be inserted medial to the artery, then pushed laterally and advanced further into the vein. This technique, however, requires ultrasound guidance, as seen in **Fig. 2**C.

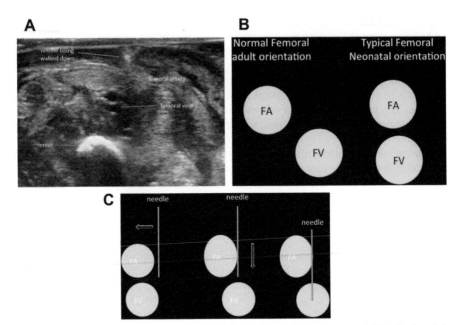

Fig. 2. Femoral access. (*A*) Ultrasound view of femoral vessels in a neonate. (*B*) Unlike in adults in whom the femoral vein (FV) lies medial to the femoral artery (FA), the femoral vein in the neonate tends to lie directly deep to the artery. (*C*) The femoral vein can be accessed in neonates by inserting the needle just medial to the femoral artery under ultrasound guidance. Once the tip of the needle is just deep to the artery, the needle can be moved laterally to push the artery aside and align the tip over the femoral vein.

Ultrasound use

Ultrasound can be immensely helpful in accurate vascular access, and the American College of Surgeons recommends use of real-time ultrasound for central venous catheter placement.[14] Like any technical skill, however, ultrasound-guided line placement requires training and practice. With enough experience, ultrasound increases the safety, accuracy, and success of central venous catheter placement.

Ultrasound displays 3-D structures in 2 dimensions. Therefore, when trying to access a vessel, the operator must choose to view the vessel transversely (as a cross-section or circle) or longitudinally (as a line). The third dimension can be obtained by moving the transducer perpendicular to its linear axis. This requires constant spatial reconstruction, however, within an operator's mind and complicates needle placement for anyone but an experienced surgeon. The procedure is simplified by using ultrasound in 1 of 2 orientations: transverse or in-line.

Transverse orientation The transducer head is oriented perpendicular to the vessel and needle axis, producing a cross-sectional view of both. The needle is inserted at a 45° angle at the midpoint of the transducer, producing excellent left-right resolution. Because the needle is seen in cross-section, however, it appears as only a small point on the display, with the location/depth of the needle tip unknown. This can be remedied by regularly sliding the transducer down the trajectory of the needle past the tip until it disappears and then back until it reappears, so that the tip location is known as the needle is walked down into the vessel. Use of the transverse orientation for IJ access is seen in **Fig. 3**A, B and for PICC placement in a neonate in **Fig. 3**C.

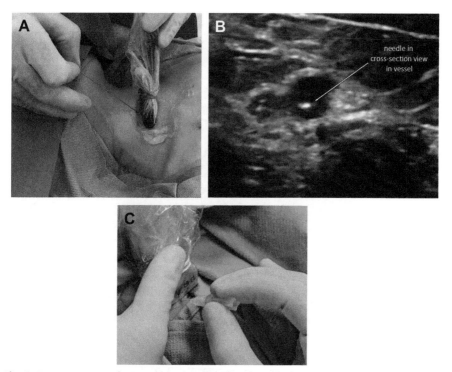

Fig. 3. Transverse transducer orientation. (*A*) The ultrasound transducer is oriented perpendicular to the vessel (here the IJ) and the needle placed under the center of the probe. (*B*) The needle is seen in cross-section within the vessel lumen. Therefore the full length is not visualized. (*C*) The needle is inserted at 45° to the skin at the midpoint of the transducer. The transducer is walked down the needle to identify the tip.

In-line orientation The ultrasound probe is oriented parallel to the needle axis. This enables visualization of the entire length of the needle. The needle can then be advanced with the tip's location known relative to nearby major structures. This orientation is ideal for IJ access, because inadvertent puncture of the carotid artery or lung can be avoided (**Fig. 4**). A common mistake using this approach is to lose sight of the needle itself and to instead view the movement of the surrounding tissue. Losing clear visualization of the needle tip defeats the purpose of in-line orientation yet is easy to do with subtle movement of the transducer. This approach requires patience, because fine adjustments of the transducer head keep it aligned directly over the needle trajectory.

Tunneling technique
When durable, long-term central access is required, tunneled IJ venous catheter placement is the procedure of choice. A subcutaneous tunnel is created from the point of access (the lateral IJ just superior to the clavicle) laterally over the clavicle and inferiorly to the anterior chest to either an external hub or to a subcutaneous port. The course of the tunnel is important, because an acute bend can lead to kinking and occlusion of the catheter, whereas tracking too high in the neck can lead to catheter malposition with head movement.

Access to the IJ is obtained using the in-line probe orientation to allow full visualization of the needle (see **Fig. 4**). The linear array, hockey-stick probe is placed just superior to the clavicle, revealing the distal IJ, subclavian vessels, the carotid artery, and

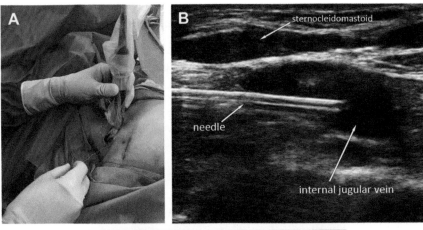

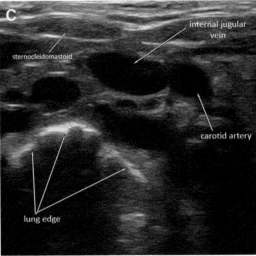

Fig. 4. In-line transducer orientation. (*A*) The needle is inserted parallel to the transducer head, starting from the end opposite the hand when using a hockey stick probe. In this case, the target vessel is the IJ. (*B*) In-line orientation allows visualization of the length of the needle. For IJ access, the needle is inserted lateral to the sternocleidomastoid muscle and advanced deep to the muscle into the vein. (*C*) Ultrasound can be used in in-line orientation to identify and avoid damage to surrounding structures. The IJ lies anterolateral to the carotid artery. The apex of the lung is seen as a bright interface between soft tissue and air.

often the brachiocephalic vessels. The needle is advanced in-line, taking care to avoid damage to the lung, carotid, or external jugular vein. Once the needle is intraluminal, the wire is advanced. With the lateral approach, occasionally the wire is advanced cephalad up the IJ, which can be seen on fluoroscopy. If this occurs, the needle tip should be confirmed to remain intraluminal with ultrasound, and, if so, the wire can be withdrawn and the needle angled inferiorly down the IJ. The needle then guides the wire in the proper direction with readvancement, again confirmed with fluoroscopy.

With the wire in place, the subcutaneous tunnel is created from the chest wall incision to the neck incision. Care is taken to avoid any sharp angles in the tunnel course, instead taking a gentle curve (**Fig. 5**A, B). Using a low, lateral neck access incision facilitates this.

Ideal catheter position is with the tip at the cavoatrial junction. This can be approximated on fluoroscopy as 1.5 to 2 vertebral bodies inferior to the carina (**Fig. 5**C). Therefore, before placement through the introducer into the IJ, the catheter is placed through the subcutaneous tunnel, and the appropriate length assessed by laying the catheter on the patient's chest while using fluoroscopy. The catheter is then cut to length and advanced through the introducer. The introducer is removed, and proper position is confirmed with fluoroscopy.

Peripheral vascular access

A similar technique can be used for both peripheral venous and arterial access. In general, the transverse ultrasound orientation is used. A helpful technique in aligning the needle is to generously apply gel to the skin overlying the vessel and then place the needle flat against the skin directly under the transducer. This creates a shadow under the needle that can be aligned directly over the vessel (**Fig. 6**). Once this appropriate

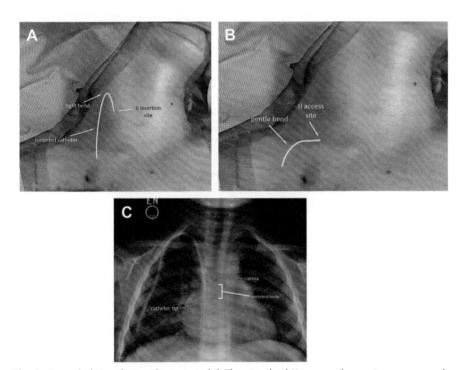

Fig. 5. Tunneled IJ catheter placement. (*A*) The standard IJ approach uses transverse probe orientation and a craniocaudal needle approach. This results in an acute angle of the tunneled catheter high in the neck and risks kinking of the catheter. (*B*) Using a lateral IJ approach with in-line transducer orientation allows for a low insertion, just above the clavicle, and a gentle curve of the tunneled catheter. (*C*) The postprocedure chest radiograph using this low lateral approach to the IJ confirms a gentle curve to the tunneled catheter without kinking. The tip of the catheter is seen at the cavoatrial junction, 1.5 to 2 vertebral bodies below the carina.

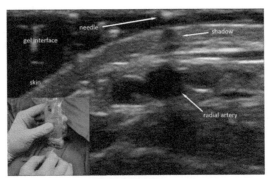

Fig. 6. Peripheral access. Using transverse transducer orientation, the needle can be placed flat against the skin directly against the skin under the midpoint (inset) of the probe. This creates a shadow, which, once aligned over the target vessel, increases the accuracy of insertion when the needle is advanced through the skin.

needle orientation is established, the needle can be angled down 45° into the skin and advanced. The tip of the needle can then be walked down to and into the target vessel with the transducer, as described previously.

Peripherally inserted central catheter

PICCs are long, thin, flexible catheters that provide added versatility because they are functionally central venous catheters but are inserted peripherally. They are made in a variety of sizes, as small as 1.9F (26 g) and can be placed through a peel-away sheath introduced with a 23-g needle in modified Seldinger fashion. They can be placed into essentially any vein into which a peripheral IV can be inserted, provided the catheter is long enough to reach the central venous compartment from that location. The basilic vein is a common target for PICC placement, because it empties directly into the axillary vein without any acute angles, allowing ease of catheter passage (see **Fig. 1**).

Immediate Postprocedural Care

In the immediate postprocedure period, any early complications must be assessed for. For vascular access procedures performed in the operating room, a brief period in the postanesthesia care unit enables close observation to rule out complications related to bleeding or anesthesia. In cases of IJ and subclavian access, regardless of where the procedure was performed, a potential early complication is pneumothorax. Therefore, routine chest radiograph should be obtained after these procedures. The chest radiograph also provides confirmation that the tip of the catheter remains in the appropriate location. In general, the line can be used immediately after placement.

REHABILITATION AND RECOVERY
Recovery

Perhaps with the exception of cut-down procedures, vascular access is minimally invasive and well tolerated. Pain is generally mild, and there are few or no limitations on routine activity. If a patient is going to be discharged with the line, the family should be educated well about care of the site as well as how to handle common issues, such as catheter damage or occlusion. These complications are discussed later.

Removal

Indications for catheter removal depend on the type of catheter and its intended use. Line infection or damage may require removal and are discussed later. Peripheral IVs and CVLs should be removed prior to hospital discharge. In general, other lines may be removed when they are no longer needed.

The complexity of catheter removal also depends on the type. Percutaneous CVLs and PICCs can generally be removed simply by pulling them out with the patient bearing down and then holding gentle pressure to ensure hemostasis. Cuffed CVLs require local anesthesia at the insertion site (children often also require sedation or general anesthesia), because the cuff induces scar formation and must be dissected free from the catheter, which can cause pain. Ports often require general anesthesia in children because removal is more invasive, requiring surgical excision of the subcutaneous port, which is sutured to the pectoralis fascia.

Occasionally, a long-standing catheter is unable to be extracted. This indicates that the catheter has adhered to the venous endothelium. If the catheter cannot be removed by gentle, constant pulling, the surgeon should immediately place a wire down the catheter, ideally with the tip of the wire well into the inferior vena cava, before using any aggressive moves to remove it. If the catheter breaks, the wire maintains vessel access and can aid in retrieval with snare in interventional radiology. Although there is some suggestion that catheters that break on removal are secured and do not embolize to the lung, the authors' experience has shown the contrary on multiple occasions and, therefore, these catheters should be retrieved when possible.

POTENTIAL COMPLICATIONS/MANAGEMENT
Early Complications

Early complications of vascular access procedures generally involve damage to nearby structures. Because the IJ, subclavian, and femoral veins are all accompanied by major arteries, arterial injury may result from central venous access. The risk of such complications can be reduced by using ultrasound guidance and a small access needle. If access is performed without ultrasound guidance, needle advancement should always be straight without lateral sliding or torque, and, if adjustment is needed, the needle should be withdrawn straight out. With ultrasound guidance, however, the needle can be directed at will if needle and surrounding structures are clearly visualized.

If arterial injury is suspected, management depends on the size of the needle used. A micropuncture needle can be withdrawn with subsequent pressure, which is usually adequate to obtain hemostasis. If the needle is large bore, it should be left in place, because it is likely plugging the hole and preventing more dramatic hemorrhage. Imaging should then be obtained (radiograph or fluoroscopy). If this supports arterial injury, surgical removal may be indicated to allow repair of the arteriotomy. Femoral arterial injury is more easily controlled than carotid or subclavian artery injury, so in this case the catheter may be removed and firm pressure held.

With IJ and subclavian access, the pleura may be damaged by the access needle as well. This risk is elevated in patients undergoing positive pressure ventilation, because the apex of the lung reaches the lower neck. Chest radiographs should be obtained routinely after these procedures to rule out this complication.

Late Complications

Line malfunction/damage
Damage to cuffed CVLs is common, given the exposed portion of the catheter and activity level of young children. Silastic catheters can usually be repaired using available

kits, provided the damage is at least 5 cm from the skin. A study in intestinal failure patients showed that there is no increased risk of infection with line repair.[15] If a catheter cannot be repaired, replacement may be necessary. In this case, as long as the catheter is not infected, it may be exchanged over a wire.

Line thrombosis/occlusion

Line thrombosis occurs more commonly in children with cancer. Tissue plasminogen activator may be successful in cases of catheter thrombosis. Occlusion due to lipid or mineral deposits may be cleared with 70% ethanol and hydrochloric acid, 0.1 N, respectively, with varying success. If medical therapy is ineffective, catheter removal and replacement may be necessary.

Perforation

Perforation of the superior vena cava or right atrium by a central venous catheter is extremely rare. Incidence in the literature ranges from 0.0001% to 1.4% but is likely under-reported.[16] The choice of catheter material (silastic vs polyurethane) does not seem to affect perforation risk.[17] The risk of perforation, however, is slightly higher with PICCs than with CVLs inserted via the IJ or subclavian.[18] Placement in the right IJ provides least risk of this terrible complication due to its straight course, because the side of the catheter tends to contact the vessel wall as opposed to the tip. Perforation below the pericardial reflection can cause tamponade but above the reflection can cause exsanguination into the pleural space. It is likely the whipping of the catheter during systole that causes erosion and perforation, so the tip should be placed near the cavoatrial junction.

Vessel thrombosis/stenosis

Vessel thrombosis due to central venous catheters can occur, especially in children with cancer. When possible, treatment involves removal of the offending line. Venous stenosis is uncommon, but more likely to occur with subclavian than IJ access.

Infection

There are 3 types of infection associated with central venous catheters: exit-site infection, tunnel or pocket infection, and CLABSI.[1]

- Exit-site infection: involves skin at the exit site of the catheter. Generally the causative organism is a skin pathogen. This usually can be treated with antibiotics and local wound care.
- Tunnel/pocket infection: more serious than an exit-site infection, this involves infection of the subcutaneous tunnel. Signs include erythema, induration, and excessive tenderness along the tract as well as expression of pus from the exit site. Antibiotic penetration is generally poor and lack of treatment can progress to systemic sepsis, so line removal is usually indicated.
- CLABSI: the most serious of the catheter-related infections, CLABSI can lead to systemic sepsis. External signs may be absent, and cultures from both the central line and peripheral site(s) are necessary.

CLABSI represents a major concern in patients with indwelling central access. Risk factors include neutropenia and TPN.[19] It was previously thought that femoral lines bore a higher risk of CVL infection. Recent studies, however, including a Cochrane review in adult patients, do not support this claim.[6,20] A 2011 systematic review identified the following strategies for preventing CLABSI in children:

- Chlorhexidine skin preparation and chlorhexidine-impregnated dressing
- Use of heparin and antibiotic-impregnated central venous catheters

- Use of ethanol lock or vancomycin lock therapy[21]

In cases of a suspected infected catheter, peripheral and central blood cultures should be drawn prior to initiating empiric antibiotics. Antibiotics are sometimes sufficient treatment. If bacteremia has not cleared after 72 hours of therapy, however, the catheter should be removed. Catheter removal is also required if the causative organism is *Staphylococcus aureus, Bacillus cereus,* fungus, or other resistant organisms.

If a catheter is removed due to infection, a new line should not be placed until at least 48 hours after the first negative blood culture and should be placed at a new site. In rare cases, if preservation of the catheter is critical and bacteremia has responded to antibiotics, the line may be exchanged over a wire. This practice, however, remains controversial.

SUMMARY

Vascular access procedures in children are a mainstay of the pediatric surgeons practice. Most procedures can be performed percutaneously by the Seldinger or modified Seldinger approaches. Although vascular access can be challenging, the use of imaging technology, such as ultrasound and fluoroscopy, increases the safety and ease of these procedures. Ultrasound, in particular, decreases complications associated with vascular access but requires patience and experience. Today's pediatric surgeon should be comfortable performing these procedures using this technology and should be able to diagnose and treat the common complications.

REFERENCES

1. Zeller KA, Petty JK. Vascular access procedures. In: Ziegler MM, Azizkhan RG, Allmen DV, et al, editors. Operative pediatric surgery. New York: McGraw-Hill Education; 2014. Available at: http://accesssurgery.mhmedical.com/content.aspx?bookid=959&Sectionid=53539574. Accessed September 19, 2016.
2. Ishii S, Shime N, Shibasaki M, et al. Ultrasound-guided radial artery catheterization in infants and small children. Pediatr Crit Care Med 2013;14(5):471–3.
3. Tang L, Wang F, Li Y, et al. Ultrasound guidance for radial artery catheterization: an updated meta-analysis of randomized controlled trials. PLoS One 2014;9(11): e111527.
4. Chiao FB, Resta-Flarer F, Lesser J, et al. Vein visualization: patient characteristic factors and efficacy of a new infrared vein finder technology. Br J Anaesth 2013; 110(6):966–71.
5. Guillon P, Makhloufi M, Baillie S, et al. Prospective evaluation of venous access difficulty and a near-infrared vein visualizer at four French haemophilia treatment centres. Haemophilia 2015;21(1):21–6.
6. Freeman JJ, Gadepalli SK, Siddiqui SM, et al. Improving central line infection rates in the neonatal intensive care unit: Effect of hospital location, site of insertion, and implementation of catheter-associated bloodstream infection protocols. J Pediatr Surg 2015;50(5):860–3.
7. Sigaut S, Skhiri A, Stany I, et al. Ultrasound guided internal jugular vein access in children and infant: a meta-analysis of published studies. Paediatric Anaesth 2009;19(12):1199–206.
8. Brass P, Hellmich M, Kolodziej L, et al. Ultrasound guidance versus anatomical landmarks for subclavian or femoral vein catheterization. Cochrane Database Syst Rev 2015;(1):CD011447.

9. Bruzoni M, Slater BJ, Wall J, et al. A prospective randomized trial of ultrasound- vs landmark-guided central venous access in the pediatric population. J Am Coll Surg 2013;216(5):939–43.

10. Hind D, Calvert N, McWilliams R, et al. Ultrasonic locating devices for central venous cannulation: meta-analysis. BMJ 2003;327(7411):361.

11. Rodriguez CJ, Bolanowski A, Patel K, et al. Classical positioning decreases the cross-sectional area of the subclavian vein. Am J Surg 2006;192(1):135–7.

12. Seldinger SI. Catheter replacement of the needle in percutaneous arteriography; a new technique. Acta radiologica 1953;39(5):368–76.

13. Costantino TG, Parikh AK, Satz WA, et al. Ultrasonography-guided peripheral intravenous access versus traditional approaches in patients with difficult intravenous access. Ann Emerg Med 2005;46(5):456–61.

14. ACS Committee on Perioperative Care. Revised statement on recommendations for use of real-time ultrasound guidance forplacement of central venous catheters. Bull Am Coll Surg 2011;96(2):36–7.

15. McNiven C, Switzer N, Wood M, et al. Central venous catheter repair is not associated with an increased risk of central line infection or colonization in intestinal failure pediatric patients. J Pediatr Surg 2016;51(3):395–7.

16. Booth SA, Norton B, Mulvey DA. Central venous catheterization and fatal cardiac tamponade. Br J Anaesth 2001;87(2):298–302.

17. Goutail-Flaud MF, Sfez M, Berg A, et al. Central venous catheter-related complications in newborns and infants: a 587-case survey. J Pediatr Surg 1991;26(6): 645–50.

18. Kayashima K. Factors affecting survival in pediatric cardiac tamponade caused by central venous catheters. J Anesth 2015;29(6):944–52.

19. Chen IC, Hsu C, Chen YC, et al. Predictors of bloodstream infection associated with permanently implantable venous port in solid cancer patients. Ann Oncol 2013;24(2):463–8.

20. Marik PE, Flemmer M, Harrison W. The risk of catheter-related bloodstream infection with femoral venous catheters as compared to subclavian and internal jugular venous catheters: a systematic review of the literature and meta-analysis. Crit Care Med 2012;40(8):2479–85.

21. Huang EY, Chen C, Abdullah F, et al. Strategies for the prevention of central venous catheter infections: an American Pediatric Surgical Association Outcomes and Clinical Trials Committee systematic review. J Pediatr Surg 2011; 46(10):2000–11.

Incarcerated Pediatric Hernias

Sophia A. Abdulhai, MD, Ian C. Glenn, MD, Todd A. Ponsky, MD*

KEYWORDS

- Incarcerated pediatric hernia • Inguinal hernia • Umbilical hernia • Spigelian hernia
- Femoral hernia

KEY POINTS

- Indirect inguinal hernias are the most commonly incarcerated hernias in children, with a higher incidence in low birth weight and premature infants.
- Contralateral groin exploration to evaluate for a patent processus vaginalis or subclinical hernia is controversial, even laparoscopically, given that most never progress to clinical hernias.
- Most indirect inguinal hernias can be reduced nonoperatively. Given the high risk of recurrence and morbidity, it is recommended to repair them in a timely fashion, even in premature infants.
- Laparoscopic repair of incarcerated inguinal hernia repair is considered a safe and effective alternative to conventional open herniorrhaphy.
- Other incarcerated pediatric hernias (umbilical, femoral, spigelian, epigastric, lumbar, and direct inguinal), which are extremely rare, may be managed effectively with laparoscopy.

INTRODUCTION

Indirect inguinal hernias are the most common incarcerated pediatric inguinal hernias, although incarceration of other pediatric hernias, such as femoral, umbilical, spigelian, epigastric, direct inguinal, and lumbar, has been reported in the literature. This article discusses the current literature on the diagnosis and management of incarcerated hernias.

INDIRECT INGUINAL HERNIA
Epidemiology

Indirect inguinal hernia is one of the most common surgical conditions seen by pediatric surgeons.[1] The overall incidence of indirect inguinal hernias ranges from 0.8% to 5% in full-term infants,[2,3] but the risk is significantly increased in low birth weight (<1 kg) and premature infants, with a prevalence up to 30%.[3,4] The risk of incarceration

Division of Pediatric Surgery, Akron Children's Hospital, One Perkins Square, Akron, OH 44308, USA
* Corresponding author.
E-mail address: TPonsky@chmca.org

Surg Clin N Am 97 (2017) 129–145
http://dx.doi.org/10.1016/j.suc.2016.08.010
0039-6109/17/© 2016 Elsevier Inc. All rights reserved.

surgical.theclinics.com

in children ranges from 3% to 16%, although it is as high as 31% in premature infants, with most occurring within the first year of life.[5,6] Inguinal hernias are more common in boys compared with girls (5:1 ratio), but girls have a higher incidence of bilateral inguinal hernias compared with boys (25.4% vs 12.9%). There does not seem to be a difference in rate of incarceration between boys and girls.[2,7]

Anatomy

An indirect inguinal hernia is a congenital abnormality from the failure of the processus vaginalis to close. The processus vaginalis is an outpouching of peritoneum that, along with the gubernaculum, guides the testes in their descent through the inguinal ring into the scrotum. In girls, the canal of Nuck, which is functionally similar to the processus vaginalis, terminates in the labia majora and assists in guiding the ovaries to their final location in the pelvis. The processus vaginalis and canal of Nuck both close between 36 and 40 weeks of gestation. The left testis descends before the right and commonly closes first, resulting in a higher incidence of right-sided inguinal hernias (60%).[1,8]

Clinical Presentation/Diagnosis

Most inguinal hernias are asymptomatic, and they are often found during routine physical examination, or by a parent. It presents as intermittent bulging in the groin, scrotum, or labia, often with straining. An incarcerated hernia presents as an irreducible nonfluctuant bulge that is tender and may be erythematous. The child is usually inconsolable, and may have obstructive symptoms such as nausea/vomiting, lack of bowel function, and abdominal distention. If incarceration progresses to strangulation, the child may have peritonitis, bloody stools, and hemodynamic instability.

Other conditions may be confused for an incarcerated hernia, such as a retractile testis, lymphadenopathy, and hydrocele.[8] Although ultrasonography has been described as a tool to help differentiate these causes,[9] physical examination can help make the correct diagnosis. For example, if the clinician's fingers can discretely feel the upper edge of the bulge in the scrotum, then it is likely a hydrocele because a hernia has bowel going up into the inguinal canal. Also, a hydrocele should not be tender. Abdominal radiograph may show dilated loops of bowel and/or air fluid levels consistent with a bowel obstruction.

Nonoperative Management

Unless there is evidence of bowel compromise, peritonitis, or hemodynamic instability, nonoperative reduction should be attempted because 70% to 95% of incarcerated inguinal hernias are successfully reduced.[5,10,11] Reduction attempts are usually performed using sedation and analgesics, although there is not a standardized protocol, and pharmacotherapy should be at the discretion of the provider.[12]

The following is the preferred technique of the authors for nonoperative reduction. The patient is placed in the supine position. One hand should be placed above the external ring, with fingers around the hernia neck to keep it fixed in place and prevent the hernia contents from sliding over the external ring. The other hand should provide simultaneous moderate and steady pressure on the hernia contents toward the abdominal cavity along the axis of the inguinal canal and internal ring. Continuous pressure may help push out some of the bowel edema and regular, delicate movement of the fingers on the hernia sac may move the hernia contents, both aiding in reduction.[13] It may take several minutes to successfully reduce the hernia.

If the inguinal hernia is unable to be reduced, or there is concern for an incomplete reduction, then operative reduction should be performed emergently. Although it is unlikely to reduce gangrenous bowel successfully, it has been reported to be possible in the literature, so there should be close observation of the patient afterward.[14]

Timing of Surgery

Many children presenting with incarcerated hernias have a previously diagnosed inguinal hernia. Stylianos and colleagues[5] found that 35% of patients presenting with incarcerated hernias had a previously diagnosed inguinal hernia. Similarly, Niedzielski and colleagues[15] reported that 52.9% of their 153 patients with incarcerated inguinal hernias had a prior episode of incarceration. The risk of postoperative complications such as testicular atrophy, bowel ischemia, wound infections, and hernia recurrence are increased in incarcerated hernias (4.5%–33% compared with 1% in elective hernia repairs in healthy, full-term infants), with the highest risk being in those with irreducible inguinal hernias.[5,15–17] Given the risk of recurrent incarceration after a successful reduction, it is recommended that herniorrhaphy be performed during the same hospitalization after a period of time, from 24 hours to within 5 days, to allow edema to resolve.[5,15,18,19] Some clinicians choose to discharge home with a reliable family with plans for hernia repair in the very near future.

Premature and low birth weight infants

There is controversy as to the optimal timing of herniorrhaphy in premature and low birth weight infants. The current practice, according to a survey of pediatric surgeons by Antonoff and colleagues,[20] is that 63% operate before discharge from the neonatal intensive care unit (ICU), 18% operate depending on patient age and weight, and 5% operate when it is convenient. As stated earlier, premature and low birth weight infants have the highest risk of infarction, but they also have a risk of anesthesia-related postoperative cardiopulmonary issues such as apnea, bradycardia, and even cardiopulmonary arrest. This risk was initially reported to be as high as 49%, but more recent data show the risk closer to 5%, with these complications mainly occurring in patients with preexisting apnea.[21] Alternatively, by waiting, the patient has a higher risk of incarceration, with one study reporting double the risk after 40 weeks of age compared with those repaired before 39 weeks.[4] There is also a higher risk of postoperative complications with incarcerated hernias, although there are some data to suggest that prematurity may be a bigger risk factor for developing complications.[18,22,23]

There is no clear consensus on the optimal time for surgery in low birth weight and premature infants, so the decision needs to be made on a case-by-case basis by the surgeon.

Anesthesia/Preoperative Planning

General anesthesia is more commonly used for inguinal herniorrhaphy, especially for acutely incarcerated and laparoscopic cases. Spinal anesthesia is being used in preterm infants, and, per a recent Cochrane Review, it may have a lower risk of postoperative cardiopulmonary issues when used without sedation.[24] Regional and local anesthetic may be used for postoperative pain control.

Patients need adequate intravenous access for fluid resuscitation and consideration of placement of a Foley catheter for close monitoring of urine output. A nasogastric tube should be placed before induction if the patient has symptoms of a bowel obstruction.

Open Repair

The technique is similar to an elective open repair with high ligation of the sac, except a longer skin incision is usually needed with incarcerated hernias to adequately reduce and inspect the hernia contents.

The patient is placed in the supine position and the external landmarks, pubic tubercle, and anterior superior iliac spine are identified to approximate the location of the inguinal canal. A skin incision is made along the inguinal crease superior and lateral to the pubic tubercle. The layers of the abdominal wall are dissected down until reaching the external oblique muscle. In incarcerated and strangulated hernias, the tissue may be extremely edematous and friable so extra care in identifying the cord structures is necessary. The external oblique muscle is then divided through the external ring, exposing the hernia sac and the cord structures. After clearing the superior and inferior flaps of the external oblique muscle using blunt dissection, the sac should be carefully dissected away from the cord structures up to the internal ring. The sac should then be opened to evaluate the hernia contents. If the bowel appears viable, it should be replaced intraperitoneally. If the internal ring appears widened from repeat episodes of incarceration, then it may need to be closed to minimize the potential for future episodes of recurrence. The incision is then closed in multiple layers and dressed according to the surgeon's preference.

Pitfalls

Irreducible hernia contents If the hernia contents are unable to be reduced after opening the sac, consider placing the patient in Trendelenburg position and using gentle, steady pressure to again attempt to reduce the hernia. If the hernia contents are still irreducible, this may be secondary to a constricting internal ring, which needs to be divided. The ring should be divided sharply on the lateral edge to avoid injuring the inferior epigastric vessels and cord structures. Consider placement of your finger or an instrument through the internal ring to help dilate the ring, protect the hernia sac contents, and also guide the ligating instrument. The internal ring requires repair before the completion of the procedure.

Nonviable hernia contents If there is a question about the viability of the bowel post-reduction, then it is reasonable to cover it with moist, warm gauze and to reevaluate it after a few minutes. If it does not appear viable, then bowel resection with primary anastomosis may be performed through various approaches, including through the inguinal incision, a right lower quadrant incision, or midline laparotomy.

When performing the bowel resection through the inguinal incision, additional bowel proximal and distal to the necrotic section needs to be pulled out through the inguinal ring for inspection and also to allow for a tension-free anastomosis. The internal ring may need to be divided for ease of removal and subsequent reduction of the bowel, with the new anastomosis, back into the abdomen.

A right lower quadrant incision, such as a La Roque incision, may also be performed as an extension of the existing inguinal incision. A La Roque incision is a gridiron incision through the abdominal wall muscles and transversalis fascia above the internal ring.[25] This incision is performed by extending the incision laterally to the McBurney point through the external oblique muscle and then splitting the internal oblique, transversalis muscle, and fascia in a separate incision 2 to 3 cm above the internal ring, so as to prevent disrupting the entire inguinal floor.[26] This incision allows visualization of the hernia entering the internal ring directly above it, and provides sufficient exposure to perform a bowel resection.

Other options are a midline laparotomy and laparoscopy-assisted minilaparotomy, the latter resulting in a smaller midline incision but still allowing for a thorough inspection of the bowel.

A right lower quadrant incision, midline laparotomy, and laparoscopy-assisted minilaparotomy may be considered if there is concern about adequate width of the internal ring to allow for proper inspection of the bowel and also reduction of the new anastomosis back into the abdomen without putting it at risk of injury. Resecting the compromised bowel through the inguinal incision and then transitioning to one of these other methods, such as the laparoscopy-assisted minilaparotomy, to perform the anastomosis is also an option.

Spontaneous reduction of hernia contents before inspection Placing the patient in reverse Trendelenburg during induction may avoid spontaneous reduction of the hernia contents. If the hernia contents do reduce before they can be fully inspected, it is reasonable to continue with the hernia repair and closely observe the patient for peritonitis postoperatively, unless there is evidence of foul-smelling or bloody fluid intraoperatively.[16] Laparoscopy through the hernia sac may also be used as an adjunct to evaluate the bowel in this situation.[27]

Girls
Uterine adnexa are found in 15% to 31% of inguinal hernia sacs.[28] Incarceration risk is estimated to be between 4% and 15%, with strangulation occurring in 2% to 33% of incarcerated ovaries.[7,28–30] Unlike the mechanism of testicular infarction, which primarily occurs from compression of the gonadal vessels at the internal ring by incarcerated bowel, ovarian infarction primarily occurs secondary to ovarian torsion.[29,31] This higher risk of torsion in incarcerated ovaries is attributed to narrowing of the angle between the suspensory ligament of the ovary and the ovarian ligament, creating a bell-clapper–like deformity, so the ligaments are no longer able to properly support the ovary, predisposing it to twisting.[29]

There is no clear consensus on how urgently an asymptomatic incarcerated ovary requires surgery. Some studies recommend urgent intervention (within 24–48 hours),[32,33] whereas other studies recommend emergent intervention of all incarcerated ovaries, including asymptomatic and chronic incarcerations, given the higher risk of torsion.[29,34,35] Based on a 2005 survey of pediatric surgeons, 50% operate at the next available opportunity, whereas 32% operate urgently or emergently.[20]

Girls also have a higher risk of sliding hernias involving the uterus, fallopian tubes, ovaries, and/or bladder, so a more distal ligation of the hernia sac may be required to avoid injury to these structures. Goldstein and Potts[37] described a technique in which the portion of the sac that contains the sliding hernia is dissected along its border creating a flap, which is then folded and placed intraperitoneally. The remaining sac is closed with a purse-string suture.[8,16,36,37]

Management of necrotic gonads
The appearance of necrotic ovaries and testes at the time of operation does not necessarily signify irreversible damage or predict future functionality. Multiple studies report that, even with evidence of ovarian ischemia (black or blue discoloration with failure to improve after detorsion), most ovaries are viable on follow-up with evidence of follicular development.[38–40] Similarly, ischemic-appearing testes after reduction of an incarcerated hernia may survive in 25% to 50% of cases.[41] Testicular atrophy is reported to result in 2.3% to 15% of incarcerated hernias (manually and operatively reduced), although some of these cases may be a result of the surgery.[11] Given the potential for retained functionality, the current recommendation is for close postoperative monitoring with avoidance of testicular resection, unless there is frank necrosis present.[7,8]

Laparoscopic Repair

Laparoscopy is now seen as a safe approach to the management of incarcerated inguinal hernias, and there are multiple laparoscopic intraperitoneal and extraperitoneal techniques being used.

Intraperitoneal approach

A Veress needle is often placed through an infraumbilical incision. Once the desired intra-abdominal pressure is achieved (usually 10–12 mm Hg), a laparoscope is inserted through a port at the umbilicus. Two additional trocars or 3-mm stab incisions are placed in the left and right lower quadrants. The hernia is then reduced using blunt graspers and possibly external compression. Insufflation may also make reduction technically easier because it widens the internal ring.[42] The abdominal cavity and bowel are then inspected. Bowel resection is performed intracorporeally or through a small umbilical incision extracorporeally as needed. Afterward, the herniorrhaphy is performed.

There are multiple techniques described to close the defect. High ligation and closure of the ring may be performed using a variety of suturing techniques, including a Z stitch, a purse-string suture, running suture, and interrupted sutures.[43–46] Endoloop ligation has also been used to perform high ligation, but this is used in girls only, because there is a high risk of injury to the cord structures.[47] There is also the flip-flap technique, which is performed by raising a peritoneal flap anterolateral to the inguinal ring and rotating it medially over the ring and suturing it.[48] Resection of the hernia sac without ligation has also been described, and it is performed by dissecting the hernia sac away from the cord structures and then resecting the entire processus vaginalis with a rim of surrounding peritoneum. The defect is not closed and it is thought that peritoneal scarring closes the inguinal ring. Riquelme and colleagues[49] performed this procedure in 91 patients, excluding those who had a wide inguinal ring (>1 cm), and had no evidence of inguinal hernia recurrence during a follow-up period of 5 months to 4 years.

Percutaneous/extracorporeal

Single-port and 2-port techniques have both been described in repair of the inguinal ligament. The SEAL (subcutaneous endoscopically assisted ligation) and PIRS (percutaneous internal ring suturing) techniques are both variations of a single-port technique with placement of a laparoscope through the umbilicus and percutaneous placement of a suture around the internal ring.[44,50,51]

Variations of the single-port technique are the hook method and the author's variation of the PIRS technique, which include placement of a 3-mm grasper through a stab incision without placement of a trocar. The hook method is performed by using a hook to bluntly dissect around the internal ring and then looping a suture around the internal ring, which is then tied down to ligate the hernia sac.[52] The variation of the PIRS technique that is used by the author is described in detail elsewhere.[53] It involves cauterization of the internal ring using a 3-mm Maryland dissector, avoiding the portion near the cord structures. This variation, in theory, leads to scarring, which reinforces the closure and decreases the risk of recurrence. Hydrodissection is then performed using either saline or local anesthetic to create a plane between the cord structures and peritoneum. Using a combination of a curved needle and looped sutures, a double-suture ligation is performed around the inguinal ring. Two-port techniques are similar to these techniques but a trocar is placed to pass the additional instruments through.[44,54]

Single-port, 2-port, and 3-port techniques have all been effectively used in incarcerated inguinal hernia management.[42,54–57]

Outcomes

Recurrence

Recurrence rates of elective open inguinal hernia repair have been reported between 0.3% and 3.8%, with a more recent case series showing a recurrence rate of

1.2%.[7,30,58,59] Recurrence rates for laparoscopic repair are reported between 0.73% and 4.1%.[60–63] Incarcerated inguinal hernias have higher recurrence rates, reported between 1.2% and 20%.[15,30,64]

Complications

Perioperative complications (ischemia of testis, ovary, or bowel; surgical site infection; injury to surrounding structures) are reported between 4.5% and 33% in incarcerated hernias compared with between 0.6% and 1% in elective hernia repairs in healthy full-term infants.[5,15–17] Testicular atrophy after testicular infarction is estimated between 2.3% and 15%[5,11] compared with 0.3% in elective hernia repairs.[7] Wound infection rates are between 0.8% and 2%,[5,7,65] with higher rates in incarcerated hernias. Other complications include injury to surrounding structures, such as the vas deferens and bladder, which are reported to be higher in incarcerated hernias because of the edema, which may increase the difficulty of the dissection.[10]

Laparoscopic Versus Open Repair

Both techniques have been compared in the management of incarcerated inguinal hernias and have similar outcomes[66]; however, laparoscopy may have advantages compared with the conventional open repair. These advantages include easier reduction because of mechanical widening of the internal ring from pneumoperitoneum, direct visualization of the bowel to ensure complete reduction and viability, and easier visualization of the contralateral groin. It is also described as technically easier because it requires minimal dissection of the edematous tissue.[42] Laparoscopy has also been associated with a shorter hospital stay, decreased postoperative pain, and better cosmetic results,[56] although other studies report comparable hospital stays and postoperative complications.[66] There are also data suggesting possible decreased recurrence rates in laparoscopic resection compared with open resection, which is attributed to the lack of dissection of the friable hernia sac.[64,67]

Contralateral Groin Exploration

The incidence of a contralateral inguinal hernia is cited as between 5.6% and 31%, with higher incidences found in younger children (aged <2 years) and premature infants.[3,7,10,30,68,69] There is ongoing debate about whether contralateral groin exploration should be performed, especially in premature infants, given their high incidence of a contralateral hernia or patent processus vaginalis (PPV). Routine exploration evaluates for and treats a subclinical contralateral hernia and PPV, avoiding a repeat operation and future risk of incarceration. However, because not all PPVs develop into clinical hernias and there is currently no way of predicting which ones are at risk, this may result in a large number of unnecessary operations and expose patients to unnecessary surgical risks.

The incidence of PPV in infants is reported between 48% and 63%, with the highest incidence found in patients within the first 2 months of life. Rowe and colleagues[70] studied the incidence of contralateral PPV during routine open exploration and found that the incidence of PPV decreased with age. Based on this, they concluded that up to 40% of PPVs close within the first few months of life, and a subsequent 20% close by 2 years of age. Surana and Puri[71] also showed a similar trend with open explorations. Some investigators argue that open exploration may overestimate the incidence of PPV, but laparoscopic explorations also found a similar incidence of 46% to 48% in children less than 2 years of age,[72–74] also showing a decreasing incidence in older children. Furthermore, PPV is less frequently found in adults (15%–37% in autopsy studies[75] and 12% in laparoscopic studies[76]), which further supports that they may close. In addition, multiple studies have reported a low risk of developing a contralateral inguinal hernia. Clark and colleagues[77] found, in a retrospective review of more than 7000 patients, that only 3.8% develop a contralateral inguinal hernia at 10 years. Similarly, Ron and colleagues[78] found that 14 contralateral explorations are required to prevent 1 hernia. Given this, routine contralateral open groin exploration is not recommended.[75,79–83]

Laparoscopic evaluation (transumbilical or transinguinal) for a contralateral PPV has been described as a safe and effective alternative to open exploration because it does not require a separate incision and minimally increases the overall operation time.[72,74,84,85] Laparoscopic evaluation has been found to have a high sensitivity and specificity in diagnosing a contralateral PPV and hernia (99.4% and 99.5% respectively[85]), but has poor predictive value in identifying which PPV will develop into clinical hernias (11%[86]). Given this poor positive predictive value, and the potential risk of cord injury in boys, there is debate about laparoscopic repair of a PPV. Burd and colleagues[87] argue that the risks of observation, which are morbidity from incarceration and repeat anesthesia exposure, are less than the risk of perioperative complications that may occur from laparoscopic repair. Lee and colleagues[88] alternatively argue that laparoscopic repair of a contralateral PPV is more cost-effective to the patient compared with a subsequent repair, although it does subject some patients to unnecessary operations. Despite these risks, if given the option, most parents prefer to have the contralateral PPV repaired at the time of the initial operation, mainly citing convenience as the reason.[89] At this time, there does not seem to be agreement on routine laparoscopic repair of contralateral PPV, except in patients at a higher risk of developing a contralateral hernia (ie, those with left-sided hernia, connective tissue disorders, higher intra-abdominal pressure) and in patients with a higher anesthesia risk (ie, cardiopulmonary issues).[68,83,85]

Postoperative Care

Most patients are discharged home on postoperative day 0 to 1 unless additional interventions, such as bowel resection, were performed. Close monitoring for postoperative apnea is recommended in premature infants, with overnight ICU care recommended in high-risk patients.[21]

UMBILICAL HERNIA
Anatomy and Pathophysiology

The classic description of in utero intestinal development states that the primitive intestine herniates through the umbilical ring where it elongates and rotates 270° before returning to the abdominal cavity.[90–92] Following this, the physiologic diastasis recti gradually resolves as the left and right rectus abdominis muscles migrate medially to occlude the umbilical ring. Disruptions to this process are thought to cause umbilical hernia.[93]

Clinical Presentation and Evaluation

Although umbilical hernia is a common entity in children,[94] the overall rate of incarceration is traditionally thought to be extremely low, estimated at 0.07% to 0.3%.[95–97] However, the rate of incarceration in some African populations has been observed to be as high as 40%.[98–100]

Presenting symptoms of umbilical hernia incarceration are those seen commonly with bowel obstruction, namely abdominal pain, nausea, and vomiting. Physical examination shows umbilical hernia, abdominal distention, and abdominal tenderness to palpation. There may be skin changes, such as erythema, associated with the umbilicus.[94],[101–104] Although the traditional presentation is that of acute umbilical hernia incarceration, some patients have been observed to experience symptomatic, recurrent incarceration of umbilical hernia followed by spontaneous reduction.[100]

Diagnosis

Diagnosis of incarcerated umbilical hernia may be made via history and physical examination alone. However, plain abdominal radiographs may show radiographic evidence of bowel obstruction.[104],[105]

Surgical Timing

In patients with peritonitis or evidence of perforated or gangrenous bowel, surgery should not be delayed. Otherwise, reduction of the incarcerated bowel from the umbilical hernia should be performed and the surgery performed at the earliest convenience. Surgery should also be performed in an emergent fashion if attempts at hernia reduction fail.[100]

Surgical Technique

The technique for repair of umbilical hernia is straightforward and has been well described.[106],[107] The presence of incarcerated material does not necessarily change this technique.

The patient is placed in the supine position. The entire abdomen should be draped and prepped in case a larger incision is required. An infraumbilical or paraumbilical incision is performed. Dissection, either sharply or with electrocautery, is carried down to the level of the hernia sac. The umbilical hernia may contain preperitoneal adipose tissue, omentum, small bowel, large bowel, or a combination of these.[104],[105] The viability of any involved bowel must be determined. This, along with any bowel resection and anastomosis, may be possible through the initial incision, or may require enlarging the fascial opening and skin incision. The hernia sac is freed circumferentially from the fascia and subcutaneous tissues, before it and its contents are reduced into the abdomen. There is no proven benefit to resection of the hernia sac.[108] The linea alba is closed in a simple fashion and the skin is closed over this. Umbilicoplasty may be performed for improved cosmetic results, particularly for very large hernias.

Minimally invasive technique for repair has been described,[109] but this technique requires modification to fully assess the bowel and/or perform a bowel resection and anastomosis.

Postoperatively, patients may benefit from a period of nil per os with nasogastric decompression, particularly if an ileus is anticipated (eg, in patients who underwent bowel resection, those with significantly dilated bowel, or individuals who experienced delayed diagnosis and treatment).

FEMORAL HERNIA

A femoral hernia is a protrusion through the femoral ring into the femoral canal. These hernias make up less than 1% of groin hernias[110] and there have only been a limited number of case reports published describing incarceration.[111] Diagnosis can be challenging, with femoral hernia often misdiagnosed as inguinal hernia, because both may present with groin pain and bulge.[112] Definitive diagnosis sometimes may only occur at the time of surgery.[113]

Open repair occurs via an inguinal incision. The femoral defect is closed by suturing the inguinal ligament to the pectineal ligament.[114] Laparoscopic repair may be accomplished by dissecting the hernia sac from the femoral canal followed by patch and plug with prosthetic material. If the defect is very large, the iliopubic tract may be approximated to the pectineal ligament with intracorporeal suture and prosthetic patch placement over this.[115] Similarly, a laparoscopic percutaneous extracorporeal closure needle may be used to percutaneously suture the pectineal ligament to the iliopubic tract.[116] In addition, repair may be accomplished in a laparoscopic-assisted fashion with 1 abdominal incision and 1 groin incision.[117,118]

SPIGELIAN HERNIA

Spigelian hernia, also known as lateral ventral hernia, is a rare entity in pediatric surgery. Herniation occurs through the aponeurosis of the transverse abdominis, between the rectus abdominis muscle medially and the linea semilunaris laterally.[119] Patients typically present with complaints of abdominal pain and abdominal tenderness to palpation on examination. Patients may have a history of abdominal trauma.[120] Repair is effected by incision directly over, or in close proximity to, the hernia with evaluation of the bowel and a subsequent tissue repair to close the hernia defect.[120,121]

EPIGASTRIC HERNIA

Epigastric hernia typically occurs in the midline, superior to the umbilicus. These lesions tend to be solitary, but may be multiple. They comprise up to 4% of pediatric abdominal wall hernias.[122] There are no reports of bowel incarceration within an epigastric hernia, possibly because of the falciform ligament covering the visceral side of the fascial defect.[109] However, incarcerated preperitoneal fat may be encountered.[109,123,124]

Whether repaired in an open or laparoscopic fashion, the epigastric hernia must be marked at the skin level before induction of anesthesia, otherwise the hernia may become difficult to identify intraoperatively. Open repair is achieved by transverse skin incision over the hernia, reduction of any incarcerated fat and hernia sac, and primary closure of the fascial defect.[109] Laparoscopic repair may be accomplished via intracorporeal suturing of the defect[109] or percutaneous suturing.[123,124]

DIRECT INGUINAL HERNIA

Direct inguinal hernia, which is a herniation through the Hesselbach triangle, comprises less than 1% of pediatric inguinal hernias. Diagnosis is difficult, both preoperatively and intraoperatively.[125–127] Furthermore, incarcerated pediatric direct inguinal hernia is extremely rare.[128]

Open techniques for repair are similar to those described in adults, using a tissue-only approach. Laparoscopic approaches have also been described.[127,129]

LUMBAR

Fewer than 100 cases of congenital lumbar hernia have been described[130] with only 1 case of incarceration.[131] Repair may be performed in an open fashion, with incision over the hernia,[130] or laparoscopically.[132]

SUMMARY

Indirect inguinal hernias are the most commonly incarcerated pediatric hernias, with a high risk of recurrence and increased perioperative morbidity compared with elective hernia repair. Laparoscopy is increasingly being used in the management of incarcerated pediatric hernias with similar outcomes to open surgery.

REFERENCES

1. Brandt ML. Pediatric hernias. Surg Clin North Am 2008;88(1):27–43.
2. Chang S-J, Chen JY-C, Hsu C-K, et al. The incidence of inguinal hernia and associated risk factors of incarceration in pediatric inguinal hernia: a nationwide longitudinal population-based study. Hernia 2016;20(4):559–63.
3. Burgmeier C, Dreyhaupt J, Schier F. Comparison of inguinal hernia and asymptomatic patent processus vaginalis in term and preterm infants. J Pediatr Surg 2014;49(9):1416–8.
4. Lautz TB, Raval MV, Reynolds M. Does timing matter? A national perspective on the risk of incarceration in premature neonates with inguinal hernia. J Pediatr 2011;158(4):573–7.
5. Stylianos S, Jacir NN, Harris BH. Incarceration of inguinal hernia in infants prior to elective repair. J Pediatr Surg 1993;28(4):582–3.
6. Rajput A, Gauderer MWL, Hack M. Inguinal hernias in very low birth weight infants: incidence and timing of repair. J Pediatr Surg 1992;27(10):1322–4.
7. Ein SH, Njere I, Ein A. Six thousand three hundred sixty-one pediatric inguinal hernias: a 35-year review. J Pediatr Surg 2006;41(5):980–6.
8. Fraser JD, Snyder CL. Inguinal hernias and hydroceles. In: Ashcraft KW, Holcomb GW, Murphy JP, et al, editors. Ashcraft's pediatric surgery. 6th edition. London: Saunders/Elsevier; 2014. p. 679–86.
9. Mishra DS, Magu S, Sharma N, et al. Imaging in acute abdomen. Indian J Pediatr 2003;70(1):15–9.
10. Lau ST, Lee Y-H, Caty MG. Current management of hernias and hydroceles. Semin Pediatr Surg 2007;16(1):50–7.
11. Puri P, Guiney EJ, O'Donnell B. Inguinal hernia in infants: the fate of the testis following incarceration. J Pediatr Surg 1984;19(1):44–6.
12. Goldman RD, Balasubramanian S, Wales P, et al. Pediatric surgeons and pediatric emergency physicians' attitudes towards analgesia and sedation for incarcerated inguinal hernia reduction. J Pain 2005;6(10):650–5.
13. Ibrahim AM, Ponsky TA. Inguinal hernia. In: Pachl M, De La Hunt MN, Jawaheer G, editors. Key clinical topics in paediatric surgery. London: JP Medical; 2014. p. 176–8.
14. Strauch ED, Voigt RW, Hill JL. Gangrenous intestine in a hernia can be reduced. J Pediatr Surg 2002;37(6):919–20.
15. Niedzielski J, Kr I R, Gawłowska A. Could incarceration of inguinal hernia in children be prevented? Med Sci Monit 2003;9(1):CR16–8.
16. Kurkchubasche AG, Tracy TF. Inguinal hernia/hydrocele. Operat Tech Gen Surg 2004;6(4):253–68.
17. Rescorla FJ, Grosfeld JL. Inguinal hernia repair in the perinatal period and early infancy: clinical considerations. J Pediatr Surg 1984;19(6):832–7.
18. Vaos G, Gardikis S, Kambouri K, et al. Optimal timing for repair of an inguinal hernia in premature infants. Pediatr Surg Int 2010;26(4):379–85.
19. Gahukamble D, Khamage A. Early versus delayed repair of reduced incarcerated inguinal hernias in the pediatric population. J Pediatr Surg 1996;31(9):1218–20.
20. Antonoff MB, Kreykes NS, Saltzman DA, et al. American Academy of Pediatrics section on surgery hernia survey revisited. J Pediatr Surg 2005;40(6):1009–14.

21. Murphy JJ, Swanson T, Ansermino M, et al. The frequency of apneas in premature infants after inguinal hernia repair: do they need overnight monitoring in the intensive care unit? J Pediatr Surg 2008;43(5):865–8.
22. Baird R, Gholoum S, Laberge J-M, et al. Prematurity, not age at operation or incarceration, impacts complication rates of inguinal hernia repair. J Pediatr Surg 2011;46(5):908–11.
23. Nagraj S, Sinha S, Grant H, et al. The incidence of complications following primary inguinal herniotomy in babies weighing 5 kg or less. Pediatr Surg Int 2006; 22(6):500–2.
24. Jones LJ, Craven PD, Lakkundi A, et al. Regional (spinal, epidural, caudal) versus general anaesthesia in preterm infants undergoing inguinal herniorrhaphy in early infancy. In: The Cochrane Collaboration, editor. Cochrane database of systematic reviews. Chichester (United Kingdom): John Wiley; 2015. p. 1–38. Available at: http://doi.wiley.com/10.1002/14651858.CD003669.pub2. Accessed July 25, 2016.
25. Banks SB, Cotlar AM. Classic groin hernia repair...lest we forget. Curr Surg 2005;62(2):249–52.
26. Williams C. Repair of sliding inguinal hernia through the abdominal (Laroque) approach. Ann Surg 1947;126(4):612–23.
27. Lin E, Wear K, Tiszenkel HI. Planned reduction of incarcerated groin hernias with hernia sac laparoscopy. Surg Endosc 2002;16(6):936–8.
28. Cascini V, Lisi G, Di Renzo D, et al. Irreducible indirect inguinal hernia containing uterus and bilateral adnexa in a premature female infant: report of an exceptional case and review of the literature. J Pediatr Surg 2013;48(1):e17–9.
29. Boley SJ, Cahn D, Lauer T, et al. The irreducible ovary: a true emergency. J Pediatr Surg 1991;26(9):1035–8.
30. Erdoğan D, Karaman İ, Aslan MK, et al. Analysis of 3776 pediatric inguinal hernia and hydrocele cases in a tertiary center. J Pediatr Surg 2013;48(8):1767–72.
31. Merriman TE, Auldist AW. Ovarian torsion in inguinal hernias. Pediatr Surg Int 2000;16(5–6):383–5.
32. Takehara H, Hanaoka J, Arakawa Y. Laparoscopic strategy for inguinal ovarian hernias in children: when to operate for irreducible ovary. J Laparoendosc Adv Surg Tech A 2009;19(Suppl 1):s129–31.
33. van Heurn LWE, Pakarinen MP, Wester T. Contemporary management of abdominal surgical emergencies in infants and children: abdominal surgical emergencies in infants and children. Br J Surg 2014;101(1):e24–33.
34. Houben CH, Chan KWE, Mou JWC, et al. Irreducible inguinal hernia in children: how serious is it? J Pediatr Surg 2015;50(7):1174–6.
35. El Gohary A. Sliding ovary inside a hernia sac; a true emergency. J Pediatr Surg Case Rep 2014;2(12):522–3.
36. Fowler CL. Sliding indirect hernia containing both ovaries. J Pediatr Surg 2005; 40(9):e13–4.
37. Goldstein IR, Potts WJ. Inguinal hernia in female infants and children. Ann Surg 1958;148(5):819–22.
38. Parelkar SV, Mundada D, Sanghvi BV, et al. Should the ovary always be conserved in torsion? A tertiary care institute experience. J Pediatr Surg 2014; 49(3):465–8.
39. Aziz D, Davis V, Allen L, et al. Ovarian torsion in children: is oophorectomy necessary? J Pediatr Surg 2004;39(5):750–3.
40. Çelik A, Ergün O, Aldemir H, et al. Long-term results of conservative management of adnexal torsion in children. J Pediatr Surg 2005;40(4):704–8.

41. Hill MR, Pollock WF, Sprong DH. Testicular infarction and incarcerated inguinal herniae. Arch Surg 1962;85:351–4.
42. Kaya M, Hückstedt T, Schier F. Laparoscopic approach to incarcerated inguinal hernia in children. J Pediatr Surg 2006;41(3):567–9.
43. Chan KL, Tam PK. A safe laparoscopic technique for the repair of inguinal hernias in boys. J Am Coll Surg 2003;196(6):987–9.
44. Saranga Bharathi R, Arora M, Baskaran V. Minimal access surgery of pediatric inguinal hernias: a review. Surg Endosc 2008;22(8):1751–62.
45. Schier F. Laparoscopic surgery of inguinal hernias in children—initial experience. J Pediatr Surg 2000;35(9):1331–5.
46. Gorsler CM, Schier F. Laparoscopic herniorrhaphy in children. Surg Endosc 2003;17(4):571–3.
47. Zallen G, Glick PL. Laparoscopic inversion and ligation inguinal hernia repair in girls. J Laparoendosc Adv Surg Tech A 2007;17(1):143–5.
48. Yip KF, Tam PKH, Li MKW. Laparoscopic flip-flap hernioplasty: an innovative technique for pediatric hernia surgery. Surg Endosc 2004;18(7):1126–9.
49. Riquelme M, Aranda A, Riquelme- QM. Laparoscopic pediatric inguinal hernia repair: no ligation, just resection. J Laparoendosc Adv Surg Tech A 2010; 20(1):77–80.
50. Patkowski D, Czernik J, Chrzan R, et al. Percutaneous internal ring suturing: a simple minimally invasive technique for inguinal hernia repair in children. J Laparoendosc Adv Surg Tech A 2006;16(5):513–7.
51. Harrison MR, Lee H, Albanese CT, et al. Subcutaneous endoscopically assisted ligation (SEAL) of the internal ring for repair of inguinal hernias in children: a novel technique. J Pediatr Surg 2005;40(7):1177–80.
52. Tam YH, Lee KH, Sihoe JDY, et al. Laparoscopic hernia repair in children by the hook method: a single-center series of 433 consecutive patients. J Pediatr Surg 2009;44(8):1502–5.
53. Ostlie DJ, Ponsky TA. Technical options of the laparoscopic pediatric inguinal hernia repair. J Laparoendosc Adv Surg Tech A 2014;24(3):194–8.
54. Shalaby R, Moniem Shams A, Mohamed S, et al. Two-trocar needlescopic approach to incarcerated inguinal hernia in children. J Pediatr Surg 2007; 42(7):1259–62.
55. Chan KWE, Lee KH, Tam YH, et al. Laparoscopic inguinal hernia repair by the hook method in emergency setting in children presenting with incarcerated inguinal hernia. J Pediatr Surg 2011;46(10):1970–3.
56. Zhou X, Peng L, Sha Y, et al. Transumbilical endoscopic surgery for incarcerated inguinal hernias in infants and children. J Pediatr Surg 2014;49(1):214–7.
57. Koivusalo A, Pakarinen MP, Rintala RJ. Laparoscopic herniorrhaphy after manual reduction of incarcerated inguinal hernia. Surg Endosc 2007;21(12): 2147–9.
58. Grosfeld JL, Minnick K, Shedd F, et al. Inguinal hernia in children: factors affecting recurrence in 62 cases. J Pediatr Surg 1991;26(3):283–7.
59. Tiryaki T, Baskin D, Bulut M. Operative complications of hernia repair in childhood. Pediatr Surg Int 1998;13(2–3):160–1.
60. Schier F. Laparoscopic inguinal hernia repair—a prospective personal series of 542 children. J Pediatr Surg 2006;41(6):1081–4.
61. Parelkar SV, Oak S, Gupta R, et al. Laparoscopic inguinal hernia repair in the pediatric age group—experience with 437 children. J Pediatr Surg 2010; 45(4):789–92.

62. Schier F, Montupet P, Esposito C. Laparoscopic inguinal herniorrhaphy in children: a three-center experience with 933 repairs. J Pediatr Surg 2002;37(3): 395–7.
63. Takehara H, Yakabe S, Kameoka K. Laparoscopic percutaneous extraperitoneal closure for inguinal hernia in children: clinical outcome of 972 repairs done in 3 pediatric surgical institutions. J Pediatr Surg 2006;41(12):1999–2003.
64. Esposito C, Turial S, Alicchio F, et al. Laparoscopic repair of incarcerated inguinal hernia. A safe and effective procedure to adopt in children. Hernia 2013;17(2):235–9.
65. Meier AH, Ricketts RR. Surgical complications of inguinal and abdominal wall hernias. Semin Pediatr Surg 2003;12(2):83–8.
66. Mishra PK, Burnand K, Minocha A, et al. Incarcerated inguinal hernia management in children: "a comparison of the open and laparoscopic approach". Pediatr Surg Int 2014;30(6):621–4.
67. Dutta S, Albanese C. Transcutaneous laparoscopic hernia repair in children: a prospective review of 275 hernia repairs with minimum 2-year follow-up. Surg Endosc 2009;23(1):103–7.
68. Tackett LD, Breuer CK, Luks FI, et al. Incidence of contralateral inguinal hernia: a prospective analysis. J Pediatr Surg 1999;34(5):684–7 [discussion: 687–8].
69. Nataraja RM, Mahomed AA. Systematic review for paediatric metachronous contralateral inguinal hernia: a decreasing concern. Pediatr Surg Int 2011; 27(9):953–61.
70. Rowe MI, Copelson LW, Clatworthy HW. The patent processus vaginalis and the inguinal hernia. J Pediatr Surg 1969;4(1):102–7.
71. Surana R, Puri P. Fate of patent processus vaginalis: a case against routine contralateral exploration for unilateral inguinal hernia in children. Pediatr Surg Int 1993;8(5):412–4.
72. Lazar DA, Lee TC, Almulhim SI, et al. Transinguinal laparoscopic exploration for identification of contralateral inguinal hernias in pediatric patients. J Pediatr Surg 2011;46(12):2349–52.
73. Toufique Ehsan M, Ng ATL, Chung PHY, et al. Laparoscopic hernioplasties in children: the implication on contralateral groin exploration for unilateral inguinal hernias. Pediatr Surg Int 2009;25(9):759–62.
74. Yerkes EB, Brock JW, Holcomb GW, et al. Laparoscopic evaluation for a contralateral patent processus vaginalis: part III. Urology 1998;51(3):480–3.
75. Shabbir J, Moore A, O'Sullivan JB, et al. Contralateral groin exploration is not justified in infants with a unilateral inguinal hernia. Ir J Med Sci 2003;172(1): 18–9.
76. van Veen RN, van Wessem KJP, Halm JA, et al. Patent processus vaginalis in the adult as a risk factor for the occurrence of indirect inguinal hernia. Surg Endosc 2007;21(2):202–5.
77. Clark JJ, Limm W, Wong LL. What is the likelihood of requiring contralateral inguinal hernia repair after unilateral repair? Am J Surg 2011;202(6):754–8.
78. Ron O, Eaton S, Pierro A. Systematic review of the risk of developing a metachronous contralateral inguinal hernia in children. Br J Surg 2007;94(7):804–11.
79. Maillet OP, Garnier S, Dadure C, et al. Inguinal hernia in premature boys: should we systematically explore the contralateral side? J Pediatr Surg 2014;49(9): 1419–23.
80. Ballantyne A, Jawaheer G, Munro FD. Contralateral groin exploration is not justified in infants with a unilateral inguinal hernia. Br J Surg 2001;88(5):720–3.

81. Chertin B, De Caluwé D, Gajaharan M, et al. Is contralateral exploration necessary in girls with unilateral inguinal hernia? J Pediatr Surg 2003;38(5):756–7.

82. Marulaiah M, Atkinson J, Kukkady A, et al. Is contralateral exploration necessary in preterm infants with unilateral inguinal hernia? J Pediatr Surg 2006;41(12): 2004–7.

83. Ikeda H, Suzuki N, Takahashi A, et al. Risk of contralateral manifestation in children with unilateral inguinal hernia: should hernia in children be treated contralaterally? J Pediatr Surg 2000;35(12):1746–8.

84. Saad S, Mansson J, Saad A, et al. Ten-year review of groin laparoscopy in 1001 pediatric patients with clinical unilateral inguinal hernia: an improved technique with transhernia multiple-channel scope. J Pediatr Surg 2011;46(5):1011–4.

85. Miltenburg DM, Nuchtern JG, Jaksic T, et al. Laparoscopic evaluation of the pediatric inguinal hernia–a meta-analysis. J Pediatr Surg 1998;33(6):874–9.

86. Maddox MM, Smith DP. A long-term prospective analysis of pediatric unilateral inguinal hernias: should laparoscopy or anything else influence the management of the contralateral side? J Pediatr Urol 2008;4(2):141–5.

87. Burd RS, Heffington SH, Teague JL. The optimal approach for management of metachronous hernias in children: a decision analysis. J Pediatr Surg 2001; 36(8):1190–5.

88. Lee SL, Sydorak RM, Lau ST. Laparoscopic contralateral groin exploration: is it cost effective? J Pediatr Surg 2010;45(4):793–5.

89. Holcomb GW, Miller KA, Chaignaud BE, et al. The parental perspective regarding the contralateral inguinal region in a child with a known unilateral inguinal hernia. J Pediatr Surg 2004;39(3):480–2.

90. Kim WK, Kim H, Ahn DH, et al. Timetable for intestinal rotation in staged human embryos and fetuses. Birth Defects Res A Clin Mol Teratol 2003;67(11):941–5.

91. Metzger R, Wachowiak R, Kluth D. Embryology of the early foregut. Semin Pediatr Surg 2011;20(3):136–44.

92. Soffers JH, Hikspoors JP, Mekonen HK, et al. The growth pattern of the human intestine and its mesentery. BMC Dev Biol 2015;15(1):31.

93. Mekonen HK, Hikspoors JPJM, Mommen G, et al. Development of the ventral body wall in the human embryo. J Anat 2015;227(5):673–85.

94. Papagrigoriadis S, Browse DJ, Howard ER. Incarceration of umbilical hernias in children: a rare but important complication. Pediatr Surg Int 1998;14(3):231–2.

95. Crump EP. Umbilical hernia. I. Occurrence of the infantile type in Negro infants and children. J Pediatr 1952;40(2):214–23.

96. Mestel AL, Burns H. Incarcerated and strangulated umbilical hernias in infants and children. Clin Pediatr (Phila) 1963;2:368–70.

97. Blumberg NA. Infantile umbilical hernia. Surg Gynecol Obstet 1980;150(2): 187–92.

98. Mawera G, Muguti GI. Umbilical hernia in Bulawayo: some observations from a hospital based study. Cent Afr J Med 1994;40(11):319–23.

99. Ameh EA, Chirdan LB, Nmadu PT, et al. Complicated umbilical hernias in children. Pediatr Surg Int 2003;19(4):280–2.

100. Chirdan LB, Uba AF, Kidmas AT. Incarcerated umbilical hernia in children. Eur J Pediatr Surg 2006;16(1):45–8.

101. Vrsansky P, Bourdelat D. Incarcerated umbilical hernia in children. Pediatr Surg Int 1997;12(1):61–2.

102. Okada T, Yoshida H, Iwai J, et al. Strangulated umbilical hernia in a child: report of a case. Surg Today 2001;31(6):546–9.

103. Keshtgar AS, Griffiths M. Incarceration of umbilical hernia in children: is the trend increasing? Eur J Pediatr Surg 2003;13(1):40–3.

104. Brown RA, Numanoglu A, Rode H. Complicated umbilical hernia in childhood. S Afr J Surg 2006;44(4):136–7.

105. Fall I, Sanou A, Ngom G, et al. Strangulated umbilical hernias in children. Pediatr Surg Int 2006;22(3):233–5.

106. Kokoska E, Weber TR. Umbilical and supraumbilical disease. In: Ziegler MM, Azizkhan RG, Von Allmen D, et al, editors. Operative pediatric surgery. 2nd edition. 2014. Available at: http://accesssurgery.mhmedical.com/book.aspx?bookid=959. Accessed July 25, 2016.

107. Ashcraft KW, Holcomb GW, Murphy JP, et al, editors. Umbilical and other abdominal wall hernias. In: Ashcraft's pediatric surgery. 6th edition. London: Saunders/Elsevier; 2014.

108. Alvear DT, Pilling GP. Management of the sac during umbilical hernia repair in children. Am J Surg 1974;127(5):518–20.

109. Albanese CT, Rengal S, Bermudez D. A novel laparoscopic technique for the repair of pediatric umbilical and epigastric hernias. J Pediatr Surg 2006;41(4): 859–62.

110. Al-Shanafey S, Giacomantonio M. Femoral hernia in children. J Pediatr Surg 1999;34(7):1104–6.

111. Tsushimi T, Takahashi T, Gohra H, et al. A case of incarcerated femoral hernia in an infant. J Pediatr Surg 2005;40(3):581–3.

112. De Caluwé D, Chertin B, Puri P. Childhood femoral hernia: a commonly misdiagnosed condition. Pediatr Surg Int 2003;19(8):608–9.

113. Temiz A, Akcora B, Temiz M, et al. A rare and frequently unrecognised pathology in children: femoral hernia. Hernia 2008;12(5):553–6.

114. Ollero Fresno JC, Alvarez M, Sanchez M, et al. Femoral hernia in childhood: review of 38 cases. Pediatr Surg Int 1997;12(7):520–1.

115. Lee SL, DuBois JJ. Laparoscopic diagnosis and repair of pediatric femoral hernia: initial experience of four cases. Surg Endosc 2000;14(12):1110–3.

116. Tainaka T, Uchida H, Ono Y, et al. A new modification of laparoscopic percutaneous extraperitoneal closure procedure for repairing pediatric femoral hernias involving a special needle and a wire loop. Nagoya J Med Sci 2015;77(3):531–5.

117. Adibe OO, Hansen EN, Seifarth FG, et al. Laparoscopic-assisted repair of femoral hernias in children. J Laparoendosc Adv Surg Tech A 2009;19(5):691–4.

118. Tan SY, Stevens MJ, Mueller CM. A novel laparoscopic-assisted approach to the repair of pediatric femoral hernias. J Laparoendosc Adv Surg Tech A 2013; 23(11):946–8.

119. Skandalakis PN, Zoras O, Skandalakis JE, et al. Spigelian hernia: surgical anatomy, embryology, and technique of repair. Am Surg 2006;72(1):42–8.

120. Losanoff J, Richman B, Jones J. Spigelian hernia in a child: case report and review of the literature. Hernia 2002;6(4):191–3.

121. Vaos G, Gardikis S, Zavras N. Strangulated low spigelian hernia in children: report of two cases. Pediatr Surg Int 2005;21(9):736–8.

122. Coats RD, Helikson MA, Burd RS. Presentation and management of epigastric hernias in children. J Pediatr Surg 2000;35(12):1754–6.

123. Babsail AA, Abelson JS, Liska D, et al. Single-incision pediatric endosurgical epigastric hernia repair. Hernia 2014;18(3):357–60.

124. Moreira-Pinto J, Correia-Pinto J. Scarless laparoscopic repair of epigastric hernia in children. Hernia 2015;19(4):623–6.

125. Viidik T, Marshall DG. Direct inguinal hernias in infancy and early childhood. J Pediatr Surg 1980;15(5):646–7.
126. Wright JE. Direct inguinal hernia in infancy and childhood. Pediatr Surg Int 1994; 9(3):161–3.
127. Schier F. Direct inguinal hernias in children: laparoscopic aspects. Pediatr Surg Int 2000;16(8):562–4.
128. Gnidec AA, Marshall DG. Incarcerated direct inguinal hernia containing uterus, both ovaries, and fallopian tubes. J Pediatr Surg 1986;21(11):986.
129. Schier F. Laparoscopic herniorrhaphy in girls. J Pediatr Surg 1998;33(10): 1495–7.
130. Sharma A, Pandey A, Rawat J, et al. Congenital lumbar hernia: 20 years' single centre experience: congenital lumbar hernia. J Paediatr Child Health 2012; 48(11):1001–3.
131. Hancock BJ, Wiseman NE. Incarcerated congenital lumbar hernia associated with the lumbocostovertebral syndrome. J Pediatr Surg 1988;23(8):782–3.
132. Zwaveling S, van der Zee D. Laparoscopic repair of an isolated congenital bilateral lumbar hernia in an infant. Eur J Pediatr Surg 2012;22(04):321–3.

Intestinal Rotation Abnormalities and Midgut Volvulus

Jacob C. Langer, MD

KEYWORDS

- Malrotation • Nonrotation • Heterotaxia • Intestinal obstruction • Bilious vomiting

KEY POINTS

- Rotation abnormalities represent a spectrum from non-rotation to normal rotation.
- Malrotation may result in lethal midgut volvulus. Any child with bilious vomiting must be assumed to have midgut volvulus until proven otherwise.
- The gold standard for the diagnosis of a rotation abnormality is an upper gastrointestinal contrast study looking for the location of the duodenojejunal junction.
- A laparoscopic approach is useful for children without midgut volvulus. Infants, and older children with suspected midgut volvulus should undergo laparotomy.

INTRODUCTION: NATURE OF THE PROBLEM

Intestinal rotation abnormalities constitute a spectrum of conditions that occur during the normal embryologic process of intestinal rotation. In some patients the rotation abnormality is asymptomatic, but others experience a variety of symptoms, including obstruction, lymphatic and venous congestion, and misdiagnosis of appendicitis in an abnormally positioned appendix **Box 1**. The most important form of obstruction is midgut volvulus, which may be fatal. For this reason, it is important for all surgeons to have an understanding of rotation abnormalities, and to have a high index of suspicion in any patient with signs and symptoms of intestinal obstruction.

RELEVANT EMBRYOLOGY AND ANATOMY

Intestinal rotation occurs during the fourth through twelfth weeks of gestation.[1] During the fourth to fifth week postconception, the straight tube of the primitive embryonic intestinal tract begins to elongate more rapidly than the embryo, causing it to buckle ventrally and force the duodenum, jejunum, ileum, and the ascending and transverse colon to extend into the umbilical cord. The duodenum curves downward and to the right of the axis of the artery, initially completing a 90° counterclockwise turn. Over the next 3 weeks, the duodenum continues to rotate so that, by the end of 8 weeks, it has

Division of General and Thoracic Surgery, Hospital for Sick Children, University of Toronto, Room 1524, 555 University Avenue, Toronto, Ontario M5G1X8, Canada
E-mail address: jacob.langer@sickkids.ca

Surg Clin N Am 97 (2017) 147–159
http://dx.doi.org/10.1016/j.suc.2016.08.011
0039-6109/17/© 2016 Elsevier Inc. All rights reserved.

surgical.theclinics.com

Box 1
Signs and symptoms of intestinal rotation abnormalities

Nonrotation

  Asymptomatic

  Associated motility disorder

  Associated condition (eg, abdominal wall defect, diaphragmatic hernia, heterotaxia)

  Appendicitis in abnormal location

Malrotation without volvulus

  Asymptomatic

  Bilious vomiting caused by Ladd bands or associated duodenal web

  Associated medical condition (eg, heterotaxia syndrome)

  Appendicitis in abnormal location

Malrotation with volvulus

  Bilious vomiting

  Abdominal pain

  Hematochezia

  Peritonitis

  Death

Malrotation with partial or intermittent volvulus

  Protein-losing enteropathy

  Abdominal pain

  Failure to thrive

  Malnutrition

  Occult gastrointestinal bleeding

---

undergone 180° rotation. During the tenth gestational week the intestines return to the abdomen. The cecum is the final portion of the intestine to return and does so by rotating superiorly and anteriorly around the superior mesenteric artery (SMA). This sequence of return causes the duodenum and proximal jejunum to be pushed superiorly and to the left posterior to the SMA so that they become fixed in a 270° rotation from their initial position. Fixation of the intestines in this position takes place over the fourth and fifth months of gestation.

DEFINITIONS OF INTESTINAL ROTATION ABNORMALITIES

The spectrum of intestinal rotation abnormalities arises from perturbations in the sequence of herniation, rotation, and fixation of the midgut. If the cecocolic loop returns to the abdomen before the return of the proximal foregut, the duodenum and jejunum are not pushed superior-laterally and undergo only 180° of rotation. In this scenario, the cecum does not undergo proper fixation and the colon remains on the left side of the abdomen, whereas the midgut fills in the space on the right and the duodenum descends directly along the course of the SMA. This condition is termed nonrotation and, because it is associated with a wide-based mesentery, does not put the child at risk for midgut volvulus. Classic malrotation occurs as a result of failed extracelomic rotation. It is most commonly characterized by a duodenal-jejunal junction (DJJ) located in the right upper quadrant and a cecum located in the middle to upper abdomen, which is fixed in place by adhesive bands to the gallbladder, duodenum, and right-sided abdominal wall (Ladd bands). Most importantly, classic malrotation results in a narrowed mesenteric base, which predisposes the child to potentially fatal midgut volvulus (**Fig. 1**). Less commonly, the bowel makes a 90° turn clockwise, rather than counterclockwise, resulting in reverse rotation, in which the duodenum lies anterior to the SMA and the colon lies posteriorly, producing a retroarterial tunnel, which may be associated with partial mesenteric arterial, venous, and lymphatic obstruction. If the mesoderm does not fuse to the retroperitoneum during the fourth and fifth months of gestation, paraduodenal or paracolic hernias may form.

CLINICAL PRESENTATION

The reported incidence of rotation abnormalities varies widely, depending largely on how they are defined. Autopsy series suggest an incidence of 0.5%. A population-based study estimated an incidence of approximately 15 per 1 million in children less than 1 year old and 10 per 1 million in children aged 1 to 2 years,[2] with a decreasing incidence after that. Associated congenital abnormalities are found in approximately 30% to 60% of cases and may include intestinal atresia or web (the most common associated anomaly), Meckel diverticulum, intussusception, Hirschsprung disease, mesenteric cyst, and anomalies of the extrahepatic biliary system. Congenital diaphragmatic hernia and abdominal wall defects such as omphalocele and gastroschisis are typically associated with an intestinal rotation abnormality, usually nonrotation, because the intestine is in an abnormal location during the time it should be undergoing rotation. Many children with intestinal motility disorders have associated rotation abnormalities. In addition, rotation abnormalities are commonly associated with congenital heart disease, often in the context of one of the various heterotaxia syndromes (HS).

The classic presentation of malrotation is bilious vomiting in a newborn infant, and every child with bilious vomiting should be assumed to have malrotation until proved otherwise. Bilious vomiting may occur for 3 reasons (which are not necessarily mutually exclusive): obstructive compression of the duodenum by Ladd bands, an associated duodenal atresia or web, or (more ominously) midgut volvulus. Midgut volvulus occurs around the narrow-based mesenteric pedicle, causing twisting of the SMA and superior mesenteric vein (SMV). The abdomen is not distended initially because the obstruction is very proximal. As the intestine becomes ischemic, the patient may develop hematochezia, irritability, pain, abdominal distension, and peritonitis. Ultimately, abdominal wall erythema, septic shock, and death may occur as the midgut becomes necrotic. Many of these findings are similar to those found in neonates with necrotizing enterocolitis; the presence of bilious vomiting or nasogastric tube aspirates should suggest the possibility of midgut volvulus as part of the differential diagnosis. In older children, chronic, partial, or intermittent volvulus may present with crampy abdominal pain, intermittent vomiting, diarrhea, occult gastrointestinal bleeding, protein-losing enteropathy caused by lymphatic obstruction, failure to thrive, or malnutrition. Distension is frequently present, although it may be intermittent.

Although volvulus associated with malrotation represents the condition's most acute, dramatic, and urgent presentation, duodenal obstruction may also be caused by Ladd (or other congenital) bands, even without midgut volvulus. In neonates, these bands can cause incomplete obstruction with feeding intolerance with or without bilious vomiting. Older children more commonly present with intermittently colicky abdominal pain associated with bilious emesis. An internal hernia associated with

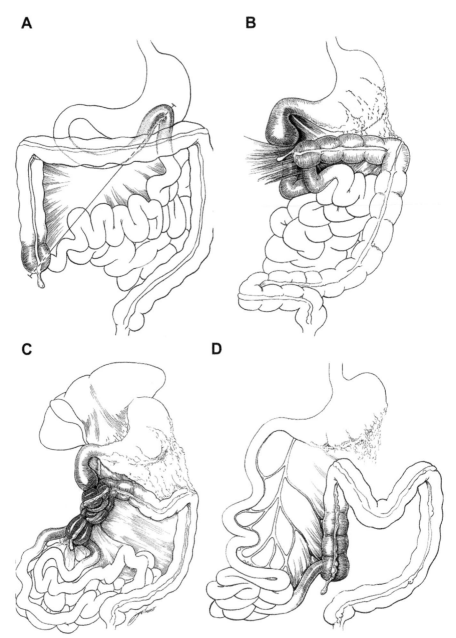

Fig. 1. (*A*) Normal intestinal rotation, (*B*) malrotation without volvulus, (*C*) malrotation with volvulus, (*D*) nonrotation.

inappropriate intestinal fixation may present in a similar fashion. Chronically symptomatic patients commonly present with recurrent respiratory symptoms, including asthma and aspiration. In addition, it is important to remember that children with a rotation abnormality may also have duodenal or jejunal atresia or web, which may be missed if the surgeon is not specifically looking for it.

RADIOLOGIC DIAGNOSIS

Prenatal diagnosis of isolated rotational abnormality is very uncommon, but fetal ultra-sonography may show the sequelae of prenatal midgut volvulus, such as bowel dilatation, meconium peritonitis, and/or fetal ascites.

Postnatally, most children with vomiting have plain abdominal radiography, which is nonspecific for the diagnosis of rotation abnormalities. Proximal obstruction caused by Ladd bands, incomplete volvulus, or associated duodenal atresia or web may present with a double bubble and a paucity of distal air. Infants with established intestinal ischemia may have pneumatosis intestinalis, which may lead to confusion with a diagnosis of necrotizing enterocolitis. Although unusual, a pattern of distal bowel obstruction consisting of multiple dilated bowel loops with air-fluid levels may be seen. Most importantly, children with rotation abnormalities, including malrotation with volvulus, may initially present with a normal bowel gas pattern (**Fig. 2**).

The current gold standard for the diagnosis of a rotation abnormality is upper gastrointestinal contrast radiography (UGI) to evaluate the position of the DJJ, which should be located to the left of the vertebral body at the level of the inferior margin of the duodenal bulb on an anteroposterior projection and must travel posteriorly on the lateral projection.[3] If the DJJ does not show these radiographic characteristics, a diagnosis of rotation abnormality should be entertained. However, conditions such as splenomegaly, renal or retroperitoneal tumors, gastric overdistension, liver transplant, small bowel obstruction, and scoliosis may cause the DJJ to be medially or inferiorly displaced. The group at the University of Arkansas attempted to define risk of malrotation, ischemic volvulus, and internal hernia in a group of consecutive patients undergoing operation for rotation abnormalities based on the positioning of the DJJ on initial UGI series.[4] The rotation abnormality was described as typical if the DJJ was positioned to the right of the midline or if it was absent, and atypical if the DJJ was at or to the left of the midline and the DJJ was low-lying. At the time of operation, volvulus had occurred in 12 of 75 typical patients versus 2 of 101 atypical patients. Internal hernias were also more common in typical than in atypical patients. Moreover, this group found that 11% to 13% of atypical patients had persistent postoperative symptoms compared with 0% of typical patients. Given the cited postoperative bowel obstruction rate following Ladd procedure (8%–12%) and the fairly high incidence of continued symptoms, the investigators advocated careful discussion in patients with atypical radiological findings. In this group a laparoscopic approach might be particularly useful (discussed later).

If the UGI is confusing or equivocal, a small bowel follow-through or a contrast enema to visualize the cecum should also be done. A short distance between the DJJ and the cecum strongly suggests the presence of malrotation with a narrow-based mesentery, and therefore a risk of midgut volvulus. However, there is a wide range of variability in normal cecal positioning and fixation, especially in neonates, and therefore a cecum located in the right lower quadrant cannot definitively rule out malrotation, and a cecum located in the right upper quadrant or epigastrium is not diagnostic of malrotation. Examples of contrast studies in the diagnosis of intestinal rotation abnormalities are shown in **Fig. 3**.

More recently, identification of an abnormal orientation of the SMA and SMV on ultrasonography has been advocated as a noninvasive way to screen for malrotation.[5] In addition, the presence of a whirlpool sign on Doppler ultrasonography has been correlated with the presence of midgut volvulus. However, the sensitivity and specificity of ultrasonography are not sufficient for it to replace UGI for a definitive diagnosis. In children with peritonitis who are too unstable to have UGI, in which midgut volvulus is part

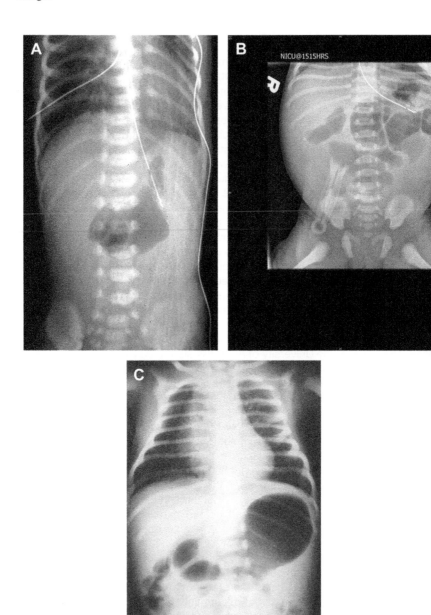

Fig. 2. The varying appearances of malrotation on plain film. (*A*) Gasless abdomen with dilated gastric bubble; (*B*) dilated small bowel suggestive of a distal obstruction; (*C*) normal film with slightly dilated duodenum.

of the differential diagnosis, a normal SMA/SMV orientation and absence of a whirl-pool sign may provide reassurance that the diagnosis is not midgut volvulus.

Although radiographic techniques are important diagnostic aids in the nonacute setting, infants who present in extremis with a history of bilious emesis and findings of peritonitis should be aggressively resuscitated, decompressed via nasogastric

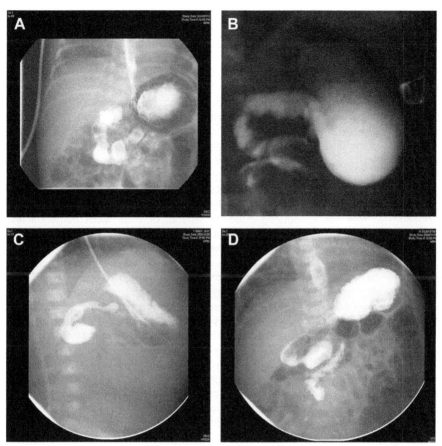

Fig. 3. UGI series with small bowel follow-through. (*A*) Normal contrast study showing the duodenal C loop crossing the midline. (*B*) Lateral view of malrotation, showing corkscrew appearance of jejunum. (*C*) Lateral view suggestive of duodenal obstruction secondary to Ladd bands or volvulus. (*D*) False-positive study; duodenal-jejunal junction is pushed rightward by large multicystic kidney.

tube, and taken for an emergent exploratory laparotomy even without a radiological diagnosis.

SURGICAL TECHNIQUE

The operative correction of malrotation was initially described by William Ladd, and has changed little since then. Most surgeons begin an open approach to a Ladd procedure via a transverse supraumbilical incision with the patient placed in the supine position. In neonates a circumumbilical omega incision affords the same access to the midgut and mesentery with a considerable cosmetic benefit.[6] On entering the abdomen, rotation and fixation of the bowel are assessed by delivering the entire midgut into the operative field. The presence of chylous ascites may indicate chronic lymphatic obstruction caused by partial midgut volvulus. If volvulus is encountered, the involved loops of bowel are gently detorsed by counterclockwise rotation until the mesentery is unfurled. At this time, the bowel is assessed for viability. Reperfusion and delineating of viable from nonviable bowel may take several minutes. During this period, the bowel should be covered with a warm, damp laparotomy pad or towel to help prevent evaporative losses and vasoconstriction. Following this, a Ladd procedure is performed. This operation consists of 4 discreet steps, the goal of which is to place the bowel into a position of nonrotation, with the small bowel on the right side of the abdomen and the colon on the left: (1) division of any abnormal bands (Ladd bands) fixing the bowel to the right upper quadrant retroperitoneal or intra-abdominal structures; (2) mobilization and rotation of the colon toward the left, taking care not to injure the colonic mesentery in the process, so that the entire colon sits on the left side of the abdomen; (3) mobilization and straightening of the duodenum so that it heads inferiorly and all the small bowel sits on the right side of the abdomen; (4) broadening of the base of the mesentery by dividing the congenital bands along the SMA and SMV. If the child has presented with duodenal obstruction, duodenal patency should be tested by milking gastric contents from the proximal to the distal duodenum to rule out associated duodenal atresia or web. Most surgeons also perform an appendectomy, either by excision or using an inversion technique (**Fig. 4**).

Before closing the abdomen, small bowel viability should be reassessed. Any frankly necrotic sections should be resected. If the rest of the bowel is completely viable, a primary anastomosis can be performed, and, if not, stomas should be created. If there are large sections of bowel in which viability is still unclear, resection should not be done, and a second-look laparotomy should be planned for 24 to 48 hours later. More ethically problematic is the situation in which the entire midgut is clearly necrotic, and resection of the bowel will result in short bowel syndrome. Options include closing the abdomen without resection and offering palliative care, or performing a massive resection and creating intestinal failure, with long-term need for total parenteral nutrition. Although historically the prognosis for neonatal intestinal failure was dismal because of the extremely high incidence of fatal cholestatic liver failure, improvements in intestinal rehabilitation and small bowel transplantation have resulted in new management paradigms for children with extreme short bowel and, in selected cases, massive intestinal resection may be a reasonable option.[7]

A laparoscopic approach to the Ladd procedure can also be used.[8] In most cases, laparoscopy should only be used for malrotation not associated with midgut volvulus, because the bowel in patients with volvulus can be friable and subject to perforation.[9] In addition, surgery must be done as quickly as possible in patients with volvulus to maximize the chance of survival, and laparoscopy may waste precious time. The operation begins with the placement of an umbilical trocar and abdominal insufflation, followed by the placement of 2 additional trocars in the right lower quadrant and left midabdomen (depending on the size of the child). A fourth port may be placed in the right upper quadrant to assist with retraction. Careful exploration of the abdomen is then performed and the specific anatomy of the patient delineated. If midgut volvulus is present, the bowel must be detorsed, which can be difficult, especially if the bowel is distended or fragile. If this is the case, the operation should be converted to an open approach. If there is no volvulus, the next step is determination of the length of the small bowel mesentery; that is, the distance between the DJJ and the cecum. If this distance is long (in our center this is defined as greater than half the diameter of the abdomen, although this is an arbitrary threshold that so far is not evidence based), as is seen in both near-normal rotation and in nonrotation, the patient is not considered to be at risk for midgut volvulus, and a Ladd procedure is not considered to be necessary. In this scenario, obstructing bands around the duodenum should be identified and divided (especially if the child is having symptoms that might be caused by partial duodenal obstruction), any internal hernias should be identified and repaired, and an

A

B

C

D

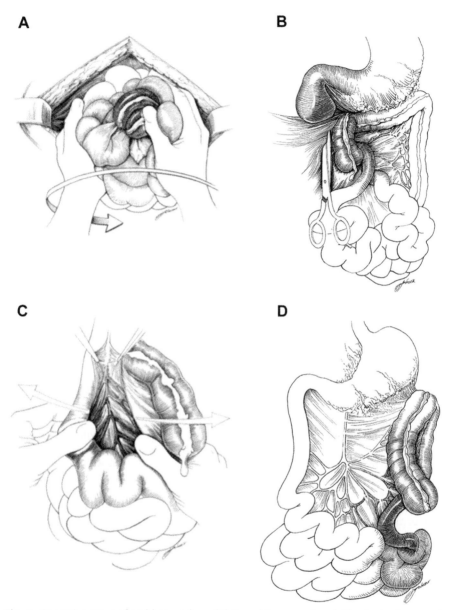

Fig. 4. Operative steps of Ladd procedure. (*A*) Bowel is assessed and, if volvulus is present, gently detorsed in a counterclockwise direction (*arrow*). (*B*) Ladd bands attaching the colon to the liver, gallbladder, or retroperitoneum are divided sharply or with electrocautery. (*C*) Adhesions to the mesentery are divided (*arrows*) and the mesenteric pedicle widened, allowing the colon to be placed on the left side of the patient and the small bowel with a straightened duodenum on the right. (*D*) Final position of the bowel contents at the completion of the Ladd procedure. An appendectomy has been performed to avoid future confusion with the presentation of atypical appendicitis in the left abdomen.

appendectomy should be considered if the appendix is in an abnormal location. If the base of the small bowel mesentery is short, the patient should be considered to be at risk for midgut volvulus, and a full Ladd procedure should be done. The steps are the same as for the open procedure, and dissection can be done using hook electrocautery, sharp scissors, or scissors attached to cautery. In larger children, a sealing device may also be used. If an appendectomy is performed, it can be done extracorporeally through the umbilical port site or intra-abdominally with an Endoloop or stapler.

Advocates of a laparoscopic approach cite decreased postoperative pain and more rapid return of bowel function (and thus shorter hospital stay) as well as an obvious cosmetic advantage. Detractors suggest that intraoperative visualization of the mesenteric pedicle is inadequate, especially in children less than 1 year of age, who are most commonly affected by malrotation. It has also been suggested that open correction of malrotation may be more effective in preventing recurrent volvulus by facilitating the formation of intra-abdominal adhesions and that the laparoscopic approach may not achieve this ancillary benefit to the same extent. Advocates of the laparoscopic approach argue that prevention of recurrent volvulus is accomplished by adequate broadening of the mesenteric base rather than by adhesions, and that adhesion formation results in a long-term risk of intestinal obstruction requiring further surgical correction. To date there have been no large-scale studies with enough longitudinal follow-up to demonstrate this theoretic benefit.

SPECIAL CONSIDERATIONS
Asymptomatic Rotation Abnormalities

Although there is general consensus that symptomatic malrotation should be addressed surgically, the role of prophylactic surgery in children with incidentally diagnosed, asymptomatic rotation abnormalities is less clear. Advocates of routine operative intervention cite reports of midgut volvulus secondary to malrotation throughout adult life and further argue that a careful history often elicits subtle symptoms of malrotation that may have been dismissed or attributed to other causes. However, population-based evidence suggests that the incidence of midgut volvulus secondary to malrotation decreases significantly after infancy and that many patients with rotation abnormalities remain asymptomatic throughout life.

Ultimately, the most important decision in asymptomatic patients is whether there is a risk of midgut volvulus or not; that is, what is the width of the small bowel mesentery? Sometimes this can be well seen on contrast imaging, and a reasonable decision can be made regarding surgical intervention. However, contrast imaging has clearly delineated false-positive and false-negative rates, and laparoscopy may be a safer and more definitive way of determining the need for a Ladd procedure. If, at the time of laparoscopy, the mesenteric base is found to be wide, the operation can be concluded, with minimal morbidity. If the mesenteric base is found to be narrow, a Ladd procedure can be done either laparoscopically or open, at the discretion of the surgeon.

Heterotaxia Syndromes

Patients with HS (defined as any arrangement of organs along the left-right body axis that is neither situs solitus nor situs inversus) are known to have a high rate of rotation anomalies, which cover the spectrum from nonrotation to classic malrotation to near-normal rotation, as well as the more uncommon rotation abnormalities such as reverse rotation. The coexistence in many cases of congenital heart disease places these children at an increased risk of operative intervention, which has resulted in controversy around the role of generalized screening for rotation abnormalities in patients with heterotaxia, and the role of intervention in asymptomatic patients with documented rotation abnormalities.[10] Although several centers have found that the morbidity and mortality associated with a Ladd procedure in patients with HS is not increased compared with a control population, others have documented a higher anesthetic and surgical risk in children with HS who have more complex cardiac disease. In addition, the Ladd procedure is associated with at least a 10% risk of postoperative bowel obstruction, and overall longer term childhood mortality in patients with HS is 23%, mainly caused by cardiac disease. In our own study following 152 asymptomatic neonates with HS, only 4 developed gastrointestinal symptoms over a median follow-up of 18 months (range, 4–216 months), and only 1 of these 4 was found to have malrotation on UGI. Of the remaining asymptomatic patients, 43% died of cardiac disease and none developed intestinal symptoms or complications. The authors have therefore adopted a more conservative approach in which asymptomatic patients with HS are not screened for rotation abnormalities unless they develop symptoms.[11] Those with documented rotation abnormalities and either mild symptoms or no symptoms are evaluated laparoscopically.

CLINICAL OUTCOMES

Outcomes for children with malrotation and midgut volvulus depend on the degree of intestinal ischemia and the need for intestinal resection. If intestinal ischemia is extensive and/or the child presents with overwhelming sepsis, death is the usual result. If massive resection is done and the child survives, outcome depends on the management of the resulting intestinal failure; however, many advances have been made in this area, including the development of intestinal rehabilitation teams and strategies for the prevention of sepsis, venous thrombosis, and cholestatic liver failure.

Surviving children with midgut volvulus who have an adequate length of small bowel, and those children without midgut volvulus, have an excellent outcome after the Ladd procedure. There is a very low rate of recurrence in those who presented with volvulus. The reported rate of adhesive intestinal obstruction is 10% to 15%, which may be lower if a laparoscopic approach is used. Some children who presented with vague symptoms may remain symptomatic, and families should be warned about that possibility before the Ladd procedure. Some persistently symptomatic children ultimately are diagnosed with an intestinal motility disorder that may not have been suspected before the Ladd procedure, and which may be difficult to differentiate from an adhesive bowel obstruction.

SUMMARY

Rotation abnormalities represent a spectrum of anomalies that may be asymptomatic or may be associated with obstruction caused by bands, midgut volvulus, or associated atresia or web. The most important goal of clinicians is to determine whether the patient has midgut volvulus with intestinal ischemia, in which case an emergency laparotomy should be done. If the patient is not acutely ill, the next goal is to determine whether the patient has a narrow-based small bowel mesentery, which may be causing nonischemic midgut volvulus, or may predispose to midgut volvulus in the future. This decision based on imaging studies or laparoscopy, and should be followed by Ladd procedure if the mesenteric base is thought to be narrow. There is still controversy around the role of laparoscopy, the management of atypical and asymptomatic rotation abnormalities, and the management of rotation abnormalities in children with HS. In general, the outcomes for children with a rotation abnormality are excellent, unless there has been midgut volvulus with significant intestinal ischemia.

Pearls and pitfalls

The gold standard for the diagnosis of a rotation abnormality is an upper gastrointestinal contrast study, specifically looking for the location of the DJJ. Ultrasonography may be useful as a screening tool.

The 3 potential causes of duodenal obstruction in children with a rotation abnormality are midgut volvulus, Ladd bands, and an intrinsic duodenal obstruction. Surgeons should look for all 3 in children undergoing surgery for a rotation abnormality with duodenal obstruction.

The distance between the DJJ and the ileocecal junction represents the length of the base of the small bowel mesentery, and can be estimated by contrast study or more accurately by laparoscopy. If this distance is less than half the width of the abdomen, the patient may be at risk for midgut volvulus and should have a Ladd procedure.

A laparoscopic approach is advantageous for older children without clinical or radiological evidence of midgut volvulus. Infants and children with midgut volvulus should be approached by laparotomy.

Controversies

Use of laparoscopy for children with a rotation abnormality

Pros

Ability to determine the length of the small bowel mesentery and potentially avoid the need for a Ladd procedure if the mesenteric base is long enough to prevent midgut volvulus

Theoretic decrease in risk of adhesive small bowel obstruction

Less pain, faster recovery, better cosmetic result

Cons

Lack of adhesions may increase the risk of recurrent rotation abnormality (assuming that adhesions are important in preventing recurrence, which is controversial)

Technically challenging in some cases, particularly infants and in children with midgut volvulus

Routine investigation for a rotation abnormality in children with heterotaxia

Pros

Many of these children have rotation abnormalities

Some of these may predispose to midgut volvulus

Cons

Risk of midgut volvulus is extremely low in asymptomatic children

Ladd procedure has a high risk in children with significant cardiac lesions

Long-term risk of adhesive bowel obstruction in children undergoing Ladd procedure

---

REFERENCES

1. Soffers JH, Hidspoors JP, Mekonen HK, et al. The growth pattern of the human intestine and its mesentery. BMC Dev Biol 2015;15:31.
2. Malek MM, Burd RS. Surgical treatment of malrotation after infancy: a population based study. J Pediatr Surg 2005;40:285–9.

3. Carrol AG, Kavanagh RG, Leifhin N, et al. Comparative effectiveness of imaging modalities for the diagnosis of intestinal obstruction in neonates and infants: a critically appraised topic. Acad Radiol 2016;23:559–68.
4. Mehall JR, Chandler JC, Mehall RL, et al. Management of typical and atypical intestinal malrotation. J Pediatr Surg 2002;37:1169–72.
5. Orzech N, Navarro OM, Langer JC. Is ultrasonography a good screening test for intestinal malrotation? J Pediatr Surg 2006;41:1005–9.
6. Suri M, Langer JC. Circumumbilical vs transverse abdominal incision for neonatal abdominal surgery. J Pediatr Surg 2011;46:1076–80.
7. Oliveira C, de Silva NT, Stanojevic S, et al. Change of outcomes in pediatric intestinal failure: use of time-series analysis to assess the evolution of an intestinal rehabilitation program. J Am Coll Surg 2016;222:1180–8.
8. Hsiao M, Langer JC. Value of laparoscopy in children with a suspected rotation abnormality on imaging. J Pediatr Surg 2011;46:1347–52.
9. Hsiao M, Langer JC. Surgery for suspected rotation abnormality: selection of open vs laparoscopic surgery using a rational approach. J Pediatr Surg 2012; 47:904–10.
10. Cullis PS, Siminas S, Losty PD. Is screening of intestinal foregut anatomy in heterotaxy patients really necessary? A systematic review in search of the evidence. Ann Surg 2015. [Epub ahead of print].
11. Choi M, Borenstein SH, Hornberger L, et al. Heterotaxia syndrome: the role of screening for intestinal rotation abnormalities. Arch Dis Child 2005;90:813–5.

Pediatric Testicular Torsion

Paul R. Bowlin, MD*, John M. Gatti, MD, J. Patrick Murphy, MD

KEYWORDS

- Testis • Torsion • Acute scrotum • Epididymitis/orchitis

KEY POINTS

- Testicular torsion is a surgical emergency and requires prompt surgical exploration and management.
- The diagnosis of testicular torsion can be made by history and physical examination alone. When suspected, surgical management should not be delayed in an effort to obtain imaging.
- When unilateral testicular torsion is discovered, a contralateral orchidopexy should be performed to reduce the risk of asynchronous testicular torsion.

OVERVIEW AND HISTORY

The pediatric patient presenting with acute scrotal pain requires prompt evaluation and management given the likelihood of testicular torsion as the underlying cause. Although other diagnoses can present with acute testicular pain, it is important to recognize the possibility of testicular torsion because the best chance of testicular preservation occurs with expeditious management.

The first published report of testicular torsion was by Delasiauve in 1840, and Taylor first described newborn torsion in 1897. Torsion of a testicular appendage was recognized in 1922 by Colt.

EPIDEMIOLOGY

Although torsion of the spermatic cord and torsion of the testicular appendages can occur at any age, it is more common to see the former in postpubertal boys and the latter in prepubertal boys.[1,2] Adolescent boys are most commonly affected, with a smaller increase in frequency seen in newborns as well.[3] There is evidence to suggest that the risk of torsion can be inherited, particularly in cases of bilateral torsion.[4] The annual incidence of torsion is estimated at 3.8 per 100,000 (0.004%) for boys age 18 years and under.[5]

Disclosures: None of the authors have any relevant disclosures.
Section of Urology, Department of Surgery, Children's Mercy Hospital, University of Missouri–Kansas City, 2401 Gillham Road, Kansas City, MO 64108, USA
* Corresponding author.
E-mail address: prbowlin@cmh.edu

Surg Clin N Am 97 (2017) 161–172
http://dx.doi.org/10.1016/j.suc.2016.08.012
0039-6109/17/© 2016 Elsevier Inc. All rights reserved.

surgical.theclinics.com

DIFFERENTIAL DIAGNOSIS

- Spermatic cord torsion
- Torsion of appendix testis/epididymis
- Tumor
- Hernia/hydrocele
- Epididymitis/orchitis
- Trauma/abuse
- Cellulitis
- Vasculitis
- Varicocele

PERINATAL TORSION

Torsion can occur during the prenatal or postnatal period and is collectively referred to as perinatal torsion. Establishing the timing of the torsion can have implications on future management but is often difficult to determine. Classically, prenatal torsion involves a twisting of the spermatic cord that occurs proximal to the tunica vaginalis—extravaginal torsion. It typically is identified at birth with a firm, discolored, and nontender hemiscrotal mass. It is often difficult to palpate the testicle separate from the scrotal skin as the inflammation causes fixation of the skin to the inflamed testicular mass. Postnatal torsion, by comparison, appears with more classic signs of torsion: acute inflammation, erythema, and tenderness. The key clinical finding that suggests postnatal torsion is the report of a previously normal scrotum and testicle at birth. Understanding this, timing is critical given that postnatal torsion should be treated as a surgical emergency with immediate exploration, detorsion, and orchidopexy of the contralateral testicle to prevent later torsion.

The management of true prenatal torsion remains debated.[6] The decision about the need for exploration, timing of exploration, and management of the contralateral testicle varies widely among practitioners. Factors that influence the decision include the age at which the torsion is diagnosed and overall health of the child. The debate exists because salvage of a prenatally torsed testicle is extremely unlikely,[7] the risk of neonatal anesthesia is higher than in older children,[8] and there is a risk of iatrogenic injury to the contralateral testicle. The age of the child at diagnosis influences the decision primarily because the tunica vaginalis becomes adherent to the surrounding dartos around 4 to 6 weeks of life. When the torsion is discovered after this 4- to 6-week age period, there is theoretically no longer a risk of asynchronous torsion and thus no need for prophylactic orchidopexy on the contralateral side. A prenatal (extravaginal) torsion event does not predispose the child to a future postpubertal (intravaginal) torsion event. **Fig. 1** outlines the authors' preferred management algorithm for perinatal torsion.

CLINICAL PRESENTATION

Testicular torsion classically presents with the sudden onset of severe unilateral scrotal pain. This pain is usually accompanied by nausea and vomiting. The pain is usually unrelenting and leads the child to immediately notify a caregiver, although very stoic children will often delay reporting the pain. Delays in recognition can also be seen in children who are unable to communicate with their caregivers.

Within hours of the torsion event, the scrotum will begin to show varying degrees of erythema, swelling, and induration. In cases where the evaluation occurs long after the

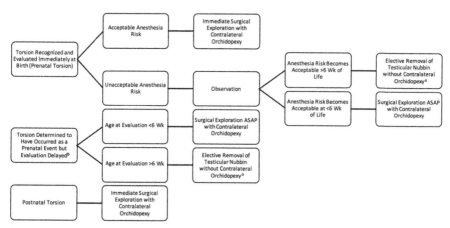

Fig. 1. Management algorithm for perinatal testicular torsion. [a]Observation is reasonable when the history and examination do not raise any concern for the presence of an intra-abdominal testicle. [b]When torsion timing is unclear, the decision of management needs to be based on a comprehensive discussion with the caregivers. ASAP, as soon as possible.

onset of symptoms, the severity of the scrotal edema can be quite severe and can make examination of the underlying testicle quite difficult.

INITIAL EVALUATION

The 2 most important components of the initial evaluation are the history and physical examination. These 2 elements alone are enough to establish the diagnosis and prompt treatment. It is important to recognize that any boy presenting with abdominal pain associated with nausea and vomiting requires a scrotal examination to evaluate for testicular torsion. Key components of the history that suggest acute testicular torsion include the following:

- Immediate onset of severe, unilateral scrotal pain
- Unrelenting pain
- Associated nausea/vomiting
- Described change in the position of the testicle

The physical examination should include a thorough investigation of the abdomen, inguinal region, penis, and scrotum. Key components of the physical examination include the following:

- Unilateral testicular tenderness
- Elevation (high-riding) of the testicle
- Transverse testicular orientation
- Palpation of the epididymis anteriorly
- Absent cremasteric reflex

The presence or absence of the cremasteric reflex is a classic teaching point in the evaluation of the acute scrotum. It is elicited by lightly stroking the inner thigh on the side of the suspected torsion. The resultant reflex occurs due to stimulation of the sensory fibers of the femoral branch of the genitofemoral nerve. This afferent input ascends to the brain, where there are superimposed cortical pathways that allow the signal to cross over and connect with motor centers that result in the efferent stimulation of the genital branch of the genitofemoral nerve, which innervates the cremaster muscle.[9] Although the cremasteric reflex is frequently absent in cases of acute torsion, the presence of the reflex does not exclude torsion.[10] The reflex is more reliable when absent on the side of pain but present on the normal side. It is less reliable when absent on both sides.

INITIAL MANAGEMENT

When the history and examination suggest testicular torsion, surgical exploration should immediately follow. If surgical care is not immediately available, an attempt at manual detorsion can be performed. Classically, this maneuver is instructed to be done in a fashion that rotates the testicle from medial to lateral, colloquially referred to as the "open book" rotation. From the perspective of the provider standing face to face with the patient, this means rotating the right testicle counterclockwise and rotating the left testicle clockwise. The success of this technique is hampered by patient discomfort, incomplete (or partial) detorsion, as well as the possibility of rotating the testicle in the wrong direction. Around one-third of testicles will be found to have rotated from medial to lateral, a situation that is only worsened when a classic "open book" detorsion maneuver is attempted.[11] In addition, the number of testicular rotations can range from 180° to 1080°, leaving open the possibility of only partial untwisting the testicle with a manual detorsion maneuver.

If manual detorsion is successful, the patient will typically have immediate relief of their pain. Although this relief may result in a longer window for testicular salvage, it should not delay prompt surgical management and fixation.

IMAGING AND LABORATORY TESTS

As stated throughout this article, clinical suspicion for acute testicular torsion mandates immediate surgical exploration. The acquisition of confirmatory imaging is generally unnecessary and typically only results in a delay in definitive management.[1] Although currently this principle remains unchanged, the advent of point-of-care ultrasound in the emergency department may ultimately lead to an environment where bedside imaging may almost be considered an extension of the physical examination with almost no delay in further management.[12]

Imaging is generally recommended only in cases where the cause of the acute scrotum is not thought to be due to acute torsion. Ultrasound with color-flow Doppler and radionuclide imaging are the 2 most commonly used imaging modalities. Although radionuclide imaging has been the historical examination of choice, the use of ultrasound with Doppler is now widely favored because of its excellent visual resolution, ability to detect the presence or absence of blood flow, availability, and lack of ionizing radiation. Ultrasound has a sensitivity and specificity of 89.9% and 98.8%, respectively, with a false-positive rate of 1% when performed by experienced providers.[13] The integration of any radiologic study, however, still needs to include the other aspects of the evaluation because false negatives can occur.[14]

Laboratory investigation in cases of suspected torsion is rarely necessary. In cases where the individual's medical history of presentation raises concern for a serious abnormality that can be demonstrated with laboratory data (anemia, coagulopathy, severe electrolyte disturbance, and so forth), laboratory investigation can be pursued. As a general principle, however, this should not delay progression to the operating room unless the risk of anesthesia is thought to be much greater than the likelihood of testicular salvage. In this unusual scenario, accepting the risk of testicular loss and theoretic risk of contralateral torsion may warrant consideration. Once the anesthetic risk is deemed acceptable, however, urgent surgical management should be undertaken.

OPERATIVE MANAGEMENT

Once surgical management is decided on, it should occur as quickly as possible. Testicular salvage rates are associated with the duration of ischemia with a "golden" window of 4 to 8 hours from the time of torsion to time of detorsion. Although an inguinal or hemiscrotal approach is reasonable, most surgeons use a midline raphe incision. Access via the midline allows each hemiscrotum to be independently explored and, once healed, the surgical scar is typically imperceptible. The general steps in the operative management of torsion are as follows:

- Midline scrotal incision
- Cautery dissection through the dartos layers of the symptomatic hemiscrotum to expose the underlying testicle
- Delivery of the testicle through the dartos
- Inspection of the tunica vaginalis and spermatic cord for extravaginal torsion (unlikely outside of newborn period)
- Incision and eversion of the tunica vaginalis to allow inspection of the testicle and epididymis
- Detorsion of the testicle noting direction and degrees of torsion
- Placement of detorsed testicle in a warm gauze sponge
- Cautery dissection through the dartos layers of the contralateral hemiscrotum to expose the underlying testicle
- Delivery of the testicle through the dartos
- Incision and eversion of the tunica vaginalis to allow inspection of the testicle and epididymis
- Fixation of the contralateral testicle
- Repeat inspection of the symptomatic testicle
  - Obviously nonviable → orchiectomy
  - Obviously viable → orchidopexy
  - Questionably viable → orchiectomy or ochidopexy

The assessment of testicular viability is a relatively subjective aspect of the surgical management. When viability is questionable, additional investigation can be performed, including incision of the tunica albuginea to inspect for active bleeding and to assess the viability of the seminiferous tubules. When no bleeding is observed and/or the tubules appear densely ischemic, orchiectomy is generally favored. In the presence of active bleeding and/or viable-appearing tubules, however, orchidopexy should be considered.

More recently there has been emerging evidence to support a third approach to the questionably viable testicle. Decompression of the tunica albuginea via a wide longitudinal incision along its surface (fasciotomy) followed by coverage of the defect with a tunica vaginalis flap has shown encouraging results as an option for testicular salvage.[15] This approach still mandates testicular fixation but theoretically allows for relief and recovery of the testicular "compartment syndrome." Although the long-term success of this option is difficult to definitively assess, it is a potentially useful option for the questionably viable testicle. The surgical technique itself has been described by Kutikov and colleagues.[16]

In cases where a torsed gonad is preserved, there has been concern raised about the possibility of damage to the contralateral testicle because of antisperm antibodies.

This debate includes cases of testicular salvage using a tunica vaginalis flap. These concerns generally arise from animal studies with the physiologic significance in humans remaining a source of debate.[17] In cases of torsion of a solitary testicle however, it is obviously recommended to make every attempt to preserve the testicle regardless of its likelihood of future atrophy. Adjuvant procedures, such as the aforementioned tunica vaginalis flap, should also be considered as a means to potentially save a gonad that would otherwise be unlikely to survive.

The techniques used to perform orchidopexy vary widely among surgeons, including debate about the following:

- Number of points of testicular fixation (typically between 1 and 3)
- Use of permanent or dissolvable suture
- Use of suture fixation versus placement of testicle within a dartos pouch alone
- Placement of fixation sutures within scrotum (medial, lateral, inferior, or a combination of all 3)

At the authors' institution, orchidopexy, in the setting of testicular torsion, is typically done in 1 of 2 ways. The first technique is to place the testicle partially back within the tunica vaginalis, leaving the anterior one-third of the surface of the testicle exposed. The edges of the tunica vaginalis are then tacked to the testicle in several places with an absorbable suture (polydioxanone or polyglactin). The second technique uses polypropylene suture to tack the tunica albuginea to the interior surface of the scrotum. This tacking is typically done inferiorly, laterally, and either anteriorly or medially for 3 total points of fixation.

FOLLOW-UP

In general, children recover well after surgery and can typically be discharged to home from the recovery room regardless of the surgical outcome (orchidopexy or orchiectomy). Outpatient follow-up several weeks after the procedure allows for evaluation of delayed atrophy. In cases where orchiectomy was performed, it also allows for discussion about future placement of a testicular prosthesis, should one be desired. Recommendations to avoid specific activities or sports are generally not given, but emphasis is given regarding the utilization of appropriate protection. Finally, it allows an opportunity to discuss the importance of testicular self-examination, a valuable topic for all male adolescents regardless of the outcome of their torsed testicle.

When counseling patients and families about torsion, it is important to remind them that the fixation of the testicle does not rule out the potential for future torsion. Recurrent torsion has been reported and requires urgent evaluation identical to an initial torsion event.[18] Similarly, studies have shown that there may be a component of heritability with testicular torsion[4] as well as a lower likelihood of testicular salvage in boys who experience an acute torsion event after having a sibling with torsion.[19] The latter phenomenon is difficult to explain but thought to potentially be related to a form of "desensitization" regarding testicular pain from the perspective of the caregiver.

INTERMITTENT TESTICULAR PAIN

Intermittent testicular pain is a frequent complaint, particularly among male adolescents. Although a history of testicular pain with spontaneous resolution should raise concern for the possibility of intermittent testicular torsion, a detailed history and examination can often elicit an alternate cause, as described in the differential diagnosis section. Anecdotally, people frequently associate testicular pain with puberty and the testicular growth that accompanies the early stages of puberty. These so-called growing pains, however, are not well described in the literature.

Individuals thought to be most at risk for intermittent testicular torsion include those with a "bell-clapper" deformity. Normally the tunica vaginalis invests upon the length of the posterior side of the testicle and epididymis, effectively fixing the testicle within the scrotum and limiting the risk of testicular torsion. When the tunical investments attach more proximally on the spermatic cord, the testicle and epididymis are allowed to hang more freely and take on a horizontal lie (**Fig. 2**), creating a narrow point of rotation that may predispose one to developing testicular torsion. The incidence of the "bell-clapper" deformity has been reported to be as high as 12% and can frequently be a bilateral process.[20] Considering that testicular torsion occurs at an incidence far lower than 12%, it is clearly not an isolated risk factor for testicular torsion. When evaluating the child with intermittent testicular pain and a "bell-clapper" deformity, it is important to counsel the patient and family about its association with testicular torsion. The risk of torsion must be weighed against the risks of anesthesia, persistent or worsened pain, and iatrogenic testicular injury or loss.

MIMICKERS OF TESTICULAR PAIN

Inflammation of the testicle and/or epididymis can occur in response to infection (viral or bacterial), trauma, torsion of the appendages, and urinary reflux into the ejaculatory duct/vas deferens, which is commonly referred to as "chemical" epididymitis/orchitis. True bacterial infections in children are generally rare. When suspected, a urine analysis and culture can be obtained. Investigation of sexually active adolescents for Gonococcus and Chlamydia is often warranted. If a true bacterial infection is diagnosed, consideration should be given to obtaining imaging of the urinary tract (renal/bladder ultrasound and/or voiding cystourethrogram) once the infection has been treated. Other anatomic abnormalities such as ectopic ureter (to the vas, ejaculatory duct, or seminal vesicle), ejaculatory duct obstruction, or posterior urethral valves may need to be considered and ruled out. Viral infections are also a rare source of testicular/epididymal inflammation. Historically, mumps orchitis, in postpubertal boys, was a common cause, which is rare today because of immunization.

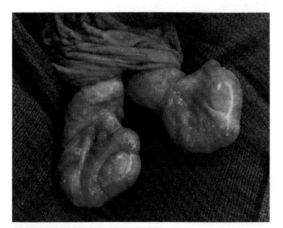

Fig. 2. Bilateral "bell-clapper" configuration of the testicles. Note the transverse testicular lie of the testicle relative to the spermatic cord. This patient underwent bilateral orchidopexy with complete resolution of his previously intermittent bilateral testicular pain.

Adenovirus, enterovirus, influenza, and parainfluenza viruses have all been implicated as infectious causes. Although viral culture and serology can be obtained, it is generally unnecessary because supportive treatment is typically all that is required.

When evaluating the child with testicular pain thought not due to acute torsion or infection, it is important to take a detailed voiding and stooling history. Children with significant constipation and/or voiding dysfunction are thought to be at an elevated risk of developing epididymitis/orchitis because of high urinary pressure that can develop in the posterior urethra. This pressure can lead to reflux of urine into the ejaculatory ducts and vasa and subsequent inflammation of the epididymis/testicle, commonly referred to as "chemical epididymitis."[21,22] Occasionally, this urinary reflux will be seen during the voiding phase of a voiding cystourethrogram.

Torsion of the appendix testis/epididymis is a common cause of acute scrotal pain and is often referred to as "the great mimicker." Embryologically, the appendages differ in origin with the appendix testicle being a Müllerian remnant and the appendix epididymis being a Wolffian remnant. It is more common to see an appendage torsion in the prepubertal boy.[23] Given the shared ischemic cause, torsion of an appendage can very closely mimic the symptoms of acute testicular torsion. Close physical inspection will occasionally reveal the ischemic and inflamed appendage to be visible through the skin. This so-called blue-dot sign is highly suggestive of a torsed appendix and is often accompanied by focal tenderness of the appendage itself (**Fig. 3**). This inflammation and tenderness can spread to the epididymis and testicle, however, depending on the duration of the appendiceal torsion. Ultrasonography can often demonstrate an enlarged and heterogenous appendage adjacent to the testicle, often with no demonstrable blood flow (**Fig. 4**). When being evaluated many hours after the onset of pain, it can be very difficult to distinguish between a torsed appendix and a

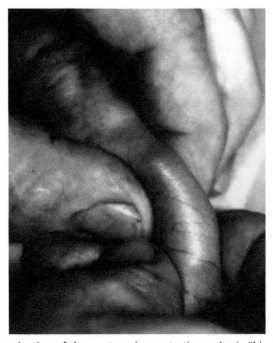

Fig. 3. Physical examination of the scrotum demonstrating a classic "blue-dot" sign.

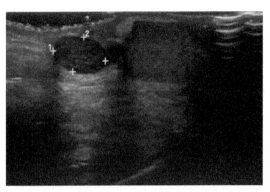

Fig. 4. Ultrasound image demonstrating torsion of the testicular appendage. Note the heterogenous appearance of the appendage relative to the normal-appearing testicle. This patient was found to have a classic "blue-dot" sign on physical examination.

torsed testicle. As with the physical examination, ultrasound can often identify a torsed appendage early on but has difficulty making this distinction later on when adjacent scrotal inflammation has progressed. Although the testis and epididymis are the most common places to find an appendage, there are potentially 5 anatomic sites where an appendage can exist (**Fig. 5**).[24,25] Surgical removal of a torsed appendage is not required because the appendage will ultimately necrose with relief of the pain. Surgical removal can occur, however, when exploration is undertaken because of concern about testicular torsion. If the torsed appendage is not removed, it may calcify

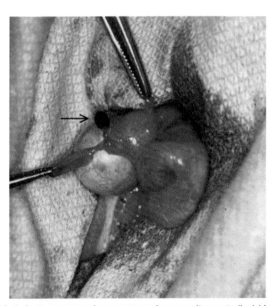

Fig. 5. Testicle with 3 distinct appendages. Normal appendix testis (held by hemostat on left side of image), torsed appendix epididymis (*black arrow*), and normal superior vas aberrans of Haller (held by hemostat at top of image).

and later be felt as a small "mass" within the scrotum. It can also end up free floating within the tunica vaginalis. When a testicular appendage is encountered incidentally in an otherwise normal testicle, most surgeons advocate for removal of all appendages to prevent the risk of future appendiceal torsion.

When counseling patients and families about a torsed appendage (or any other cause of scrotal pain), it is important to emphasize the potential of future torsion of the spermatic cord. It is critical that the patient and family understand that the diagnosis of scrotal pain due to appendiceal torsion or minor trauma may increase the risk of spermatic cord torsion during the recovery period.[26]

The appropriate management of epididymal/testicular inflammation and pain needs to include treatment of the acute inflammation as well as treatment of the underlying factors (if any) that led to development of the inflammation. Once testicular torsion and infection have been ruled out, children are often given little guidance as to how to manage their ongoing testicular pain. Repeat medical evaluation is frequently sought because of persistence of the pain. Antibiotics are frequently prescribed but rarely indicated in children in the absence of an abnormal urine analysis/culture. Similarly, narcotics can be used but are generally not required. Clinical improvement depends on relieving the inflammation. The key aspects of the management of the epididymal/testicular inflammation include the following:

- 48 to 72 hours of an age-/weight-appropriate dose of anti-inflammatory medication
- Corresponding 48- to 72-hour period of modified bed rest
- Aggressive oral hydration
- Timed voiding
- Management of constipation (if present)

The goal of the above recommendations is to help break the inflammatory cycle. Patients are recommended to limit all activities aside from normal activities of daily life (bathroom, meals, and so forth). Limiting activity has the benefit of reducing the physical movement of the scrotum and contents, which in turn allows the inflammation to subside, akin to elevating a sprained ankle. Hydration, timed voiding, and constipation management help to begin addressing any underlying issues that may have predisposed development of the inflammation. Long term, these issues may require additional directed management to fully address the problem.

Although most pediatric scrotal pain cases will be caused by one of the above issues, other less common causes exist. Vasculitic syndromes, such as Henoch-Schönlein purpura (HSP), can lead to pain, erythema, and swelling of the scrotum in up to two-thirds of patients.[27] Although rare, cases of HSP have been associated with acute testicular torsion, which reinforces the importance of always keeping torsion in mind when evaluating the acute scrotum.[28] Scrotal pain due to hernia, hydrocele, trauma, or neoplasia can also occur. Typically, a thorough history and physical examination are sufficient to differentiate these issues from acute testicular torsion.

SUMMARY

Despite being a common issue, acute scrotal pain in a child should be considered a surgical emergency until proven otherwise. History and physical examination are sufficient to confirm the diagnosis and prompt surgical exploration. When torsion is ruled out, aggressive management of the underlying cause or causes is important to provide relief of discomfort and limit the chance of recurrence.

REFERENCES

1. Baker LA, Sigman D, Mathews RI, et al. An analysis of clinical outcomes using color Doppler testicular ultrasound for testicular torsion. Pediatrics 2000;105(3 Pt 1):604–7.
2. Ballesteros Sampol JJ, Munne A, Bosch A. A vas aberrans torsion. Br J Urol 1986; 58(1):97.
3. Yang C, Song B, Tan J, et al. Testicular torsion in children: a 20-year retrospective study in a single institution. ScientificWorldJournal 2011;11:362–8.
4. Shteynshlyuger A, Yu J. Familial testicular torsion: a meta analysis suggests inheritance. J Pediatr Urol 2013;9(5):683–90.
5. Zhao LC, Lautz TB, Meeks JJ, et al. Pediatric testicular torsion epidemiology using a national database: incidence, risk of orchiectomy and possible measures toward improving the quality of care. J Urol 2011;186(5):2009–13.
6. Broderick KM, Martin BG, Herndon CDA, et al. The current state of surgical practice for neonatal torsion: a survey of pediatric urologists. J Pediatr Urol 2013;9(5): 542–5.
7. Brandt MT, Sheldon CA, Wacksman J, et al. Prenatal testicular torsion: principles of management. J Urol 1992;147(3):670–2.
8. Cohen MM, Cameron CB, Duncan PG. Pediatric anesthesia morbidity and mortality in the perioperative period. Anesth Analg 1990;70(2):160–7.
9. Bingöl-Koloğlu M, Tanyel FC, Anlar B, et al. Cremasteric reflex and retraction of a testis. J Pediatr Surg 2001;36(6):863–7.
10. Beni-Israel T, Goldman M, Bar Chaim S, et al. Clinical predictors for testicular torsion as seen in the pediatric ED. Am J Emerg Med 2010;28(7):786–9.
11. Sessions AE, Rabinowitz R, Hulbert WC, et al. Testicular torsion: direction, degree, duration and disinformation. J Urol 2003;169(2):663–5.
12. Bomann JS, Moore C. Bedside ultrasound of a painful testicle: before and after manual detorsion by an emergency physician. Acad Emerg Med 2009;16(4):366.
13. Kalfa N, Veyrac C, Baud C, et al. Ultrasonography of the spermatic cord in children with testicular torsion: impact on the surgical strategy. J Urol 2004;172(4 Pt 2):1692–5 [discussion: 1695].
14. Boettcher M, Krebs T, Bergholz R, et al. Clinical and sonographic features predict testicular torsion in children: a prospective study. BJU Int 2013;112(8):1201–6.
15. Figueroa V, Pippi-Salle JL, Braga LHP, et al. Comparative analysis of detorsion alone versus detorsion and tunica albuginea decompression (fasciotomy) with tunica vaginalis flap coverage in the surgical management of prolonged testicular ischemia. J Urol 2012;188(4 Suppl):1417–22.
16. Kutikov A, Casale P, White MA, et al. Testicular compartment syndrome: a new approach to conceptualizing and managing testicular torsion. Urology 2008; 72(4):786–9.
17. Koşar A, Küpeli B, Alçigir G, et al. Immunologic aspect of testicular torsion: detection of antisperm antibodies in contralateral testicle. Eur Urol 1999;36(6): 640–4.
18. Mor Y, Pinthus JH, Nadu A, et al. Testicular fixation following torsion of the spermatic cord–does it guarantee prevention of recurrent torsion events? J Urol 2006; 175(1):171–3 [discussion: 173–4].
19. Cubillos J, Palmer JS, Friedman SC, et al. Familial testicular torsion. J Urol 2011; 185(6 Suppl):2469–72.
20. Caesar RE, Kaplan GW. Incidence of the bell-clapper deformity in an autopsy series. Urology 1994;44(1):114–6.

21. Kiviat MD, Shurtleff D, Ansell JS. Urinary reflux via the vas deferens: unusual cause of epididymitis in infancy. J Pediatr 1972;80(3):476–9.
22. Thind P, Brandt B, Kristensen JK. Assessment of voiding dysfunction in men with acute epididymitis. Urol Int 1992;48(3):320–2.
23. Lev M, Ramon J, Mor Y, et al. Sonographic appearances of torsion of the appendix testis and appendix epididymis in children. J Clin Ultrasound 2015;43(8):485–9.
24. Favorito LA, Cavalcante AGL, Babinski MA. Study on the incidence of testicular and epididymal appendages in patients with cryptorchidism. Int Braz J Urol 2004;30(1):49–52.
25. Aworanti O, Awadalla S. An unusual cause of acute scrotum in a child. Ir Med J 2014;107(10):327–8.
26. Seng YJ, Moissinac K. Trauma induced testicular torsion: a reminder for the unwary. J Accid Emerg Med 2000;17(5):381–2.
27. Ha T-S, Lee J-S. Scrotal involvement in childhood Henoch-Schönlein purpura. Acta Paediatr 2007;96(4):552–5.
28. Søreide K. Surgical management of nonrenal genitourinary manifestations in children with Henoch-Schönlein purpura. J Pediatr Surg 2005;40(8):1243–7.

Lower Gastrointestinal Bleeding & Intussusception

 CrossMark

Benjamin E. Padilla, MD[a],*, Willieford Moses, MD[b]

KEYWORDS

- Pediatric • Gastrointestinal bleeding • Intussusception • Hydrostatic reduction
- Pneumatic reduction

KEY POINTS

- Lower gastrointestinal bleeding in children is uncommon.
- The differential diagnosis is largely guided by the age of the patient.
- Surgical emergencies in the neonatal period, such as necrotizing enterocolitis, midgut volvulus, and Hirschsprung disease, can present with gastrointestinal bleeding.
- Ileocolic intussusception is a common cause of gastrointestinal bleeding.
- Radiologic reduction of an ileocolic intussusception is first-line therapy for a patient without peritonitis or hemodynamic instability.

LOWER GASTROINTESTINAL BLEEDING
Epidemiology

Although data remain limited regarding the incidence of lower gastrointestinal (GI) bleeding (LGIB) in children, a Healthcare Cost and Utilization Project Nationwide Emergency Department Sample analysis from 2006 to 2011 estimated that there were a total of 437,000 emergency department (ED) visits associated with GI bleeding in the pediatric population (children up to 19 years old).[1] Of these visits, 20% were identified as upper GI bleeding, 30% were LGIB, and the remaining 40% were not specified. By age, 38% of the patients were younger than 5 years, 23% were between 5 and 15 years, and 39% were between 15 and 19 years. Interestingly, only 11.6% of the ED visits required hospitalization with most being treated either in the ED or as an outpatient.

Clinical Presentation and Initial Evaluation

Patients with LGIB can present with nausea, vomiting, diarrhea, and abdominal pain. A complete history should be obtained, including the duration and amount of bleeding

---

Disclosure Statement: There are no financial or commercial conflicts of interests for either author.
[a] Division of Pediatric Surgery, University of California, San Francisco, 550 16th Street, 5th Floor, Box 0570, San Francisco, CA 94158-2549, USA; [b] General Surgery, Department of Surgery, University of California, San Francisco, 513 Parnassus Avenue, S-321, San Francisco, CA 94143, USA
* Corresponding author.
E-mail address: benjamin.padilla@ucsf.edu

Surg Clin N Am 97 (2017) 173–188
http://dx.doi.org/10.1016/j.suc.2016.08.015
0039-6109/17/© 2016 Elsevier Inc. All rights reserved.

surgical.theclinics.com

and the color and consistency of the blood. Although a well-appearing infant or child is relatively reassuring, the clinical condition can deteriorate precipitously in the face of ongoing bleeding. Initial physical examination and evaluation should focus on ascertaining the child's hemodynamic condition and promptly initiating resuscitation if indicated. A thorough physical examination should be performed, including inspection for anal fissures; a rectal examination for prolapse, polyps, or masses; and stool guaiac testing. The abdomen should be assessed for peritonitis and the presence of an abdominal mass. The findings of petechiae or bruising on the skin may suggest an underlying coagulopathy.

The initial diagnostic test of choice for children presenting with LGIB largely depends on their age, clinical status, and the likelihood for various underlying pathologic conditions. If the source of the bleeding (lower vs upper tract) is unclear, a nasogastric tube can be placed for lavage. Abdominal plain radiographs, particularly in the neonatal and infant population, can aid in the diagnosis of underlying conditions such as necrotizing enterocolitis (NEC) or Hirschsprung disease. Ultrasonography is also helpful in identifying underlying conditions such as intussusception. Although endoscopy (upper and lower) requires general anesthesia, it can help in both identifying the lesion and providing an opportunity for intervention.[2] Red blood cell scintigraphy and angiography can also aid in identifying the source of bleeding, although slow bleeding is often difficult to identify with these modalities.

Differential Diagnosis

The differential diagnosis for LGIB in the pediatric population is broad. However, it can be quickly narrowed based on the age group of the patient and the clinical presentation. It is helpful to categorize the patients into 3 groups to assist in the diagnosis: neonatal, infant and toddler, and school age (**Box 1**).

NEONATAL

LGIB in the neonatal population presents a diagnostic challenge because of the broad range of etiologies, from benign conditions, such as swallowed maternal blood to more concerning conditions, such as midgut volvulus or NEC. As mentioned, the clinical presentation (well child vs distressed) and the hemodynamic status of the patient are essential to effectively diagnose and treat the underlying condition. Although not exhaustive, the following is a summary of the common conditions that can present with LGIB in the neonates.

MIDGUT VOLVULUS

One of the true surgical emergencies in pediatrics, midgut volvulus, is an obstructive condition of the small intestines caused by twisting of the bowel around the axis of the mesentery. In addition to intestinal obstruction, the mesenteric blood vessels are kinked, resulting in ischemia to the midgut that can manifest as LGIB. Bilious emesis in an infant is alarming and should prompt an expeditious workup for midgut volvulus. Midgut volvulus typically occurs in the setting of intestinal malrotation caused by failed rotation and fixation of the gut during in utero development. Melena or hematochezia is present in up to 20% of cases and is an ominous sign suggestive of gut ischemia. Similarly, abdominal wall erythema caused by bowel ischemia is a late and concerning finding. The diagnosis is established with an upper GI contrast study that shows proximal duodenal obstruction (midgut volvulus) or abnormal rotation and positioning of the duodenal-jejunal junction (malrotation).[3,4] Emergency surgical intervention with a

Box 1
Lower gastrointestinal bleeding differential diagnosis

Neonatal
- Swallowed blood
- Fissures
- Necrotizing enterocolitis
- Midgut volvulus
- Hirschsprung disease
- Vascular
- Coagulopathy
- GI duplication

Infant and Toddler
- Fissures
- Allergic colitis
- Intussusception
- Meckel diverticulum
- GI duplication

School Age
- Infections
- Polyps
- IBD
- Malignancies
- Typhlitis
- Henoch-Schonlein purpura
- Hemolytic uremic syndrome

Ladd procedure to relieve the obstruction and restore perfusion to the bowel can be lifesaving.[5,6]

Necrotizing Enterocolitis

Also considered a surgical emergency, NEC likely results from relative gut ischemia and infection of the intestines caused by bacterial translocation across the immature intestinal epithelium.[7,8] Risk factors for NEC include severe prematurity, low Apgar score, low birth weight, and hyperosmolar enteral feedings. Although most commonly occurring in the setting of prematurity, between 5% and 25% of NEC occurs in full-term infants.[9,10] Babies with gastroschisis and congenital heart defects are also at risk for NEC. Patients can present with occult or gross bleeding, often in the setting of clinical decompensation, and abdominal distension, vomiting, or diarrhea. The ileum, cecum, and right colon are most commonly involved. Findings on plain radiographs that support the diagnosis of NEC include dilated or fixed intestinal loops, pneumatosis intestinalis, portal venous gas, or pneumoperitoneum.[11] Although most patients are effectively treated with bowel rest and intravenous antibiotics, evidence of intestinal perforation or necrosis and clinical deterioration despite antibiotics are indications to operate.

Hirschsprung Disease

Hirschsprung disease (HD) is an obstructive disorder of the colon caused by incomplete cranio-caudal migration of enteric ganglion cells in the colon. The incidence is about 1 in 5000 live births with a 4:1 male/female predominance.[12,13] Although most commonly seen in newborns with delayed passage of meconium (>24 hours), some neonates and infants can present with progressively worsening constipation. Patients with HD commonly have enterocolitis that can manifest as LGIB. In fact, enterocolitis is the presenting clinical finding in up to 24% of patients with HD.[14] Hirschsprung enterocolitis can be life threatening and should be promptly treated with intravenous antibiotics, fluid resuscitation and colonic irrigation. Multiple surgical options exist for the treatment of HD, which is beyond the scope of this review.

Anal Fissures

Often associated with constipation, anal fissures are one of the most common causes of LGIB in the neonatal population.[1,15] Similar to older children and adults, the history is often notable for pain with defecation. In infants, this can present as grunting, straining, or arching of the back during defecation. Blood is typically seen around the stool and on the surface but not mixed within it. On physical examination, spreading the perianal skin will evert the anus and reveal the fissure. Treatment is usually conservative and includes dietary changes or medications depending on the patient's age.

Swallowed Maternal Blood

In a well-appearing infant without any clinical evidence of bleeding, swallowed maternal blood should be considered on the differential diagnosis for rectal bleeding. Either ingested at the time of delivery or during breast feeding, maternal blood often presents as melanotic stools or hematemesis. A history of cracked or fissured maternal nipples is common. To confirm the diagnosis, an Apt-Downey test should be performed, which distinguishes fetal hemoglobin from maternal adult hemoglobin by the degree of denaturation in the setting of alkaline solution. The more stable fetal hemoglobin will remain pinkish in color as opposed to adult hemoglobin, which turns yellowish-brown because of the higher susceptibility to denaturation.

Other Conditions

Vascular anomalies and several types of coagulopathies can all precipitate bleeding in neonates. The hemophilia syndromes along with von Willebrand disease can present in the neonatal period; however, these syndromes are rare. In addition to GI bleeding, clinical history and physical examination findings, such as unexplained bruising, petechiae, or prolonged bleeding episodes after minor trauma such as circumcision, can indicate a possible coagulation disorder.

INFANTS AND TODDLERS

The differential diagnosis for LGIB in the infant/toddler period is narrower than in neonates. Furthermore, the clinical history and presentation tend to lead toward a conclusive diagnosis. Intussusception and Meckel diverticulum often warrant the most immediate intervention, as bleeding can be indicative of a late-stage condition. Below is a summary of the most common conditions and presentations.

Meckel Diverticulum

The etiology of Meckel diverticulum is related to failed closure of the omphalomesenteric duct, also known as the vitelline duct. Embryologically, the duct serves to join the yolk sac to the lumen of the primitive midgut during early fetal development. As the placenta matures the duct no longer serves as a source of nourishment and typically obliterates by the seventh to ninth week of life. If this process fails, one of multiple congenital anomalies can occur, including but not limited to a Meckel diverticulum (most common), an umbilical sinus, an omphalomesenteric fistula, or residual fibrous cords. Despite being common, occurring in approximately 2% of the population, most patients are asymptomatic. However, painless rectal bleeding can be a common presentation because of gastric heterotopia within the diverticulum, leading to mucosal ulceration of the adjacent small intestine.[16] Although the preoperative diagnosis of a Meckel's diverticulum is often difficult, in the appropriate clinical setting, a Meckel scan can be performed in which intravenous technetium 99m concentrates in the ectopic gastric mucosa allowing for identification on scintigraphy.[17] Because the bleeding arises from ulcerations in the small bowel directly adjacent to the diverticulum, definitive therapy requires a segmental bowel resection that encompasses the Meckel diverticulum and ulcerated small bowel. Other complications that can arise from a Meckel diverticulum include intestinal obstruction, intussusception, diverticulitis, and perforation. The presentation of Meckel diverticulitis can be difficult to distinguish from acute appendicitis. If a normal appendix is encountered at the time of surgery for what was thought to be acute appendicitis, it is important to inspect the ileum for the presence of Meckel diverticulitis.

Allergic Colitis

Allergic colitis, or food protein-induced colitis, is most often caused by an inflammatory reaction to cow's milk or soy proteins. Although most commonly occurring in formula-fed infants, it can also occur in those who are breast fed owing to the lactating mother's ingestion of cow's milk. Relatively benign in nature, most infants present with loose diarrhea and occult or frank hematochezia.[18] Once other causes for lower GI bleeding have been excluded, attention should be given to identifying the precipitating agent and removing it from the diet. If formula fed, the infant should be started on a formula with an alternative protein source or amino acid composition. If breast fed, the maternal diet should be interrogated and possible causative agents removed.

Intussusception

Although classic for intussusception, the clinical triad of abdominal pain, a palpable abdominal mass, and currant jelly stools (caused by intestinal ischemia and mucosal sloughing) occurs in less than 25% of cases.[19,20] More typically, infants and toddlers present with abdominal colic: intermittent, crampy abdominal pain every 15 to 20 minutes. Intussusception is generally treated with a therapeutic enema, reserving an operation for the most difficult cases. For a more detailed understanding of intussusception, please see the following section.

SCHOOL-AGE CHILDREN

The differential diagnosis for bleeding in a school-age child (preschool and beyond) is relatively broad because of the variety of possible exposures (infections and toxins) and conditions that can present in this age group. Similar to many of the conditions discussed previously, making the diagnosis relies principally on the clinical history and presentation.

Infections

School-age children are at particular risk for infectious colitis because of their exposure to environmental pathogens (eg, daycare, school). Most food-borne infections, are self-limiting and do not often lead to lower GI bleeding. However, certain pathogens can cause significant hematochezia (eg, *Salmonella, Shigella, Campylobacter, Clostridium difficile*). The mainstay of treatment of bacterial colitis is antibiotic therapy. However, antibiotics should not be initiated if enterohemorrhagic *Escherichia coli* (strains O157:H7 or O104:H4) infection is suspected, as antibiotic treatment is associated with the development of hemolytic uremic syndrome.[21] *E coli* colitis should be suspected in patients with acute bloody diarrhea, or hemolytic uremic syndrome, particularly if associated with abdominal tenderness and the absence of fever. Antibiotic therapy for enterohemorrhagic *E coli* infection does not alter the duration of acute illnesses.[22] Thus, antibiotic therapy is not recommended for enterohemorrhagic *E coli* infections. With the exception of the immunocompromised patient, an operation for infectious colitis is rarely needed.

Inflammatory Bowel Disease

Inflammatory bowel disease (IBD), which includes Crohn disease and ulcerative colitis, is rare in early childhood. However, IBD has a peak in incidence during late adolescence. Distinguishing between the 2 entities is often difficult, as both commonly present with abdominal pain, fevers, and diarrhea. Often the diagnosis is delayed, and patients can have growth delays associated with untreated illness.[23] Gastrointestinal bleeding in the setting of IBD is typically caused by mucosal ulceration and inflammation and is, thus, more suggestive of ulcerative colitis. Malignancy is also on the differential diagnosis as patients with IBD are at higher risk for both small and large bowel malignancy. Diagnosis of IBD typically requires endoscopic evaluation (upper and lower) with biopsies for histologic diagnosis.

Malignancies

Although rare, GI malignancies do occur in the pediatric population. Primary tumors can include GI stromal tumors, lymphomas, and adenocarcinomas. Metastatic lesions to the intestines can also present with GI bleeding. Patients receiving chemotherapy for a non-GI malignancy (often hematologic malignancies) can have typhlitis caused by the neutropenia, which can lead to GI bleeding.

Polyps

Colorectal polyps are a fairly common source for bleeding in this age group. A large analysis of the Pediatric Endoscopy Database System Clinical Outcomes Research Initiative found that polyps were found in 12% of the patients with LGIB undergoing colonoscopy.[24] Most polyps found in the pediatric population are in fact juvenile hamartomatous polyps with low likelihood for malignancy. However, they can be associated with syndromes such as juvenile polyposis syndrome or familial adenomatous polyposis, which necessitate further evaluation and treatment.[25]

INTUSSUSCEPTION

Intussusception is the invagination (telescoping) of a segment of intestine into the adjacent bowel. Intussusception is the most common cause of intestinal obstruction in infants and toddlers. In addition to obstructive symptoms, intussusception often presents with hematochezia in the form of "currant jelly stool." John Hutchinson reported the successful surgical correction of an intussusception in 1873. In 1876, Hirschsprung described hydrostatic reduction of intussusception by enema, resulting in decreased mortality.[26] Contrast enema eventually became the accepted initial mode of therapy for intussusception in stable pediatric patients.

PATHOPHYSIOLOGY

The intussusceptum is the proximal inner segment of the intestine, whereas the intussuscipiens is the distal outer receiving portion (**Fig. 1**). Ileocolic intussusception is the most common location and accounts for 80% to 95% of all pediatric intussusceptions. Ileoileal, cecocolic, colocolic, and jejunojejunal intussusceptions occur with decreasing frequency. The intussusceptum drags the associated mesentery into the intussuscipiens, resulting in venous and lymphatic congestion, bowel edema, and ultimately ischemia and perforation. Although some intussusceptions spontaneously reduce, the natural history of an intussusception is to progress to perforation and sepsis unless the condition is recognized and treated appropriately.

Intussusception can occur at any age. In children, 60% occur before the age of 1 year, and 80% to 90% occur before the age of 2 years.[27] A Swiss population-based study reports yearly mean incidences of intussusception were 38, 31, and 26 cases per 100,000 live births in the first, second, and third year of life, respectively.[28] Intussusception is uncommon before 3 months and after 3 years of age. Intussusception in younger and older patients is more commonly associated with a pathologic lead point.

Idiopathic (Primary) Intussusception

Approximately 75% of intussusceptions in children do not have a pathologic lead point and are classified as idiopathic or primary intussusceptions. Idiopathic

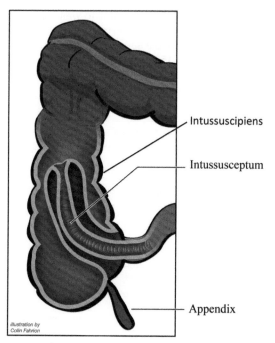

Illustration by
Colin Fahrion

Fig. 1. Ileocolic intussusception.

intussusception is most common in children between 3 months and 3 years of age. For unclear reasons, intussusception is slightly more common in boys.[28] There is an increasing body of evidence implicating the role of viral infections as the trigger for idiopathic intussusception. The putative lead point in idiopathic intussusception is attributed to hypertrophied Peyer's patches in the lymphoid-rich terminal ileum (**Box 2**).

Secondary Intussusception

An intussusception may have an identifiable abnormality in the intestine that acts as a lead point, drawing the proximal bowel into the distal bowel by peristaltic activity. These so-called secondary intussusceptions account for 10% to 25% of intussusceptions. A pathologic lead point is seen more commonly in children younger than 3 months and older than 3 years.[28,32] A Meckel diverticulum is the most common pathologic lead point followed by polyps and enteric duplication cysts. A summary of pathologic lead points is listed in **Box 3**.

CLINICAL MANIFESTATION
Presentation

Intussusception occurs most commonly in healthy, well-nourished infants and toddlers. The typical presentation is the sudden onset of severe, intermittent, crampy abdominal pain. The child is often writhing in pain and crying inconsolably, drawing the knees toward the abdomen seeking a position of comfort. The episodes can resolve as quickly as they begin and usually recur at 15- to 30-minute intervals with increasing intensity. Vomiting is a common symptom and may become bilious as the obstruction progresses. With time, the child becomes dehydrated and lethargic. Initially, bowel movements may result from evacuation of stool distal to the intussusception. Later in the course, the stool may become mucoid and blood tinged as the ischemic mucosa sloughs. It is a diagnostic pitfall to wait for these so-called currant jelly stools, as this is a late sign and is absent in nearly one-third of patients. The classically described triad of pain, a palpable sausage-shaped abdominal mass, and currant jelly stools is seen in less than 15% of patients.[33] Particularly in infants, lethargy can be the only presenting symptom, thus, intussusception should be included in the evaluation of unexplained altered consciousness.[34]

Physical Examination

Early in the course of intussusception, the child's vital signs are usually normal. When in pain, the child is often writhing and difficult to examine. During painless intervals, the

---

Box 2
Evidence implicating viral trigger in idiopathic intussusception

- Thirty percent of patients experience viral illness (upper respiratory infection, GI, otitis media) before intussusception.
- Incidence of intussusception varies directly with seasonal respiratory viral illness.[29]
- There is an 8-fold increase in intussusception among infants vaccinated with early form of rotavirus vaccine.[30]
- Recent adenovirus documented in up to 50% of intussusceptions.[31]

   [a] *Rotashield*, the new generation of rotavirus vaccine, has not been implicated in intussusception.[30]
   Data from Refs.[29–31]

Box 3
Pathologic lead points in children

Benign focal bowel abnormalities
- Meckel diverticulum
- Polyps
- Enteric duplication cysts
- Vascular malformation
- Foreign body

Malignant lead points
- Lymphoma
- Melanoma
- Lymphosarcoma
- Bowel tumor

Systemic diseases
- Henoch-Schonlein purpura resulting in small bowel wall hematomas
- Cystic fibrosis
- Crohn disease
- Celiac disease
- Hemolytic uremic syndrome

---

belly is typically not tender. An abdominal mass may be palpable or even visible in a thin child. Rectal examination may yield blood or bloody mucus. As the obstruction worsens and the intussusceptum becomes more ischemic, the child may become febrile, hypovolemic, and tachycardic. Hypotension and peritonitis are ominous findings owing to bowel perforation and sepsis, thus, prompt diagnosis, resuscitation, and operation are imperative for survival.

DIAGNOSIS
Laboratory Studies

No specific laboratory studies point to the diagnosis of intussusception. Late in the disease process there may be electrolyte abnormalities caused by hypovolemia and anemia. There may be a leukocytosis caused by gut ischemia.

Ultrasonography

Ultrasonography for the evaluation of intussusception has been in use since the 1970s and has become the method of choice for detecting intussusception at most institutions.[35] Ultrasonography is an ideal screening modality because it avoids radiation exposure, and in experienced hands has a sensitivity and specificity approaching 100%. The intussusception is usually detected in the right side of the abdomen. The classic finding is referred to as the *target sign*, in which concentric alternating rings of low and high echogenicity are seen, representing the layers of intestine and mesenteric fat within the intestine (**Fig. 2**). Ultrasonography can also detect the rare case of ileoileal intussusception and is effective at identifying a pathologic lead point when present. More recently, ultrasonography is used to monitor the success of intussusception reduction procedures.[36]

Abdominal Radiographs

Plain radiographs are often obtained as part of the routine evaluation of patients with abdominal symptoms (**Fig. 3**). Plain radiographs are much less sensitive than ultrasonography at detecting intussusception. Thus, if there is a high clinical suspicion

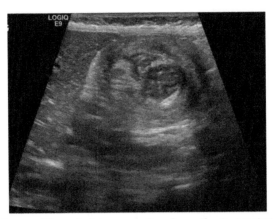

Fig. 2. Ultrasound scan of ileocolic intussusception shows the target sign.

for intussusception, ultrasonography, not plain radiographs, should be the first diagnostic maneuver. Radiographic findings suggestive of intussusception are listed in **Box 4**.[37]

Computed Tomography and MRI

An intussusception can be identified on both computed tomography (CT) and MRI. However, neither modality is routinely used to evaluate for intussusception because they cannot reduce the intussusception, often require sedation in young children, and can be time consuming. CT also exposes the child to a considerable dose of radiation. Small bowel intussusceptions that are detected on CT or MRI are usually transient and clinically insignificant.

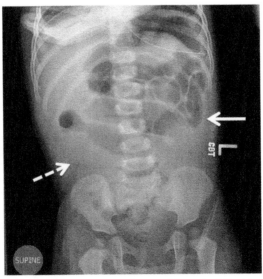

Fig. 3. Abdominal plain film shows concern for small bowel obstruction with multiple air-filled loops of dilated small bowel (*solid arrow*) with the absence of gas in the right lower quadrant (*dashed arrow*).

Box 4
Radiographic findings concerning for intussusception

- Signs of intestinal obstruction (dilated small bowel and air-fluid levels)
- Abdominal mass
- Target sign
- Absence of air in cecum
- Obscured liver margin
- Lateralization of the ileum

Contrast Enema

The availability of ultrasonographic expertise is limited at many institutions. Therefore, some institutions use contrast enema under fluoroscopy to establish the diagnosis of intussusception. In the presence of an intussusception, the study is converted to a therapeutic hydrostatic reduction of the intussusception.

TREATMENT

Stable patients with a high clinical suspicion or radiographic evidence of intussusception should undergo nonoperative reduction as the first-line therapy. Evidence of intestinal perforation, peritonitis, or hemodynamic instability is an absolute contraindication to nonoperative reduction and warrants an emergency operation. Before attempting reduction, the patient should be adequately resuscitated with intravenous fluids.

NONOPERATIVE REDUCTION

Nonoperative reduction of an ileocolic intussusception using hydrostatic or pneumatic pressure enema is effective and safe in children. Both reduction techniques can be performed under sonographic or fluoroscopic guidance. Although ultrasound scan avoids radiation exposure, sonographic and fluoroscopic guidance techniques have comparable success rates.[38] In practice, the choice between hydrostatic or pneumatic reduction and between sonographic or fluoroscopic guidance is largely dictated by the expertise of the individual performing the procedure.

Although the risk of intestinal perforation is only about 1%,[39] the surgical team should be notified that reduction is being attempted in the event of perforation or failed reduction. Bowel perforation during attempted pneumatic reduction can result in massive pneumoperitoneum and respiratory compromise from abdominal compartment syndrome. Emergency decompression of the pneumoperitoneum with an angiocatheter can relieve the compartment syndrome until the perforation and intussusception can be definitively repaired. The utility of antibiotics before reduction to prevent bacterial translocation or as preemptive treatment in the event of perforation has not been established.[40] Fevers are common after reduction of an intussusception because of bacterial translocation or the release of endotoxin and cytokines. The intussusceptum is edematous after reduction, which may itself act as a lead point and lead to recurrent intussusception in the short term. After successful reduction of an intussusception, the patient should be observed for 12 to 24 hours or until tolerating a normal diet.

Hydrostatic Reduction

Hydrostatic reduction was historically performed with barium under fluoroscopic guidance. Today, water-soluble contrast is commonly used because of the potential hazards of barium peritonitis in the event of intestinal perforation. The standard technique is to place a large, lubricated catheter into the rectum and tape the buttocks together to prevent leakage. Balloon catheters are generally avoided. As described in **Box 5**, the contrast reservoir is placed 3 feet above the patient to generate a hydrostatic column of pressure. Under fluoroscopy or ultrasound guidance, the contrast agent is instilled until a concave filling defect is seen (**Fig. 4**). Hydrostatic pressure is administered as long as the intussusceptum is reducing. Reduction is complete when contrast flows freely into the terminal ileum. Successful reduction rates range from 80% to 95%.[41]

Pneumatic Reduction

Pneumatic reduction of intussusceptions gained popularity in the 1980s. Air enemas reduce the intussusception more easily and are more effective than hydrostatic enemas. A recent meta-analysis showed the success rate of reducing an intussusception with an air enema was 83% compared with 70% for hydrostatic enema.[42] A large catheter is placed into the rectum and the buttocks are taped closed. A sphygmomanometer is used to monitor the intracolonic pressure, typically not to exceed 120 mm Hg. The colon is pressurized under fluoroscopy or ultrasonography, monitoring for the reflux of air into the terminal ileum and disappearance of the mass at the ileocecal valve that indicates complete reduction of the intussusception (**Fig. 5**). Carbon dioxide can be used instead of air because it is rapidly absorbed and may be less uncomfortable.

Several studies found improved reduction rates with delayed, repeated attempts at nonoperative reduction in clinically stable patients. In one large series, delayed repeated attempts at reductions were made in 15% of cases and were successful in 50% of cases.[43] Protocols call for a 30-minute to 24-hour interval between attempts at reducing an intussusception.[44,45]

RECURRENCE

Intussusception recurs in approximately 10% of patients after successful reduction. The recurrence rate is similar for the different modes of reduction. About one-third of recurrent intussusceptions occur within the first 24 hours, often after initiation of feedings.[46,47] The parents are most closely attuned to the signs of intussusception in their child and should be on the lookout for evidence of recurrence. Recurrence does not mandate operative reduction. Each recurrence should be treated as if it were an initial episode of intussusception.[44,48] However, multiple recurrences should heighten the concern for the presence of a pathologic lead point (**Box 6**).

Box 5
Rule of 3s for hydrostatic reduction

1. Hydrostatic column 3 feet above the patient

2. No more than 3 attempts at reduction

3. Each attempt less than 3 minutes long

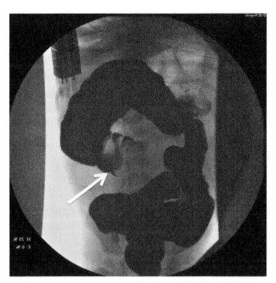

Fig. 4. Hydrostatic contrast enema. Arrow shows the leading edge of the intussusceptum.

OPERATIVE TREATMENT
Open Reduction

Operative reduction of the intussusception is indicated when enema reduction has failed, there is peritonitis, or there is evidence for a pathologic lead point. An open exploration is typically performed via a transverse right lower quadrant incision, as intussusception most commonly involves the terminal ileum and cecum. The classical teaching is to avoid pulling the intussusceptum and intussuscipiens apart but rather push the leading edge of the intussusceptum from distal to proximal. Once the

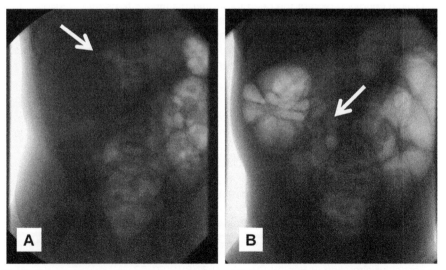

Fig. 5. Pneumatic reduction of intussusception. (*A*) Arrow shows the leading edge of the intussusceptum. (*B*). Successful reduction of intussusception. Arrow marks air in the terminal ileum.

> **Box 6**
> **Clinical summary of nonoperative reduction of intussusception**
>
> - Pneumatic reduction is superior to hydrostatic reduction.
> - Ultrasonography and fluoroscopy are comparable for guiding reduction.
> - If initial attempts at reduction fail, delayed repeat enema may be successful.
> - Intussusception recurs in about 10%.
> - Each recurrence should be treated as if it were an initial episode of intussusception.

intussusception is reduced, the bowel should be evaluated for viability, perforation, and pathologic lead point. The bowel is generally ischemic and edematous. In the absence of a pathologic lead point, bowel resection is rarely required.[49]

Laparoscopic Reduction

Laparoscopy was initially used as a diagnostic adjunct in intussusception to either confirm the diagnosis or search for a pathologic lead point. Several recent studies describe the laparoscopic reduction of intussusception through 3 small abdominal ports.[50] Unlike the open operation, it is necessary to place gentle traction on the intussusceptum and intussuscipiens. It is important to evaluate for traumatic injury to the bowel after reduction. Little is lost by first attempting laparoscopic reduction. If this cannot be accomplished safely, the operation should be converted to a laparotomy. About 30% of attempted laparoscopic reductions are converted to laparotomy.[50,51]

SUMMARY

The differential diagnosis for LGIB in children is broad; however, the age of the patient helps narrow the diagnosis. Although most episodes of LGIB are benign and do not warrant hospitalization or surgical intervention, physical examination findings and the clinical condition dictate the need for further diagnostic tests and possible intervention. Intussusception is most common in children younger than 3 years. The diagnosis of intussusception is typically made with ultrasonography. Nonoperative reduction, either hydrostatic or pneumatic, should be attempted in a clinically stable patient without evidence of perforation, peritonitis, or hemodynamic instability.

REFERENCES

1. Pant C, Olyaee M, Sferra TJ, et al. Emergency department visits for gastrointestinal bleeding in children: results from the Nationwide Emergency Department Sample 2006-2011. Curr Med Res Opin 2015;31(2):347–51.
2. Balkan E, Kiriştioğlu I, Gürpinar A, Ozel I, Sinmaz K, Dogruyol H. Sigmoidoscopy in minor lower gastrointestinal bleeding. Arch Dis Child 1998;78(3):267–8.
3. Applegate KE. Evidence-based diagnosis of malrotation and volvulus. Pediatr Radiol 2009;39(Suppl 2):S161–3.
4. Long FR, Kramer SS, Markowitz RI, et al. Radiographic patterns of intestinal malrotation in children. Radiographics 1996;16(3):547–56 [discussion: 556–60].
5. Mehall JR, Chandler JC, Mehall RL, et al. Management of typical and atypical intestinal malrotation. J Pediatr Surg 2002;37(8):1169–72.
6. Ladd WE. Surgical diseases of the alimentary tract in infants. N Engl J Med 1936; 215(16):705–8.

7. Emami CN, Petrosyan M, Giuliani S, et al. Role of the host defense system and intestinal microbial flora in the pathogenesis of necrotizing enterocolitis. Surg Infect (Larchmt) 2009;10(5):407–17.
8. Petrosyan M, Guner YS, Williams M, et al. Current concepts regarding the pathogenesis of necrotizing enterocolitis. Pediatr Surg Int 2009;25(4):309–18.
9. Lin PW, Stoll BJ. Necrotising enterocolitis. Lancet 2006;368(9543):1271–83.
10. Ng S. Necrotizing enterocolitis in the full-term neonate. J Paediatr Child Health 2001;37(1):1–4.
11. Muller A, Schurink M, Bos AF, et al. Clinical importance of a fixed bowel loop in the treatment of necrotizing enterocolitis. Neonatology 2014;105(1):33–8.
12. Amiel J, Sproat-Emison E, Garcia-Barcelo M, et al. Hirschsprung disease, associated syndromes and genetics: a review. J Med Genet 2008;45(1):1–14.
13. Badner JA, Sieber WK, Garver KL, et al. A genetic study of Hirschsprung disease. Am J Hum Genet 1990;46(3):568–80.
14. Austin KM. The pathogenesis of Hirschsprung's disease-associated enterocolitis. Semin Pediatr Surg 2012;21(4):319–27.
15. O'Connor JJ. Pediatric proctology. Dis Colon Rectum 1975;18(2):126–7.
16. Cserni G. Gastric pathology in Meckel's diverticulum. Review of cases resected between 1965 and 1995. Am J Clin Pathol 1996;106(6):782–5.
17. Sagar J, Kumar V, Shah DK. Meckel's diverticulum: a systematic review. J R Soc Med 2006;99(10):501–5.
18. Willetts IE, Dalzell M, Puntis JW, et al. Cow's milk enteropathy: surgical pitfalls. J Pediatr Surg 1999;34(10):1486–8.
19. Applegate KE. Intussusception in children: evidence-based diagnosis and treatment. Pediatr Radiol 2009;39(Suppl 2):S140–3.
20. Harrington L, Connolly B, Hu X, et al. Ultrasonographic and clinical predictors of intussusception. J Pediatr 1998;132(5):836–9.
21. Freedman SB, Xie J, Neufeld MS, et al. Shiga toxin-producing escherichia coli infection, antibiotics, and risk of developing hemolytic uremic syndrome: a meta-analysis. Clin Infect Dis 2016;62(10):1251–8.
22. Proulx F, Turgeon JP, Delage G, et al. Randomized, controlled trial of antibiotic therapy for Escherichia coli O157:H7 enteritis. J Pediatr 1992;121(2):299–303.
23. Sawczenko A, Sandhu BK. Presenting features of inflammatory bowel disease in Great Britain and Ireland. Arch Dis Child 2003;88(11):995–1000.
24. Thakkar K, Alsarraj A, Fong E, et al. Prevalence of colorectal polyps in pediatric colonoscopy. Dig Dis Sci 2012;57(4):1050–5.
25. Thakkar K, Fishman DS, Gilger MA. Colorectal polyps in childhood. Curr Opin Pediatr 2012;24(5):632–7.
26. Hirschsprung H. 107 falle van darmin agination bei kindern, behandelt inkoningin louisin-kinderhospital in Kopenhagen wahrend der jahre 1871-1904. Mitt Grenzgeb Medezin Chir 1905;14:555–74.
27. Mandeville K, Chien M, Willyerd FA, et al. Intussusception: clinical presentations and imaging characteristics. Pediatr Emerg Care 2012;28(9):842–4.
28. Buettcher M, Baer G, Bonhoeffer J, et al. Three-year surveillance of intussusception in children in Switzerland. Pediatrics 2007;120(3):473–80.
29. West K, Grossfeld JL. Intussusception. In: Wyllie R, Hyams JS, editors. Pediatric gastrointestinal disease: pathophysiology, diagnosis and management. Philadelphia: Saunders; 1999. p. 427.
30. Weintraub ES, Baggs J, Duffy J, et al. Risk of intussusception after monovalent rotavirus vaccination. N Engl J Med 2014;370(6):513–9.

31. Bines JE, Liem NT, Justice FA, et al. Risk factors for intussusception in infants in Vietnam and Australia: adenovirus implicated, but not rotavirus. J Pediatr 2006; 149(4):452–60.
32. Rubinstein JC, Liu L, Caty MG, et al. Pathologic leadpoint is uncommon in ileo-colic intussusception regardless of age. J Pediatr Surg 2015;50(10):1665–7.
33. Yamamoto LG, Morita SY, Boychuk RB, et al. Stool appearance in intussuscep-tion: assessing the value of the term "currant jelly". Am J Emerg Med 1997; 15(3):293–8.
34. Kleizen KJ, Hunck A, Wijnen MH, et al. Neurological symptoms in children with intussusception. Acta Paediatr 2009;98(11):1822–4.
35. Ko HS, Schenk JP, Troger J, et al. Current radiological management of intussus-ception in children. Eur Radiol 2007;17(9):2411–21.
36. Di Renzo D, Colangelo M, Lauriti G, et al. Ultrasound-guided Hartmann's solution enema: first-choice procedure for reducing idiopathic intussusception. Radiol Med 2012;117(4):679–89.
37. Saverino BP, Lava C, Lowe LH, et al. Radiographic findings in the diagnosis of pediatric ileocolic intussusception: comparison to a control population. Pediatr Emerg Care 2010;26(4):281–4.
38. Hadidi AT, El Shal N. Childhood intussusception: a comparative study of nonsur-gical management. J Pediatr Surg 1999;34(2):304–7.
39. Maoate K, Beasley SW. Perforation during gas reduction of intussusception. Pe-diatr Surg Int 1998;14(3):168–70.
40. Al-Tokhais T, Hsieh H, Pemberton J, et al. Antibiotics administration before enema reduction of intussusception: is it necessary? J Pediatr Surg 2012;47(5):928–30.
41. Flaum V, Schneider A, Gomes Ferreira C, et al. Twenty years' experience for reduction of ileocolic intussusceptions by saline enema under sonography con-trol. J Pediatr Surg 2016;51(1):179–82.
42. Sadigh G, Zou KH, Razavi SA, et al. Meta-analysis of air versus liquid enema for intussusception reduction in children. AJR Am J Roentgenol 2015;205(5):W542–9.
43. Navarro OM, Daneman A, Chae A. Intussusception: the use of delayed, repeated reduction attempts and the management of intussusceptions due to pathologic lead points in pediatric patients. AJR Am J Roentgenol 2004;182(5):1169–76.
44. Lautz TB, Thurm CW, Rothstein DH. Delayed repeat enemas are safe and cost-effective in the management of pediatric intussusception. J Pediatr Surg 2015; 50(3):423–7.
45. Pazo A, Hill J, Losek JD. Delayed repeat enema in the management of intussus-ception. Pediatr Emerg Care 2010;26(9):640–5.
46. Daneman A, Alton DJ, Lobo E, et al. Patterns of recurrence of intussusception in children: a 17-year review. Pediatr Radiol 1998;28(12):913–9.
47. Gray MP, Li SH, Hoffmann RG, et al. Recurrence rates after intussusception enema reduction: a meta-analysis. Pediatrics 2014;134(1):110–9.
48. Niramis R, Watanatittan S, Kruatrachue A, et al. Management of recurrent intussus-ception: nonoperative or operative reduction? J Pediatr Surg 2010;45(11):2175–80.
49. Banapour P, Sydorak RM, Shaul D. Surgical approach to intussusception in older children: influence of lead points. J Pediatr Surg 2015;50(4):647–50.
50. Bonnard A, Demarche M, Dimitriu C, et al. Indications for laparoscopy in the man-agement of intussusception: a multicenter retrospective study conducted by the French Study Group for Pediatric Laparoscopy (GECI). J Pediatr Surg 2008; 43(7):1249–53.
51. Apelt N, Featherstone N, Giuliani S. Laparoscopic treatment of intussusception in children: a systematic review. J Pediatr Surg 2013;48(8):1789–93.

Overview of Wound Healing and Management

Dylan R. Childs, MD[a], Ananth S. Murthy, MD[b],*

KEYWORDS

- Wound • Healing • Management • Skin • Soft tissue injuries

KEY POINTS

- Wound repair is a coordinated series of phases that have predictable cell types and microenvironments.
- Wound healing is divided into inflammatory, proliferative and maturation phases.
- The pathway of healing is determined by characteristics of the wound on presentation.
- Wounds can heal via primary, secondary or delayed primary healing.
- Debridement and negative pressure wound therapy (NPWT) are important adjuncts to treat contaminated or chronic wounds.
- Soft tissue injuries should be assessed for blood supply, hypoxia, infection, edema and foreign body contamination; and treated based on these characteristics.

PHASES OF WOUND HEALING

Wound healing is a complex, highly developed chain of events that allows people to interact with their environment. The skin is a protective organ, and it provides vital functions like temperature modulation, moisture regulation, as well as sensation, reception, and transmission. The ability to repair and regenerate is central to these functions. Wound repair is a coordinated series of phases that have predictable cell types and microenvironment preparations.

Inflammatory Phase

The initial event when a wound occurs is a platelet plug that limits bleeding and begins cytokine signaling. This event initiates the coagulation cascade and promotes amplification and recruitment of cells for the debridement of nonviable tissue. The platelets create the plug in response to exposed collagen, which then releases ADP promoting continued platelet aggregation. Aggregation is accompanied by release

[a] Division of Plastic Surgery, Summa Health System, 525 E Market Street, Akron, OH 44304, USA; [b] Division of Plastic Surgery, Akron Children's Hospital, 215 W Bowery Street, Akron, OH 44308, USA
* Corresponding author. Plastic & Reconstructive Surgery, Akron Children's Hospital, 215 West Bowery Street, Suite 3300, Akron, OH 44308-1062.
E-mail address: amurthy@chmca.org

Surg Clin N Am 97 (2017) 189–207
http://dx.doi.org/10.1016/j.suc.2016.08.013
0039-6109/17/© 2016 Elsevier Inc. All rights reserved.
surgical.theclinics.com

of platelet-derived growth factor (PDGF) and transforming growth factor beta (TGF-β), which is chemotactic for neutrophils in the blood.[1,2]

Neutrophils are drawn to and trapped in the platelet plug in response to PDGF.[1] They are the initial scavengers for debridement. They serve initially to phagocytize dead tissue and bacterial particles as well as create a wound hostile to bacteria by using reactive oxygen species. Neutrophils also provide a key proinflammatory cytokine in interleukin (IL)-1, which has dual effects as a proinflammatory cytokine and a stimulus for proliferation of keratinocytes.[3] The local environment also changes; initially, there is severe vasoconstriction secondary to catecholamine release. This vasoconstriction abates shortly after and there is subsequent vasodilation in response to histamine release from circulating mast cells[4,5] (**Fig. 1**).

As the inflammatory phase progresses, macrophages become the dominant cell type within 24 to 72 hours. Their role in the orchestration of wound healing is critical and changes as wound healing progresses.[6–8] It is widely accepted that macrophages play a central role and their response is key to establishing homeostasis within the wound and downregulating the inflammatory state to avoid pathologic inflammation (**Fig. 2**).

Proliferative Phase

The proliferative phase occurs from days 4 to 21, and is representative of angiogenesis, extracellular matrix (ECM) formation, and epithelialization.[9,10] Although there is considerable overlap between the phases of wound healing, the ability to transition into the next phase can determine whether a wound heals appropriately. ECM formation likely starts with platelet degranulation, because PDGF is a known promoter of proteoglycan and collagen formation. Local fibroblasts respond to PDGF by

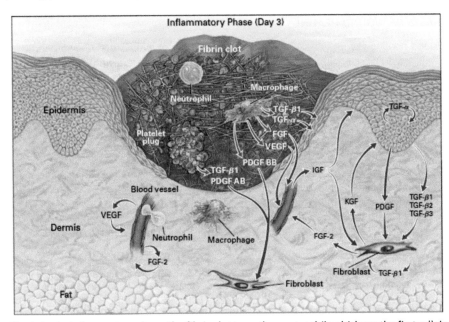

Fig. 1. In the inflammatory phase, the fibrin clot traps the neutrophils which are the first cells in the wound. It invites the macrophage which is involved in orchestrating the process of wound healing. FGF, fibroblast growth factor; KGF, keratinocyte-derived growth factor; VEGF, vascular endothelial growth factor. (*From* Singer AJ, Clark RAF. Cutaneous wound healing. N Engl J Med 1999;341(10):739; with permission. Copyright © 1999 Massachusetts Medical Society.)

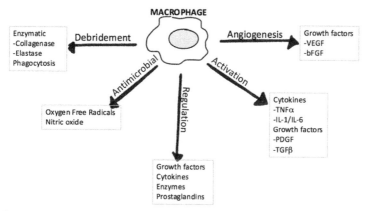

Fig. 2. The macrophage has multiple actions, such as debridement, antimicrobial action, wound regulation, cellular activation via cytokines, and angiogenesis via growth factors. It is the most critical cell involved, and without the action of macrophages there would be no progression in wound healing. bFGF, basic fibroblast growth factor. (*Data from* Broughton G, Janis J, Attinger C. Wound healing: an overview. Plast Reconstr Surg 2006;117:1e-s.)

producing collagen as well as transforming into myofibroblasts to promote wound contraction. Fibroblasts also secrete keratinocyte-derived growth factor (KGF), which stimulates epithelialization from keratinocytes,[11] and endothelial cells produce vascular endothelial growth factor (VEGF), and basis fibroblast growth factor (bFGF) to promote ingrowth of blood vessels. A hallmark of normal wound healing physiology is the ability to cease ongoing collagen production, with maximum deposition at approximately 21 days (**Fig. 3**).

Maturation Phase

Remodeling phase occurs from 3 weeks to 1 year after injury. It is characterized by wound contraction and collagen remodeling. Macrophages are the principal cell

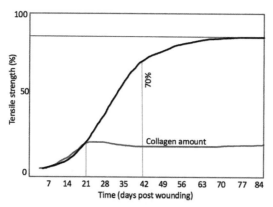

Fig. 3. Collagen accumulation steadily increases till 3 weeks after injury. However, the strength of the wound closure continues to increase after 3 weeks secondary to the cross-linking and alignment of collagen fibers. This strength reaches 70% at 6 weeks and reaches about 80% to 90% at full maturation. (*Data from* Geever EF, Stein JM, Levenson SM. Variations in breaking strength in healing wounds of young guinea pigs. J Trauma Acute Care Surgery 1965;5(5):624–35.)

type in proliferation, and fibroblasts are the principle cell type in remodeling. The hallmark process is the conversion of type III collagen to type I.[12] Equilibrium between type I and type III occurs after approximately 30 days, and maximum strength occurs after roughly 42 to 60 days, hence the traditional recommendation of activity restriction after 6 weeks (see **Fig. 3**). Successful wound healing is contingent on adequate tissue oxygenation at the wound edges. Poor oxygenation can generally be attributed to local strangulation from excessive tension or poor delivery of oxygen to distal tissues. Local measures can be undertaken to improve tissue mobility, because excessive tension is a clinical miscalculation that inevitably fails.

HEALING PROCESSES AND PROBLEMS WITH WOUND HEALING

Wounds generally heal without issue and progress through one of 3 different pathways. The pathway of healing is determined by characteristics of the wound on initial presentation, and it is vital to select the appropriate method to treat the wound based on its ability to avoid hypoxia, infection, excessive edema, and foreign bodies. These factors create an environment that interrupts healing and creates a cycle of hypoxia, inflammation, necrosis, and infection, creating a chronic wound.

Surgical incisions are an example of primary healing, which is an immediate reapproximation of the skin edges, with subsequent epithelialization reconstituting the barrier within 48 to 72 hours. The key component of success with primary healing is limiting tension at the incision line, which can be accomplished by elevating deeper layers, placing progressive tension sutures to distribute the stress, with local tissue rearrangement. If there is too much tension at the suture line, breakdown occurs as a result of local tissue ischemia and necrosis.

Secondary healing is a process that uses contraction and epithelialization to restore the epithelial barrier. The wound is left open, or is in discontinuity, typically because of tension or contamination. The wound bed is kept clean and optimized for keratinocyte migration, which is generally accomplished by using hydrogels and transparent films that are waterproof and impermeable to bacteria. Once again, optimizing the wound bed to prevent hypoxia, necrosis, and infections is key to secondary healing.

Delayed primary healing is used in poorly delineated or contaminated wounds. The principle is to convert a hostile wound into a favorable one that subsequently permits surgical closure. Often adjuncts such as debridement, dressing changes, and placement of negative pressure wound therapy (NPWT) form a bridge to definitive reestablishment of an epithelial barrier. Often this method is used to treat wounds with tissue transfer; however, this can also be used as a bridge to close the wound edges.[13,14] The bridging options that are available depend on the underlying structures (**Fig. 4**).

Molecular Requirements for Wound Healing

Poor oxygenation caused by inadequate delivery is a common occurrence and is often the sequela of patient-derived factors such as smoking, peripheral vascular disease, or poorly controlled diabetes. Although these diseases have a higher prevalence in the adult population, the significance of distal oxygenation must be appreciated in the pediatric population as well. Oxygen is central to many levels of wound healing and can be described as an enzymatic subcellular nutrient critical to oxidative phosphorylation and leukocyte respiratory burst, and integral for collagen synthesis.[15,16]

Proper nutrition is also critical, because wound healing is an anabolic process with increased metabolic demand. Although the physiologic reserve of children is often astounding, establishing and maintaining adequate nutritional stores should be one

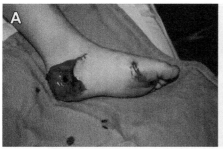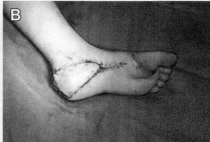

Fig. 4. (*A*) This child had a heel injury secondary to a lawnmower accident with exposed calcaneus. The wound was first debrided to normal, viable tissue and underwent dressing changes for 3 weeks with NPWT. Wound closure should not be attempted in the acute setting in cases of extensive contamination. (*B*) After obtaining a clean wound, a sensate, medial plantar artery flap was used to cover the calcaneus.

of the first interventions when dealing with a chronic wound. In the pediatric burn population, it was shown that early excision and aggressive feeding improved outcomes.[17] It has also been shown in animal models that the tensile strength of wounds is significantly less than that of controls secondary to poor nutrition.[18]

Although protein stores are central to healing, there are specific vitamin and mineral deficiencies that can negatively affect it. The best known is vitamin C because of its role in scurvy. It is a required cofactor for collagen cross-linking but is also implicated in reducing oxidative stress.[19] A deficiency of vitamin C has been associated with a greater susceptibility to wound infection.[20] Vitamin A has been shown to reverse the deleterious effects of steroid use on wound healing, and has demonstrable benefit in other conditions, such as diabetic wound care and tumors.[21,22] Zinc (Zn) is an essential cofactor in DNA and RNA synthesis, and deficiencies lead to poor wound healing. However, the importance of Zn in wound healing was further confirmed when the structure of matrix metalloproteinases was found to have Zn as a cofactor. Zn benefits can be shown topically, but supplementation when levels are normal does not augment healing.[23]

Genetic Disorders in Wound Healing

There are heritable derangements in wound healing. These derangements are generally part of a larger spectrum of disease so effects on healing may be multifactorial. Pseudoxanthoma elasticum is a disease that has both autosomal dominant and recessive pathways. It is characterized by abnormal calcium depositions with hallmark yellowish papules over flexure sites. There can be associated cardiac and ocular disturbances as well as a tendency to form keloids with delayed wound healing.[24] Ehlers-Danlos syndrome is characterized by hyperelastic skin and hypermobile joints. There are 6 major types of Ehlers-Danlos and all but 1 is a heritable disorder of collagen, the exception being a heritable disorder of tenascin.[25,26] It is an autosomal dominant condition often associated with mitral valve prolapse. Because of innate errors in collagen production, wound healing is delayed and disturbed (**Fig. 5**). Type IV is a vascular subtype that has high association with arterial, bowel, and uterine rupture and often results in premature death.[27] Cutis laxa is an inborn error in elastin resulting in severely drooping skin folds. The skin abnormalities are accompanied by cardiovascular and pulmonary comorbidities, all of which result from a nonfunctioning elastase inhibitor.[28]

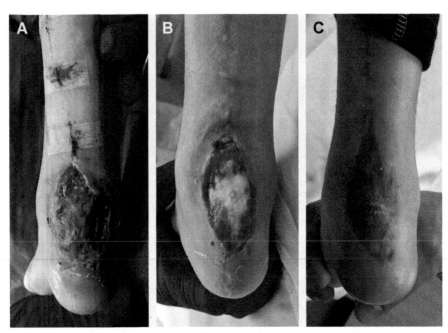

Fig. 5. (*A*) A young woman with Ehlers-Danlos syndrome presented with a complex open wound over the Achilles tendon after trauma. (*B*) After debridement and NPWT for 3 weeks, a bilayer wound matrix (Integra) was used as a bridge to achieving closure. The use of Acticoat (nanocrystalline silver) along with NPWT provides antibacterial coverage and enhances angiogenesis into the scaffold. (*C*) Final outcome with coverage of Achilles tendon. Patients with Ehlers-Danlos have a heritable disorder of collagen and require longer-than-usual times for achieving wound closure.

There are some inherited disorders that are contraindications for elective surgery. Werner syndrome (adult progeria) is autosomal recessive and has plaque-ridden, variably pigmented skin. Affected patients generally are short of stature with premature graying hair or baldness, trophic ulcers, and hypogonadism.[29] The pathologic mutation is of DNA helicase, which leads to chromosomal instability and early death. The error leads to difficulty healing because of poor fibroblast function secondary to poor response to growth factors PDGF and fibroblast growth factor (FGF).[30] Elastoderma is an exceptionally rare disease of excessive elastin fibers in the reticular dermis. It generally presents in young female patients, and the excess skin can be described as pendulous.[31] These conditions are associated with enough morbidity that elective surgery is generally discouraged.

Hypertrophic Scars and Keloids

Common wound healing disorders include hypertrophic scarring and keloids. It is typically taught that if the scar remains within the border of the wound, it is a hypertrophic scar, and if it exceeds the border of the wound it is a keloid. On microscopic examination keloids possess thick eosinophilic collagen bundles,[32] as well as a thickened epidermis and increased mesenchymal density. Often there is a difference in presenting wounds, with hypertrophic scars arising in major incisions or lacerations, whereas keloids arise from minor skin trauma. There is also an increase predilection for both in sites that are exposed to more mechanical forces, such as the sternum, shoulder, and knee. Foreign bodies and infection also seem to be contributing factors, secondary to lengthening of a proinflammatory state within the wound[33,34] (**Fig. 6**).

WOUND MANAGEMENT
Suture Types and Postoperative Care

Sutures can be divided into classes based on their makeup, number of strands, and permanence. When suturing in cosmetically sensitive areas, it generally advisable to use layered closures and to use a small monofilament for the most superficial layer of closure. The length of time a suture is retained can predispose to unsightly marks (railroad tracks), because the skin can epithelialize along the suture strand. Another skin closure application is the use of a cyanoacrylate. It has advantages, such as no trauma from needles; however, it alone cannot aid in alignment or support of skin edges. When suturing wounds, using a layered closure helps with final alignment and reduces tension, minimizing scar. For pediatric patients, final closure with delicate sutures, such as 6.0 rapidly absorbable suture, is often recommended for the face or cosmetically sensitive areas. A nonreactive 6.0 nonabsorbable suture can be used, but requires removal in 4 to 6 days, and removal can be difficult in the toddler population.

Postoperative care can be optimized by using a petroleum-based emollient for the first 1 to 3 weeks. After the expected fibroplasia, scar management can be addressed.

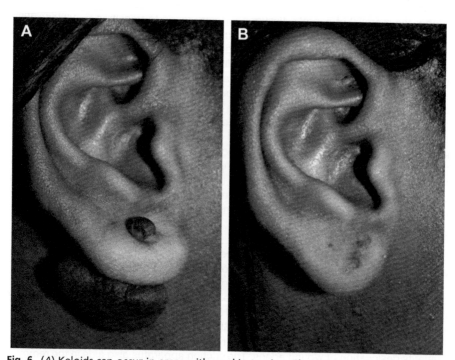

Fig. 6. (*A*) Keloids can occur in areas with no skin tension. The presence of foreign bodies, such as piercings, can be a predisposing factor. Recurrence after excision is common if no adjuvant therapy is performed. (*B*) Treatment commonly is preoperative, serial intralesional triamcinolone injections (usually 6 weeks apart), followed by excision. Low-dose radiation therapy (10–12 Gy) has been shown to ameliorate recurrent keloids that are resistant to corticosteroid therapy.

Often a protocol incorporating silicone-based products and scar massage aid in the aligning of collagen. It is important to convey to the patient that scar maturation can take between 6 and 12 months. Sunscreen during that time can be helpful. A scar initially is hyperemic and this indicates healing. Patience must be counseled to the patient and family because an early intervention rarely results in superior results. After a period of observation, interventions to improve scar appearance can be undertaken. Recently, Donelan and colleagues[35] showed improvement in facial burn scarring using a pulsed dye laser. Other modalities, such as fractional CO_2 lasers, are also being studied for scar management.

Role of Debridement

The goal for any chronic wound is to convert it to an active, healing wound, which is often accomplished by debridement. Whether this is autolytic, mechanical, or enzymatic the goal is to removal all necrotic tissue. Often, adequate debridement unmasks hidden collections, revealing a much more extensive wound than was initially presumed. By removing the necrotic tissue, the wound can optimize the regenerative potential of the bordering tissue. Preservation of the adjacent viable tissue is often critical in areas where there is limited local tissue. Operatively, a limit of debridement has often been to healthy bleeding tissue. This limit often has led to aggressive initial debridement sacrificing otherwise viable tissue. One of the adjuncts that is useful to debride atraumatically, sparing more viable tissue, is the Versajet hydrosurgery system.

After the removal of necrotic tissue, efforts are made to transition to a granulating wound. This transition is accomplished with barrier products that protect neighboring tissue. Some commonly used barrier products are petroleum jelly, zinc oxide, and Cavilon (3M Products). These products maintain peripheral moisture while limiting superficial damage from adhesives. There is an array of topical products available. The appropriate dressing should take into account the frequency of dressing changes as well as the associated edema and moisture of the wound. If the wound is exudative, a more absorbent dressing should be selected. However, if the wound is not excessively moist, using a product that dessicates will limit keratinocyte migration.[36] A dressing ideally provides a level of protection mimicking the epithelium's function. However, this is a difficult function to replicate. In infected wounds, a combination of debridement and silver application is being used in many formulations and delivery. It has broad spectrum of activity against gram-negative bacteria as well as the methicillin-resistant *Staphylococcus aureus* (MRSA) that colonize many chronic wounds.[37]

Negative Pressure Wound Therapy

Having a basic overview of the healing process allows various interventions to either augment or alter the healing process. One of the major advancements in wound healing has been NPWT, or vacuum-assisted closure. The principle of NPWT is its ability to create microdeformation of cells.[38–40] One of its benefits is stimulation of VEGF by creating an area of relative hypoxia, as well as stimulation of other proproliferative cytokines such as TGF-β and basic FGF (bFGF).[41]

NPWT also helps to keep wounds moist, relying on a semiocclusive dressing, which prevents desiccation of wound edges. The suction apparatus also aids in the removal of fluid around the wound, limiting wound edema and maceration, which limits inflammation in chronic wounds.[42] The dressing changes also provide a mechanical debridement.

The application of NPWT has found an increasing number of uses in pediatric surgery. Initially, NPWT was used to aid in closure of pediatric pilonidal disease and was described as being well tolerated and permitting an earlier return to activities.[43] Subsequent studies expanded on the anatomic regions as well as the age groups to include sternal wounds and complicated neonatal abdominal wounds, and found them to be safe and effective.[44–46]

A key benefit with NPWT is that it minimizes dressing changes. Typically, NPWT dressing changes are 3 times per week as opposed to the daily or twice-daily regimens previously used. The lessened frequency and the continued improvement in the portability of the vacuum device has also allowed faster transition from the hospital setting to home with intermittent nursing visits for dressing changes. Although the up-front cost of NPWT is higher than that of standard dressing care, the overall cost is lessened, specifically when evaluated over increasing lengths of time.[47]

Soft Tissue Wounds to the Face

Facial soft tissue injuries are often a traumatic experience, both for the child and the caregiver. Whenever encountering these injuries, the initial focus should be on identifying and stabilizing more critical issues before addressing soft tissue injuries. Once primary and secondary surveys are complete, attention can be turned to care of soft tissue wounds. An examination assessing the function of motor and sensory nerves should be undertaken as well as documentation of the length, width, depth, and any loss of tissue or presence of contamination. Tetanus vaccine should be administered and antibiotic prophylaxis should be given, especially in bite wounds, contaminated wounds, and patients with comorbidities that predispose them to infections. Initial management should center on cleaning the wound and, if possible, early closure, because delay in closure often worsens the eventual aesthetic outcome.[48] The repair in superficial wounds should be undertaken within 24 hours in areas of good oxygenation and without contamination. Contaminated wounds or regions of poor blood flow should have primary closure within 6 hours if possible.[49] With the exception of dog bites (which are generally clean), bites (cats and humans), ballistic wounds, birds, or barnyard injuries require early debridement with delayed closure to fully assess the extent of damage caused by contamination.

The scalp is a highly vascular region with anastomosis between the external and internal carotid system taking place in the loose fibrofatty region above the epicranium. This region is prone to avulsion and needs to be copiously irrigated because of the presence of emissary veins which may have connections to the dural sinus. The blood supply to the scalp often allows it to survive on a single pedicle in partial avulsion settings, but complete avulsion may require replantation.[50,51] The scalp can also be extended for primary closure using galeal scoring, which involves placing horizontal incisions through the galea to expand the area of coverage. Various rotation and advancement flaps exist for scalp closure. In some cases of cranial bone exposure, the outer cortex can be burred to the diploe space followed by skin grafting, which can be used to achieve pericranial coverage. This grafting can then be treated with subsequent tissue expansion[52] (**Fig. 7**).

Wounds to the ear are challenging, but most can be closed primarily. One of the most important considerations when repairing an ear wound is to prevent chondritis. If the perichondrium is intact, closure of the overlying skin is adequate. Any damaged cartilage should be carefully debrided. If the ear is totally avulsed, surgical replantation should be undertaken. Partial defects are candidates for delayed techniques of reconstruction using local flaps and cartilage grafts[53] (**Fig. 8**). In cases of hematoma or avulsion, it is a general practice to place a bolster to maintain compression and prevent the formation of a hematoma. Formation of a hematoma under the perichondrium can result in anomalous cartilage healing resulting in so-called cauliflower ear.

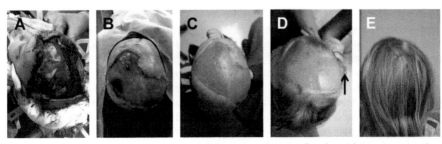

Fig. 7. (A) Severe dog bite to the scalp with avulsion of 50% of scalp with gross contamination. (B) After repeat debridements, galeal scoring was used to expand native scalp; burring of outer cortex, followed by incorporation of Integra. (C) Appearance after skin grafting over Integra. (D) Arrow point to tissue expanders in the scalp with recruitment of extra skin. (E) Full scalp coverage after 2 rounds of tissue expansion.

Traumatic nasal wounds can be problematic, because the nose has a mucosal lining, along with cartilage structural units and a soft tissue envelope. The nose can be divided into several aesthetic subunits for reconstruction. This approach aids in classification and reconstruction options with local tissue flaps.[54] Total destruction of the nose often requires an axial forehead flap based on the supratrochlear vessels (**Fig. 9**).

Cheek wounds can usually be primarily closed. However, the deeper structures must be assessed, specifically the parotid duct and the facial nerve. It is imperative

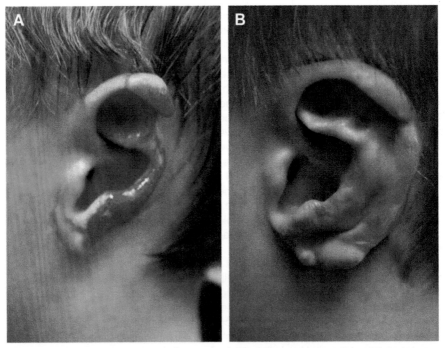

Fig. 8. (A) Dog bite with avulsion of posterior half of the ear and ear lobe. (B) Appearance after a 2-stage correction with costal cartilage graft and posteriorly based skin flap, followed by division and skin grafting to provide an auricular sulcus.

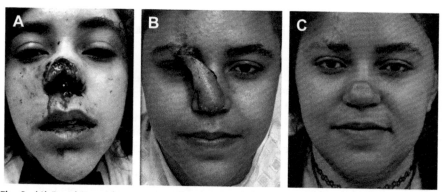

Fig. 9. (*A*) Dog bite with consequent loss of nasal tip subunit. (*B*) Reconstruction with forehead flap. (*C*) Appearance of division and inset of the forehead. The patient can benefit from thinning of the flap at a second stage.

that the branches of the facial nerve are checked for function before administering any local anesthetic. The course of the facial nerve has some variability in anatomy and branching patterns,[55] but some cardinal landmarks can be helpful (**Fig. 10**). The zygomatic and buccal branch can often be found at a line from the midpoint of the root of the helix to the lateral commissure of the mouth.[56] This nerve innervates the zygomaticus major muscle and aids in smiling. The course of the parotid ducts through the cheek has often been described as a line from the tragus to the commissure.[57] The parotid duct exits into the mouth at the level of the first molar. When duct injury is suspected, it can be cannulated with a 24-gauge angiocatheter and injected with methylene blue to assess whether a leak is present in the laceration. If present, the duct needs to be repaired over a stent.

Lip repair can involve direct repair, healing by secondary intent, rotational flaps, or microvascular replantation. Major landmarks such as the philtrum, cupid's bow, white roll, and vermilion-mucosal junction (red line) should be carefully assessed after a laceration in the lip. Discontinuity or the loss of these landmarks requires repair, because alterations of landmarks are conspicuous at conversation distances.[58,59] Small linear lacerations do not require repair because secondary healing in children

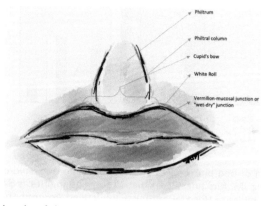

Philtrum

Philtral column

Cupid's bow

White Roll

Vermilion-mucosal junction or "wet-dry" junction

Fig. 10. Major landmarks of the lip.

can produce excellent results. Adhesive closure without sutures has also been used with success.[60] If repair of the lip is to be undertaken, accurate alignment of the landmarks is necessary.

Dog Bites

Dog bites are a common occurrence in the pediatric population. According to the US Centers for Disease Control and Prevention, approximately 4.5 million dog bites occur annually[61] and children aged 5 to 9 years are the most at risk. This number likely understates the actual numbers because some people do not seek treatment. Two large series evaluated morbidity and interventions over a 5-year period at pediatric tertiary care centers[62,63] and both found that more than half of the patients with bites had familiarity with the dog, and 1 study found that 53% were bitten by the family dog.

The location of the injury varied with age because infants and toddlers were more likely to be bitten on the face and older children were more likely to be bitten on the extremity. The studies also showed that pit bulls caused the highest percentage of bites. This finding reinforces previous studies showing that infants and young children are the most at-risk population and the most likely to incur injuries to cosmetically sensitive areas (**Fig. 11**).

Infection rates in dog bites vary, from 1.3% to 45%[64,65]; however, the route and duration of antibiotics varied in studies. It is our practice to ensure that intravenous antibiotics are administered before washout and repair, and generally patients are sent home on an oral course of amoxicillin/clavulanate, to cover the most common bacteria in a dog's mouth (*Pasteurella multocida*).[66] A meta-analysis by Cummings[67] evaluated the role of prophylactic antibiotics and showed a reduced incidence of infection with prophylactic antibiotics.

Necrotizing Fasciitis

Necrotizing fasciitis is a rapidly progressive and destructive infective process that is not frequently seen in the pediatric population; however, because of the speed and extent of injury, it is vital that pediatric practitioners maintain vigilance with soft tissue infections. The diagnosis is clinical and includes severe pain at the site out of

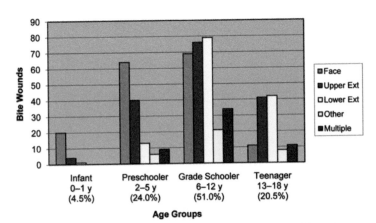

Fig. 11. Distribution of dog bite injuries by anatomic regions in children. Ext, extremities. (*From* Kaye AE, Belz JM, Kirschner RE. Pediatric dog bite injuries: a 5-year review of the experience at the Children's Hospital of Philadelphia. Plast Reconstr Surg 2009;124(2):553; with permission.)

proportion to its appearance. The patient appears toxic, and the skin may appear mottled erythematous or even ecchymotic, and this rapidly spreads. Classically, gray dishwater drainage is described, as is subcutaneous emphysema and large bullae. In children, immune deficient diseases such as acute lymphoblastic leukemia have been implicated. One of the largest case series of pediatric necrotizing fasciitis cited malnutrition as the most common predisposing factor.[68,69]

Microbiology in necrotizing fasciitis is classified into 2 types. Type 1 is polymicrobial and type II is monomicrobial. Type I is often seen after abdominal surgery, rectal perforation, or a spreading infection of the perineum (Fournier gangrene). Microbes in this population are aerobic *Staphylococcus*, *Escherichia coli*, group A *Streptococcus*, and anaerobes of *Peptostreptococcus*, *Prevotella*, *Bacteroides*, and *Clostridium*. Type II is generally *Streptococcus pyogenes*. Necrotizing fasciitis is an emergency with initial management designed for resuscitation, broad-spectrum antibiotics to include clindamycin, and emergent surgical debridement to healthy bleeding tissue.

Exposed Bone/Hardware

Degloving injuries can occur anywhere on the body. The shearing force associated with these injuries can completely denude structures or locally separate, leaving attachments proximally and distally. The initial priority is assessment and repair of deep structures (specifically orthopedic injuries) because there is a significant risk for concomitant injuries.[60] There should be a priority on maintaining any degloved skin because it can be repurposed, and viable pieces can be used as autografts. Other treatment options include tissue substitutes such as Integra and delayed skin grafting.[70]

The need to reconstruct the soft tissue barrier over exposed bone or hardware is critical to heal wounds and prevent infection. Godina[71] recognized that the ability to transfer viable tissue over an injury was beneficial in healing. He showed that coverage of fracture within 75 hours had a lower infection rate and better time to union than coverage between 3 days and 3 months or after 3 months (1.5% and 6 month vs 17.5% and 12.3 months vs 6% and 29 months respectively).[71] Pediatric free tissue transfers have been proved safe and effective.[72] Some benefits of microsurgery in children include the lack of comorbid conditions and anatomy that is generally more favorable than that of their adult counterparts. Neuroplasticity is also greatly improved in children, who have better return of function than adults.[72] It is important to remember that the fourth dimension of time needs to be accounted for in flap design, and although this is rarely a limiting factor it cannot be ignored.

Soft tissue coverage can be attempted for salvage of exposed hardware. The criteria needed for hardware salvage includes no hardware loosening, duration of exposure (<3 weeks), negative wound cultures, and location of the hardware with no signs of instability.[73] Maintaining implants in the spine is key for stability; however, in cases of exposed extremity hardware, removal with external stabilization is still the standard of care (**Fig. 12**). Reconstruction after tumor resection and radiation may result in exposure and complex wounds. Because of the effects of radiation on local tissue, free tissue transfer[74] is required for reconstruction. The benefits of a vascularized graft include accelerated healing and primary bone healing.[75]

Sternal wound infection in pediatric cardiothoracic surgery has been reported to be between 1.5% and 6.7%.[76,77] Different methods to help prevent wound infections with sternotomies have been developed, such as preoperative nasal carriage screening and treatment of MRSA, preoperative chlorhexidine bathing, and optimization of preoperative comorbidities (especially glycemic control).[78] Many of the preoperative adult practices have been adopted in pediatric practice as well.[79]

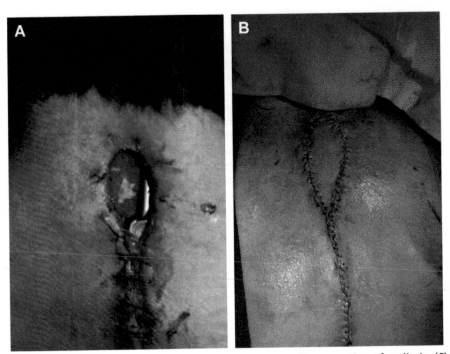

Fig. 12. (*A*) Cervical spinal hardware exposure was seen after correction of scoliosis. (*B*) Trapezius myocutaneous flap was used to cover the hardware, for salvage and stability.

Repair and coverage for sternal wound infections can use many adjacent flaps to provide good stable soft tissue coverage. A pectoralis flap has been used in infants for closure of sternal wound infections.[80,81] Any regional transfer is generally approached in a staged fashion, with initial debridement and dressing changes for a clean wound, followed by flap closure. Rectus muscle can also be used in a vertically based fashion, but the course of the internal mammary artery to the superficial epigastric may be disrupted, so the contralateral side should be used. A regional flap that can be used with success is a pedicled omental flap. Transdiaphragmatic description has been reported in the adult literature.[82]

Abdominal wall disorders such as omphaloceles have well-established protocols for management in infancy. Component separation (which involves separating and advancing certain layers of abdominal muscles, and lengthening their reach to achieve primary midline closure) and tissue expanders are being used to aid in closure of abdominal wall defects when classic methods are unsuccessful. Rohrich and colleagues[83] proposed an algorithm for management of abdominal wall reconstruction, which outlined the size of the defect and an appropriate regional flap or free tissue transfer. Other groups have reported complete reconstruction of the abdominal wall in adults using the lateral circumflex system and a conjoined tensor fascia lata and anterolateral thigh flap.[84]

In extremity reconstruction most bony defects are reconstructed using a fibula graft. Noaman[85] performed a retrospective study in adult patients with an average defect of 8 cm of bone in the extremity. They had a 93% success rate, and, as in the spine, the benefits of vascularized bone grafting included osteogenesis at the fracture site. In the pediatric population requiring lower extremity reconstruction, 75% of patients were

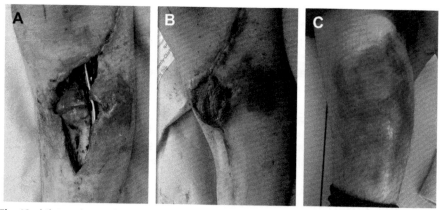

Fig. 13. (*A*) A malnourished young man had exposure of his tibial fracture and hardware. (*B*) After debridement and optimizing nutrition, salvage of hardware (which was found to be stable) was performed with a gastrocnemius muscle flap. (*C*) Final outcome.

able to achieve independent ambulation, and another 20% were able to achieve assisted ambulation.[85] Modifications can be made to the free fibular graft, such as adding cortical allografts to aid in support. Although there is the likelihood of leg length discrepancy, only 14% of patients required surgical correction[86–89] (**Fig. 13**).

Although it may never be possible to eliminate the risk of a wound, the medical armamentarium continues to expand with methods to manage it. The expanded knowledge of cell signaling within a wound may someday allow clinicians to guide healing in a normal cascade even in abnormal conditions.

REFERENCES

1. Goldman R. Growth factors and chronic wound healing: past, present, and future. Adv Skin Wound Care 2004;17(1):24–35.
2. Kim WJ-H, Gittes GK, Longaker MT. Signal transduction in wound pharmacology. Arch Pharm Res 1998;21(5):487–95.
3. Lewis T, Grant R. Vascular reaction of the skin. Part II. The liberation of histamine like substance in injured akin; The underlying cause of factitious urticarial and wheal produced by burning, and observations upon the nervous controls of certain skin reactions. Heart 1924;11:209–65.
4. O'Leary JP, Tabuenca A, Capote LR, editors. The physiologic basis of surgery. Philadelphia: Lippincott Williams & Wilkins; 2008.
5. Raja SK, Garcia MS, Isseroff RR. Wound re-epithelialization: modulating keratinocyte migration in wound healing. Front Biosci 2007;12:2849–68.
6. Schulz C, Gomez Perdiguero E, Chorro L, et al. A lineage of myeloid cells independent of Myb and hematopoietic stem cells. Science 2012;336:86–90.
7. Lech M, Anders H. Macrophages and fibrosis: how resident and infiltrating mononuclear phagocytes orchestrate all phases of tissue injury and repair. Biochim Biophys Acta 2013;1832(7):989–97.
8. Barrientos S, Stojadinovic O, Golinko MS, et al. Perspective article: growth factors and cytokines in wound healing. Wound Repair Regen 2008;16:585–601.
9. Broughton G, Janis J, Attinger C. Wound healing: an overview. Plast Reconstr Surg 2006;117:1e-s.

10. Reinke JM, Sorg H. Wound repair and regeneration. Eur Surg Res 2012;49: 35–43.

11. Thorne CH. Grabb and Smith's plastic surgery. Philadelphia: Lippincott Williams & Wilkins; 2013.

12. Romo T Pearson JM Yalamanchili H, et al. Wound healing, skin. E-medicine specialties. Available at: http://www.emedicine.com/ent/topics13.htm. Accessed May 12, 2016.

13. Atiyeh BS, Amm CA, El Musa KA. Improved scar quality following primary and secondary healing of cutaneous wounds. Aesthetic Plast Surg 2003;27(5):411–7.

14. Leininger BE, Rasmussen TE, Smith DL, et al. Experience with wound VAC and delayed primary closure of contaminated soft tissue injuries in Iraq. J Trauma 2006;61(5):1207–11.

15. Tandara AA, Mustoe TA. Oxygen in wound healing—more than a nutrient. World J Surg 2004;28(3):294–300.

16. Hopf HW, Humphrey LM, Puzziferri N, et al. Adjuncts to preparing wounds for closure: hyperbaric oxygen, growth factors, skin substitutes, negative pressure wound therapy (vacuum-assisted closure). Foot Ankle Clin 2001;6(4):661–82.

17. Hart DW, Wolf SE, Chinkes DL, et al. Effects of early excision and aggressive enteral feeding on hypermetabolism, catabolism, and sepsis after severe burn. J Trauma 2003;54(4):755–64.

18. Zaizen Y, Ford EG, Costin G, et al. Stimulation of wound bursting strength during protein malnutrition. J Surg Res 1990;49(4):333–6.

19. Padh H. Vitamin C: newer insights into its biochemical functions. Nutr Rev 1991; 49(3):65–70.

20. Arnold M, Barbul A. Nutrition and wound healing. Plast Reconstr Surg 2006; 117(7S):42S–58S.

21. Ehrlich HP, Hunt TK. Effects of cortisone and vitamin A on wound healing. Ann Surg 1968;167(3):324.

22. Lansdown ABG, Mirastschijski U, Stubbs N, et al. Zinc in wound healing: theoretical, experimental, and clinical aspects. Wound Repair Regen 2007;15(1):2–16.

23. Lebwohl M, Neldner K, Pope FM, et al. Classification of pseudoxanthoma elasticum: report of a consensus conference. J Am Acad Dermatol 1994;30(1):103–7.

24. Beighton P, De Paepe A, Steinmann B, et al. Ehlers-Danlos syndromes: revised nosology, Villefranche, 1997. Am J Med Genet 1998;77(1):31–7.

25. Burch GH, Gong Y, Liu W, et al. Tenascin-X deficiency is associated with Ehlers-Danlos syndrome. Nat Genet 1997;17(1):104–8.

26. Pepin M, Schwarze U, Superti-Furga A, et al. Clinical and genetic features of Ehlers–Danlos syndrome type IV, the vascular type. N Engl J Med 2000;342(10): 673–80.

27. Zhang M-C, He L, Giro M, et al. Cutis laxa arising from frameshift mutations in exon 30 of the elastin gene (ELN). J Biol Chem 1999;274(2):981–6.

28. Salk D. Werner's syndrome: a review of recent research with an analysis of connective tissue metabolism, growth control of cultured cells, and chromosomal aberrations. Hum Genet 1982;62(1):1–15.

29. Bauer EA, Silverman N, Busiek DF, et al. Diminished response of Werner's syndrome fibroblasts to growth factors PDGF and FGF. Science 1986;234(4781): 1240–3.

30. Patterson JW. Weedon's skin pathology. China: Elsevier Health Sciences; 2014.

31. Ogawa R, Akaishi S, Izumi M. Histologic analysis of keloids and hypertrophic scars. Ann Plast Surg 2009;62(1):104–5.

32. Butler PD, Longaker MT, Yang GP. Current progress in keloid research and treatment. J Am Coll Surg 2008;206(4):731–41.
33. Ogawa R. The most current algorithms for the treatment and prevention of hypertrophic scars and keloids. Plast Reconstr Surg 2010;125(2):557–68.
34. Attinger CE, Janis JE, Steinberg J, et al. Clinical approach to wounds: debridement and wound bed preparation including the use of dressings and wound-healing adjuvants. Plast Reconstr Surg 2006;117(7S):72S–109S.
35. Donelan MB, Parrett BM, Sheridan RL. Pulsed dye laser therapy and z-plasty for facial burn scars: the alternative to excision. Ann Plast Surg 2008;60(5):480–6.
36. Fonder MA, Lazarus GS, Cowan DA, et al. Treating the chronic wound: a practical approach to the care of nonhealing wounds and wound care dressings. J Am Acad Dermatol 2008;58(2):185–206.
37. Wright JB, Lam K, Burrell RE. Wound management in an era of increasing bacterial antibiotic resistance: a role for topical silver treatment. Am J Infect Control 1998;26(6):572–7.
38. Morykwas MJ, Argenta LC, Shelton-Brown EI, et al. Vacuum-assisted closure: a new method for wound control and treatment: animal studies and basic foundation. Ann Plast Surg 1997;38(6):553–62.
39. Ingber DE. The mechanochemical basis of cell and tissue regulation. Mech Chem Biosyst 2004;1(1):53–68.
40. Ingber DE. Mechanical control of tissue growth: function follows form. Proc Natl Acad Sci U S A 2005;102(33):11571–2.
41. Lu F, Ogawa R, Nguyen DT, et al. Microdeformation of three-dimensional cultured fibroblasts induces gene expression and morphological changes. Ann Plast Surg 2011;66(3):296.
42. Heit YI, Dastouri P, Helm DL, et al. Foam pore size is a critical interface parameter of suction-based wound healing devices. Plast Reconstr Surg 2012;129(3):589–97.
43. Bütter A, Emran M, Al-Jazaeri A, et al. Vacuum-assisted closure for wound management in the pediatric population. J Pediatr Surg 2006;41(5):940–2.
44. Pauniaho S-L, Costa J, Boken C, et al. Vacuum drainage in the management of complicated abdominal wound dehiscence in children. J Pediatr Surg 2009;44(9):1736–40.
45. Lopez G, Clifton-Koeppel R, Emil S. Vacuum-assisted closure for complicated neonatal abdominal wounds. J Pediatr Surg 2008;43(12):2202–7.
46. Othman D. Negative pressure wound therapy literature review of efficacy, cost effectiveness, and impact on patients' quality of life in chronic wound management and its implementation in the United Kingdom. Plast Surg Int 2012;2012:374398.
47. Erba P, Ogawa R, Ackermann M, et al. Angiogenesis in wounds treated by microdeformational wound therapy. Ann Surg 2011;253(2):402.
48. Quinn JV, Drzewiecki A, Li MM, et al. A randomized, controlled trial comparing a tissue adhesive with suturing in the repair of pediatric facial lacerations. Ann Emerg Med 1993;22(7):1130–5.
49. Singer AJ, Hollander JE, Quinn JV. Evaluation and management of traumatic lacerations. N Engl J Med 1997;337(16):1142–8.
50. Hurvitz KA, Kobayashi M, Evans GRD. Current options in head and neck reconstruction. Plast Reconstr Surg 2006;118(5):122e–33e.
51. Kretlow JD, McKnight AJ, Izaddoost SA. Facial soft tissue trauma. Semin Plast Surg 2010;24(4):348–56.

52. Miller GDH, Anstee EJ, Snell JA. Successful replantation of an avulsed scalp by microvascular anastomoses. Plast Reconstr Surg 1976;58(2):133–6.

53. Steffen A, Katzbach R, Klaiber S. A comparison of ear reattachment methods: a review of 25 years since Pennington. Plast Reconstr Surg 2006;118(6):1358–64.

54. Guo L, Pribaz JR, Pribaz JJ. Nasal reconstruction with local flaps: a simple algorithm for management of small defects. Plast Reconstr Surg 2008;122(5):130e–9e.

55. Tzafetta K, Terzis JK. Essays on the facial nerve: Part I. Microanatomy. Plast Reconstr Surg 2010;125(3):879–89.

56. Dorafshar AH, Borsuk DE, Bojovic B, et al. Surface anatomy of the middle division of the facial nerve: Zuker's point. Plast Reconstr Surg 2013;131(2):253–7.

57. Stringer MD, Mirjalili SA, Meredith SJ, et al. Redefining the surface anatomy of the parotid duct: an in vivo ultrasound study. Plast Reconstr Surg 2012;130(5):1032–7.

58. Rhee ST, Colville C, Buchman SR. Conservative management of large avulsions of the lip and local landmarks. Pediatr Emerg Care 2004;20(1):40–2.

59. Smith J, Maconochie I. Should we glue lip lacerations in children? Arch Dis Child 2003;88(1):83.

60. Kudsk KA, Sheldon GF, Walton RI. Degloving injuries of the extremities and torso. J Trauma 1981;21(10):835–9.

61. Available at: http://www.cdc.gov/features/dog-bite-prevention/. Accessed February 23, 2016.

62. Garvey EM, Twitchell DK, Ragar R, et al. Morbidity of pediatric dog bites: a case series at a level one pediatric trauma center. J Pediatr Surg 2015;50(2):343–6.

63. Kaye AE, Belz JM, Kirschner RE. Pediatric dog bite injuries: a 5-year review of the experience at the Children's Hospital of Philadelphia. Plast Reconstr Surg 2009;124(2):551–8.

64. Gurunluoglu R, Glasgow M, Arton J, et al. Retrospective analysis of facial dog bite injuries at a Level I trauma center in the Denver metro area. J Trauma Acute Care Surg 2014;76(5):1294–300.

65. Fleisher GR. The management of bite wounds. N Engl J Med 1999;340:138–40.

66. Bailie WE, Stowe EC, Schmitt AM. Aerobic bacterial flora of oral and nasal fluids of canines with reference to bacteria associated with bites. J Clin Microbiol 1978;7(2):223–31.

67. Cummings P. Antibiotics to prevent infection in patients with dog bite wounds: a meta-analysis of randomized trials. Ann Emerg Med 1994;23(3):535–40.

68. Ferri FF. Ferri's clinical advisor 2013: 5 Books in 1. Philadelphia: Elsevier Health Sciences; 2012.

69. Sudarsky LA, Laschinger JC, Coppa GF, et al. Improved results from a standardized approach in treating patients with necrotizing fasciitis. Ann Surg 1987;206(5):661.

70. Wolter TP, Noah EM, Pallua N. The use of Integra® in an upper extremity avulsion injury. Br J Plast Surg 2005;58(3):416–8.

71. Godina M. Early microsurgical reconstruction of complex trauma of the extremities. Plast Reconstr Surg 1986;78(3):285–92.

72. Upton J, Guo L. Pediatric free tissue transfer: a 29-year experience with 433 transfers. Plast Reconstr Surg 2008;121(5):1725–37.

73. Upton J, Guo L, Labow BI. Pediatric free-tissue transfer. Plast Reconstr Surg 2009;124(6S):e313–26.

74. Viol A, Pradka SP, Baumeister SP, et al. Soft-tissue defects and exposed hardware: a review of indications for soft-tissue reconstruction and hardware preservation. Plast Reconstr Surg 2009;123(4):1256–63.
75. Jandali S, Diluna ML, Storm PB, et al. Use of the vascularized free fibula graft with an arteriovenous loop for fusion of cervical and thoracic spinal defects in previously irradiated pediatric patients. Plast Reconstr Surg 2011;127(5):1932–8.
76. Moran SL, Bakri K, Mardini S, et al. The use of vascularized fibular grafts for the reconstruction of spinal and sacral defects. Microsurgery 2009;29(5):393–400.
77. Woodward CS, Son M, Calhoon J, et al. Sternal wound infections in pediatric congenital cardiac surgery: a survey of incidence and preventative practice. Ann Thorac Surg 2011;91(3):799–804.
78. Tabbutt S, Duncan BW, McLaughlin D, et al. Delayed sternal closure after cardiac operations in a pediatric population. J Thorac Cardiovasc Surg 1997;113(5):886–93.
79. Bryan CS, Yarbrough WM. Preventing deep wound infection after coronary artery bypass grafting. Tex Heart Inst J 2013;40(2):125–39.
80. Sung K, Jun TG, Park PW, et al. Management of deep sternal infection in infants and children with advanced pectoralis major muscle flaps. Ann Thorac Surg 2004;77(4):1371–5.
81. Falagas ME, Tansarli GS, Kapaskelis A, et al. Impact of vacuum-assisted closure (VAC) therapy on clinical outcomes of patients with sternal wound infections: a meta-analysis of non-randomized studies. PLoS One 2013;8(5):e64741.
82. Vyas RM, Prsic A, Orgill DP. Transdiaphragmatic omental harvest: a simple, efficient method for sternal wound coverage. Plast Reconstr Surg 2013;131(3):544–52.
83. Rohrich RJ, Lowe JB, Hackney FL, et al. An algorithm for abdominal wall reconstruction. Plast Reconstr Surg 2000;105(1):202–16.
84. Wong C-H, Lin CH, Fu B, et al. Reconstruction of complex abdominal wall defects with free flaps: indications and clinical outcome. Plast Reconstr Surg 2009;124(2):500–9.
85. Noaman HH. Management of upper limb bone defects using free vascularized osteoseptocutaneous fibular bone graft. Ann Plast Surg 2013;71(5):503–9.
86. Piper M, Irwin C, Sbitany H. Pediatric lower extremity sarcoma reconstruction: a review of limb salvage procedures and outcomes. J Plast Reconstr Aesthet Surg 2016;69(1):91–6.
87. Moran SL, Shin AY, Bishop AT. The use of massive bone allograft with intramedullary free fibular flap for limb salvage in a pediatric and adolescent population. Plast Reconstr Surg 2006;118(2):413–9.
88. Capanna R, Bufalini C, Campanacci M. A new technique for reconstructions of large metadiaphyseal bone defects. Orthoped Traumatol 1993;2(3):159–77.
89. Innocenti M, Abed YY, Beltrami G, et al. Biological reconstruction after resection of bone tumors of the proximal tibia using allograft shell and intramedullary free vascularized fibular graft: long-term results. Microsurgery 2009;29(5):361–72.

Pediatric Ovarian Torsion

Krista J. Childress, MD[a], Jennifer E. Dietrich, MD, MSc[b],*

KEYWORDS

- Adnexal torsion • Ovarian torsion • Pediatric • Adolescent • Surgical management

KEY POINTS

- Adnexal torsion is rare, but does account for 2.7% of all cases of abdominal pain in children and adolescents and is the fifth most common gynecologic emergency.
- The incidence in women younger than 20 years is estimated at 4.9 per 100,000 with a median age of 11 years; however, it can be seen at any age.
- The diagnosis of adnexal torsion is difficult due to the variable clinical presentation and nonspecific imaging findings. The presence or absence of Doppler flow is not diagnostic for ruling out adnexal torsion; therefore, Doppler flow cannot be used to absolutely confirm or exclude torsion.
- Adnexal torsion is a clinical diagnosis and a surgical emergency. Management should include diagnostic laparoscopy, adnexal detorsion, and ovarian or paraovarian cystectomy if indicated.
- Conservative management with ovarian preservation even in the event of a necrotic-appearing ovary is important for maintenance of ovarian function for these young women to assist in pubertal development and preservation future fertility.

INTRODUCTION

Adnexal torsion is a surgical emergency, and is reported to be the fifth most common gynecologic emergency with a prevalence of 2.7% and incidence of 4.9 per 100,000 in women younger than 20 years.[1–4] It is more likely to occur in women of reproductive age, but can be seen at any age.[5,6] Adnexal torsion in the pediatric and adolescent population accounts for approximately 15% of all cases of torsion.[7] Although adnexal torsion can occur at any age in children (infants to 18 years), up to 52% of torsion cases in children occur between the ages of 9 and 14 years of age, with a median age of 11 years. Neonatal ovarian torsion is rare, with only 16% of cases occurring in girls younger than 1 year.[7,8]

Disclosure: None.
[a] Division of Pediatric and Adolescent Gynecology, Department of Obstetrics and Gynecology, Baylor College of Medicine, 6651 Main Street, 10th Floor, Houston, TX 77030, USA; [b] Division of Pediatric and Adolescent Gynecology, Department of Obstetrics and Gynecology, Baylor College of Medicine, 6651 Main Street, Suite F1020, Houston, TX 77030, USA
* Corresponding author.
E-mail address: jedietri@texaschildrens.org

Surg Clin N Am 97 (2017) 209–221
http://dx.doi.org/10.1016/j.suc.2016.08.008
0039-6109/17/© 2016 Elsevier Inc. All rights reserved.

ANATOMY

The adnexal structures include bilateral ovaries and fallopian tubes. These structures are contained within multiple folds of the peritoneum called the broad ligament, making them relatively mobile structures. The mesometrium, mesovarium, and mesosalpinx together make up the broad ligament. The ovary has a dual blood supply from the ovarian artery coursing through the suspensory ligament, which courses through the peritoneum attaching laterally to the ovary, and the ovarian branch of the uterine artery within the cardinal ligament. These 2 arteries anastomose at the lateral margins of the uterus. The ovarian ligament attaches the uterus to the ovary medially[9] (**Fig. 1**).

Isolated ovarian torsion is twisting of the ovary alone by twisting on the mesovarium. Adnexal torsion involves twisting of all the adnexal components (fallopian tube and ovary) causing impairment of blood flow[9] (**Fig. 2**). Adnexal torsion is more common than isolated ovarian torsion, being present in up to 67% of torsion cases.[9,10] Isolated tubal torsion is defined as tubal torsion in the absence of torsion of the ovary, and is rare with an incidence of only 1.0 per 1.5 million.[11,12] Torsion is more common on the right because of the hypermobility of the cecum and ileum and the slightly longer mesosalpinx and utero-ovarian ligament on the right, allowing more mobility of the adnexa.[6,13]

PATHOPHYSIOLOGY

Up to 25% of pediatric patients with adnexal torsion may have normal ovaries. This increased propensity for adnexal torsion in this population may be due to the small size of the uterus in pediatric patients and the relatively long utero-ovarian ligaments leading to excess mobility of the adnexa.[14,15] More commonly, 51% to 84% of pediatric adnexal torsion cases occur due to adnexal pathology, including cystic teratomas or dermoids (31%), follicular or hemorrhagic ovarian cysts (23%–33%), and,

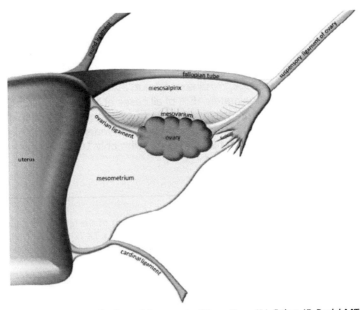

Fig. 1. Schematic drawing of adnexal ligaments. (*From* Ngo AV, Otjen JP, Parisi MT, et al. Pediatric ovarian torsion: a pictorial review. Pediatr Radiol 2015;45:1846; with permission.)

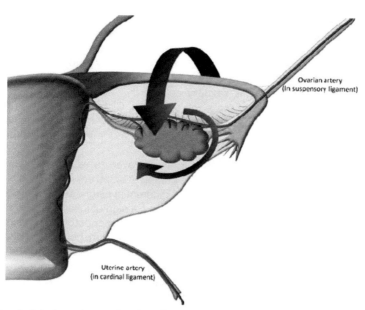

Fig. 2. True isolated ovarian torsion (*small arrow*) and adnexal torsion (*large arrow*). (*From* Ngo AV, Otjen JP, Parisi MT, et al. Pediatric ovarian torsion: a pictorial review. Pediatr Radiol 2015;45:1846; with permission.)

less frequently, paraovarian/paratubal cysts, cystadenomas, or hydrosalpinx.[15,16] The risk of adnexal torsion increases when the mass is benign and the size is 5 cm or larger. Malignancies are often fixed to adjacent tissues and thus are less likely to be associated with torsion. Polycystic ovarian syndrome can result in enlarged ovaries leading to abdominal pain; however, the increased weight and size of the ovaries also can be a risk factor for torsion. Congenital anomalies, such as agenesis, hypoplasia, or other abnormal development of müllerian structures, can lead to clinical examination findings consistent with torsion; therefore, it is important to corroborate the ultrasound and other imaging results with physical examination findings to ensure an appropriate diagnosis.[11,13,17–19]

Torsion of the ovarian pedicle first compressed venous blood flow, followed by arterial flow because the walls of arteries are thicker and more resistant to compression. The impairment in venous blood flow causes ovarian edema and enlargement of the ovary. If torsion persists, arterial blood flow is then affected due to increased pressure within the ovary, leading to ovarian ischemia and necrosis. Complications such as pelvic thrombophlebitis, hemorrhage, infection, and peritonitis can then occur, although this is extremely rare and may be more of a theoretic concern.[18,20,21]

CLINICAL PRESENTATION

Physical examination findings in patients with adnexal torsion are typically nonspecific and can include normal temperature or a low-grade fever and/or mild tachycardia. The most common symptom of adnexal torsion is the acute onset of pelvic or abdominal pain. The pain can be variable in nature, including nonradiating, constant, or intermittent (depending on whether the torsion is partial or complete); mild or intense; and of variable duration (days to months), but is often isolated to one side. The patient also may voice a history of transient episodes of similar pain indicating previous events of partial, intermittent torsion.[22] Other commonly associated symptoms include nausea and vomiting due to peritoneal reflexes, flank pain, and anorexia. Vaginal bleeding and bowel or bladder abnormalities are other rare associated symptoms. Pelvic examinations are generally not performed in this patient population unless the patient has a specific vaginal complaint or is sexually active.[6,13,23] Also, it is not necessary to perform a pelvic examination to make the diagnosis. Clinical symptoms in neonates can be difficult to interpret due to the lack of specific symptoms and limitations in assessing pain; however, they may present with an abdominal mass and/or feeding intolerance.[8,24]

There are no laboratory tests that have been proven to establish a diagnosis of adnexal torsion; however, a pregnancy test, complete blood cell count, and electrolyte values are helpful in clinical assessment and differential diagnosis. A complete blood count is useful to assess white blood cell count as a sign of inflammatory reaction or infection and a urine pregnancy test to rule out pregnancy or ectopic pregnancy. Most laboratory findings are normal in patients with adnexal torsion; however, a slight leukocytosis sometimes can occur.[22] Adnexal torsion must be differentiated from other diagnoses, including appendicitis, kidney stone, gastroenteritis, hemorrhagic ovarian cyst rupture, pelvic inflammatory disease, and ectopic pregnancy.[15,18,22] If a complex ovarian mass (septations and/or solid components) is present on imaging, serum of tumor markers, including HCG (human chorionic gonadotropin), AFP (alpha-fetoprotein), CA125 (cancer antigen 125), and LDH (lactate dehydrogenase) can be useful in assessing malignancy risk.[4]

DIAGNOSTIC PROCEDURES

The diagnosis of adnexal torsion is often difficult due to the vague and variable clinical presentation as well as nonspecific imaging findings. The most commonly used and accurate imaging study used to assist in the diagnosis of adnexal torsion in pediatric and adolescent patients is pelvic ultrasonography with color Doppler to evaluate blood flow to the ovaries. The abdominal approach for pelvic ultrasound is most often used in the pediatric and adolescent population compared with the transvaginal approach used in the adult population.[9,22,25] Ultrasound findings in adnexal torsion can include a unilaterally enlarged ovary or asymmetric ovarian enlargement, heterogeneous appearance of one ovary due to edema, the presence of a simple or complex adnexal mass, present or diminished/absent flow on color Doppler, peripherally displaced follicles due to stromal edema from ischemia, medialization of the ovary, displacement of the uterus from the midline, free pelvic fluid, and the whirlpool sign, defined as twisting of the ovarian pedicle causing twisting of vessels (**Figs. 3–6**). The most frequently observed adnexal lesions found during torsion include ovarian cystic teratomas, follicular or hemorrhagic cyst, paraovarian/paratubal cysts, cystadenoma, and hydrosalpinx. A torsed fallopian tube can appear dilated and edematous. The risk of adnexal torsion also increases when the adnexal mass is 5 cm or larger; however, children can experience adnexal torsion with completely normal size ovaries as well.[15,18,22,23,26,27]

Unfortunately, torsion cannot be absolutely confirmed or excluded based on the presence or absence of Doppler flow on ultrasound.[18,22] Although the absence of vascular flow is highly suspicious for torsion, the sensitivity of absent arterial flow is as low as 40% to 73%; however, venous compression is evident in up to 93% of torsion cases.[28] There are cases of torsion in which completely obstructed vascular flow is not present on ultrasound Doppler as well[22] (**Fig. 7**). Computed tomography and

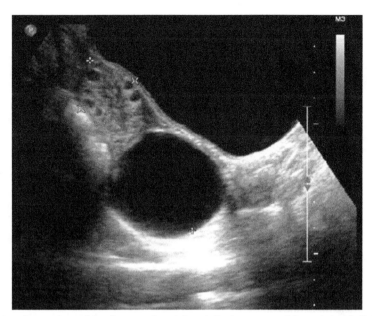

Fig. 3. Ovarian torsion with edema and peripheral displacement of the ovarian follicles. The image demonstrates an enlarged left ovary with scattered small peripheral follicles and a paraovarian cyst. The presence of peripheral follicles confirms that the structure is ovarian in origin. Unilateral ovarian enlargement with peripheral displacement of the follicles suggests torsion. (*From* Ngo AV, Otjen JP, Parisi MT, et al. Pediatric ovarian torsion: a pictorial review. Pediatr Radiol 2015;45:1849; with permission.)

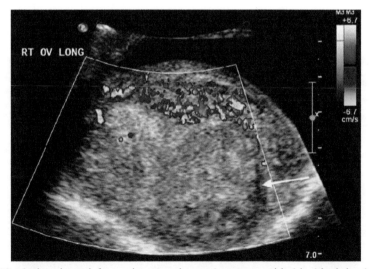

Fig. 4. Massively enlarged, featureless torsed ovary in a 4-year-old girl with abdominal pain for 1 week. Ultrasound image demonstrates a heterogeneous, hyperechoic avascular mass in the midabdomen. No peripheral follicles are present to aid in the identification of ovarian tissue. This is an example of a case in which a torsed ovary (*arrow*) became massively enlarged and edematous/necrotic, leading to loss of the normal imaging features of an ovary and making it difficult to distinguish ovarian torsion from an adnexal mass. (*From* Ngo AV, Otjen JP, Parisi MT, et al. Pediatric ovarian torsion: a pictorial review. Pediatr Radiol 2015;45:1853; with permission.)

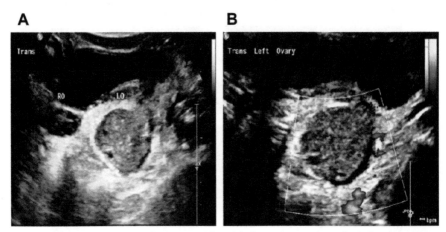

Fig. 5. (*A*) Ultrasound image of a 6-year-old with left ovarian torsion. The left ovary is larger than the right ovary. Note peripheral follicles in the left ovary from ovarian edema. (*B*) Power Doppler image of the left ovary with no intraovarian flow identified. (*From* Ngo AV, Otjen JP, Parisi MT, et al. Pediatric ovarian torsion: a pictorial review. Pediatr Radiol 2015;45:1848; with permission.)

MRI are not first-line imaging modalities, but can be used to further delineate anatomy, if ultrasound is not available, or if other pathologies remain in the differential diagnosis, such as appendicitis. MRI is the gold standard imaging modality for müllerian anomalies.[18]

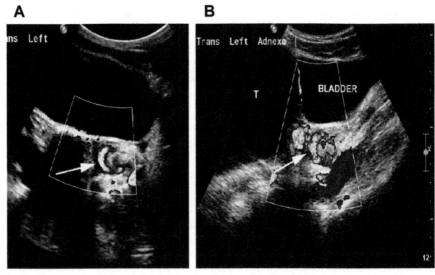

Fig. 6. Ultrasound whirlpool sign in ovarian torsion. (*A, B*) Color flow on Doppler ultrasound images demonstrates the twisted pedicle (*arrows*) in a 12-year-old girl with a large, mature cystic teratoma (T) arising from the left adnexa, representing the lead point for left adnexal torsion. (*From* Ngo AV, Otjen JP, Parisi MT, et al. Pediatric ovarian torsion: a pictorial review. Pediatr Radiol 2015;45:1849; with permission.)

A   **B**

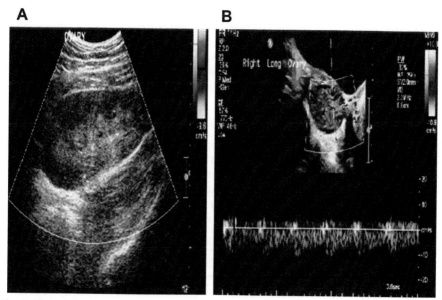

Fig. 7. Flow variation in 2 girls with surgically confirmed ovarian torsion. (*A*) Color Doppler ultrasound image demonstrates an enlarged right ovary measuring 9.7 × 9.9 × 4.8 cm for a total volume of 242 mL. No color or spectral flow is identified. (*B*) Color Doppler image with both arterial and venous flows are present in the enlarged, torsed right ovary, which measures 5.17 × 4.6 × 3.2 cm for a total volume of 39.2 mL. (*From* Ngo AV, Otjen JP, Parisi MT, et al. Pediatric ovarian torsion: a pictorial review. Pediatr Radiol 2015;45:1849; with permission.)

DIAGNOSIS AND TREATMENT

Adnexal torsion is a clinical diagnosis. If clinical features, patient history, and/or imaging suggest a high suspicion for adnexal torsion, the final diagnosis is made by immediate exploratory surgery. Prompt diagnosis and operation are beneficial so as to prevent irreversible adnexal damage, salvaging the torsed adnexa, and maximizing the success of ovarian conservation.[3,4,15,29] Pain lasting more than 10 hours is associated with an increased rate of tissue necrosis.[11] Laparoscopic surgery is considered the best diagnostic and therapeutic approach in the pediatric population[3,4,15,29] (**Fig. 8**).

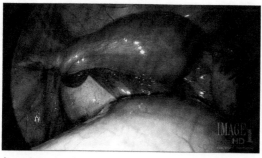

Fig. 8. Left adnexal torsion visualized during diagnostic laparoscopy on a young patient who presented with acute-onset severe abdominal pain and was found to have a left ovarian cyst.

Traditionally, surgeons performed oophorectomy in children and adolescents if a torsed ovary appeared necrotic.[30–32] There were also concerns that the inflammatory effect from the necrotic ovary could lead to adhesive disease and subsequent bowel obstruction, along with increased risk of venous thrombosis once the ovary was detorsed.[30,31,33] Evidence has shown that even necrotic-appearing ovaries, which are black-blue in color, appear to improve after detorsing, showing signs of recovery (**Fig. 9**). In addition, follow-up ultrasound postoperatively demonstrates normal Doppler flow, and follicular development after only 6 weeks.[21,22,34–36] Another commonly cited reason for oophorectomy has been due to concern for malignancy. Fortunately, ovarian malignancy in children also is extremely rare; thus, the probability of occurrence with torsion is rare. It is still important to identify malignancy risk ahead of time. Studies have reinforced that oophorectomy should be reserved for grossly abnormal ovaries and/or elevated tumor markers including HCG, AFP, and CA125 drawn preoperatively.[4,15] Recent literature supports conservative management, including detorsion, ovarian or paraovarian/paratubal cystectomy to reduce cyst recurrence (not simple drainage of the cyst), and preservation of the adnexa (ovary and fallopian tube) even if necrotic, as a safe and effective approach to the management of adnexal torsion.[16,30,33,34,37–40] Even though evidence reinforces conservative management, oophorectomy is still performed in a significant number of cases, with national data showing rates unchanged from 2000 (61%) to 2006 (58%).[41]

Ovarian or paraovarian/paratubal cystectomies as opposed to simple cyst drainage should be performed for all cysts confirmed as nonfunctional or physiologic types (hemorrhagic or follicular cyst).[42,43] Ovarian or paraovarian/paratubal cystectomy if indicated can be safely performed using a bipolar device such as the Harmonic Scalpel or a monopolar device to incise the ovarian capsule or mesosalpinx of the paraovarian/paratubal cyst, and with blunt and sharp dissection, the cyst can be easily removed from the cyst bed. Occasionally the cyst bed needs to be coagulated with electrocautery to provide hemostasis.

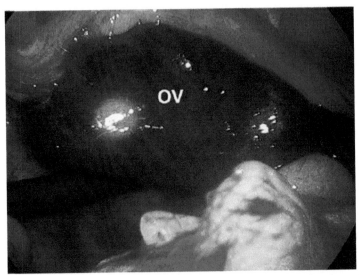

Fig. 9. Enlarged congested left ovary after detorsion. (*From* Ngo AV, Otjen JP, Parisi MT, et al. Pediatric ovarian torsion: a pictorial review. Pediatr Radiol 2015;45:1848; with permission.)

A study by Styer and Laufer[44] also advocated for ovarian bivalving after detorsion cases of severely hemorrhagic and edematous adnexa. During this procedure, they describe using a linear incision along the antimesenteric aspect of the affected ovary after untwisting. This method serves to confirm viable tissue within hemorrhagic, ischemic areas, and releases the increased pressure of the edematous ovarian capsule to facilitate lymphatic and venous drainage and allow for arterial flow, thus reducing ischemia of the ovary after detorsion.[44]

Oophoropexy after detorsing the adnexa is a controversial surgical technique that can be used to limit ovarian mobility and prevent retorsion.[3,6,45–47] Several techniques for this procedure have been described, including fixation of the ovary to the peritoneum on the pelvic sidewall, uterosacral ligaments, or round ligament, shortening the utero-ovarian ligament via plication, and suturing the ovary to the back of the uterus.[48,49] This is not a procedure that is routinely done for every case of adnexal torsion because there is no widely agreed consensus on the topic and removal of adnexal masses that could have precipitated the torsion usually prevent retorsion.[50,51] Use of this procedure can be considered in management of recurrent torsion of an affected ovary to decrease the likelihood of subsequent retorsion or can be performed if only one ovary remains due to prior oophorectomy. The only reported disadvantage of oophoropexy is the possibility of anatomic distortion between the ovary and fallopian tube and the possibility of reduced fertility due to this anatomic stability change to prevent retorsion. However, this type of fertility reduction has been described only in the lateralizing type of oophoropexy (eg, fixation to the pelvic sidewall), and thus medial oophoropexy (eg, utero-ovarian ligament plication) may be a better choice[46,52,53] (**Fig. 10**). Overall, the efficacy and safety of this ovarian fixation procedure are not well established.[16,54–56]

CLINICAL OUTCOMES

There is variability in the literature about the late effects of conservative surgical management versus more radical techniques as treatment for ovarian torsion. In the pediatric population, menstrual cycles are used to assess ovarian function. Some studies have suggested women who undergo conservative procedures show an increase in menstrual irregularity and painful menses.[57] Certain studies suggest that removal of one ovary does not significantly worsen female fertility,[58] whereas others state that resection of the affected ovary can have a negative impact on future fertility.[2] Prior studies evaluating long-term follow-up of patients with ovarian torsion managed conservatively showed rates of normal-sized ovaries and follicular function as high as 91% to 98%. These studies reinforce that most detorsed ovaries recover function and show follicular development after only 6 weeks even when they appear necrotic intraoperatively.[21,22,34–36] Despite the contradictory literature, studies overall agree that conservative management of adnexal torsion via laparoscopy is the preferred management and will preserve ovarian function in pediatric patients, allowing for subsequent normal progression through puberty and future fertility.[2,4,15,35,45,59]

Surveillance ultrasounds can be performed to monitor for cyst recurrence and ovarian integrity 3 months after a procedure for adnexal torsion and/or cystectomy and then every 6 months to 1 year for long-term surveillance. Menarchal patients with history of functional ovarian cysts (follicular or corpus luteal, which develop from the follicle containing the egg during menstrual cycle) can be placed on hormonal therapy to reduce ovulation and recurrence of ovarian cysts, thereby reducing the risk of subsequent adnexal torsion. Hormonal therapy does not reduce recurrence of paraovarian/paratubal cysts or dermoid ovarian cysts because these are not formed as a

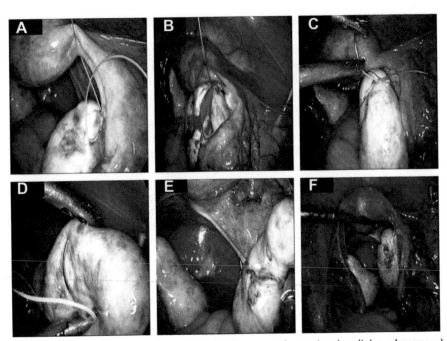

Fig. 10. (*A–C*) The technique of utero-ovarian ligament shortening (medial oophoropexy). (*D* and *E*) The technique of fixation of the left ovary to the pelvic sidewall (lateral oophoropexy). (*F*) Neutral position of the uterus, tubes, and ovaries after fixation procedure completed. (*From* Simsek E, Kilicdag E, Kalayci H, et al. Repeated ovariopexy failure in recurrent adnexal torsion: combined approach and review of the literature. Eur J Obstet Gynecol Reprod Biol 2013;170:307; with permission.)

consequence of ovulation. Therapeutic options for functional ovarian cysts include combined hormonal contraception (estrogen and progesterone) methods, such as oral contraceptive pills, patch, or vaginal ring or progesterone-only options including depo medroxyprogesterone acetate or etonogestrel implants, all of which suppress ovulation and subsequent functional cyst formation.[60,61]

SUMMARY

In summary, adnexal torsion is a surgical emergency and the fifth most common gynecologic emergency presenting with variable examination and radiologic findings. Early diagnosis and surgical intervention with diagnostic laparoscopy and conservative management with ovarian preservation are important for maintenance of ovarian function and preservation of future fertility in girls and adolescents.

REFERENCES

1. Hasdemir PS, Eskicioglu F, Pekindil G, et al. Adnexal torsion with dystrophic calcifications in an adolescent: a chronic entity? Case Rep Obstet Gynecol 2013; 2013:235459.
2. Parelkar SV, Mundada D, Sanghvi BV, et al. Should the ovary always be conserved in torsion? A tertiary care institute experience. J Pediatr Surg 2014; 49:465–8.

3. Sheizaf B, Ohana E, Weintraub AY. "Habitual adnexal torsions"–recurrence after two oophoropexies in a prepubertal girl: a case report and review of the literature. J Pediatr Adolesc Gynecol 2013;26:e81–4.

4. Yildiz A, Erginel B, Akin M, et al. A retrospective review of the adnexal outcome after detorsion in premenarchal girls. Afr J Paediatr Surg 2014;11:304–7.

5. Haskins T, Shull BL. Adnexal torsion: a mind-twisting diagnosis. South Med J 1986;79:576–7.

6. Mellor A, Grover S. Auto-amputation of the ovary and fallopian tube in a child. Aust N Z J Obstet Gynaecol 2014;54:189–90.

7. Servaes S, Zurakowski D, Laufer MR, et al. Sonographic findings of ovarian torsion in children. Pediatr Radiol 2007;37:446–51.

8. Oltmann SC, Fischer A, Barber R, et al. Cannot exclude torsion–a 15-year review. J Pediatr Surg 2009;44:1212–6 [discussion: 7].

9. Ngo AV, Otjen JP, Parisi MT, et al. Pediatric ovarian torsion: a pictorial review. Pediatr Radiol 2015;45:1845–55.

10. Chang HC, Bhatt S, Dogra VS. Pearls and pitfalls in diagnosis of ovarian torsion. Radiographics 2008;28:1355–68.

11. Erikci VS, Hosgor M. Isolated salpingeal torsion in children: a case series and review of the literature. Ulus Travma Acil Cerrahi Derg 2014;20:75–8.

12. Narayanan S, Bandarkar A, Bulas DI. Fallopian tube torsion in the pediatric age group: radiologic evaluation. J Ultrasound Med 2014;33:1697–704.

13. Blitz MJ, Appelbaum H. Management of isolated tubal torsion in a premenarchal adolescent female with prior oophoropexy: a case report and review of the literature. J Pediatr Adolesc Gynecol 2013;26:e95–7.

14. Focseneanu MA, Omurtag K, Ratts VS, et al. The auto-amputated adnexa: a review of findings in a pediatric population. J Pediatr Adolesc Gynecol 2013;26:305–13.

15. Geimanaite L, Trainavicius K. Ovarian torsion in children: management and outcomes. J Pediatr Surg 2013;48:1946–53.

16. Cass DL. Ovarian torsion. Semin Pediatr Surg 2005;14:86–92.

17. Kisku S, Thomas RJ. An uncommon twist: isolated fallopian tube torsion in an adolescent. Case Rep Surg 2013;2013:509424.

18. Lourenco AP, Swenson D, Tubbs RJ, et al. Ovarian and tubal torsion: imaging findings on US, CT, and MRI. Emerg Radiol 2014;21:179–87.

19. Visnjic S, Kralj R, Zupancic B. Isolated fallopian tube torsion with partial hydrosalpinx in a premenarcheal girl: a case report. J Med Case Rep 2014;8:197.

20. Nichols DH, Julian PJ. Torsion of the adnexa. Clin Obstet Gynecol 1985;28:375–80.

21. Rha SE, Byun JY, Jung SE, et al. CT and MR imaging features of adnexal torsion. Radiographics 2002;22:283–94.

22. Sasaki KJ, Miller CE. Adnexal torsion: review of the literature. J Minim Invasive Gynecol 2014;21:196–202.

23. Gerscovich EO, Corwin MT, Sekhon S, et al. Sonographic appearance of adnexal torsion, correlation with other imaging modalities, and clinical history. Ultrasound Q 2014;30:49–55.

24. Nussbaum AR, Sanders RC, Hartman DS, et al. Neonatal ovarian cysts: sonographic-pathologic correlation. Radiology 1988;168:817–21.

25. Naiditch JA, Barsness KA. The positive and negative predictive value of transabdominal color Doppler ultrasound for diagnosing ovarian torsion in pediatric patients. J Pediatr Surg 2013;48:1283–7.

26. Navve D, Hershkovitz R, Zetounie E, et al. Medial or lateral location of the whirlpool sign in adnexal torsion: clinical importance. J Ultrasound Med 2013;32:1631–4.

27. Appelbaum H, Abraham C, Choi-Rosen J, et al. Key clinical predictors in the early diagnosis of adnexal torsion in children. J Pediatr Adolesc Gynecol 2013;26:167–70.

28. Albayram F, Hamper UM. Ovarian and adnexal torsion: spectrum of sonographic findings with pathologic correlation. J Ultrasound Med 2001;20:1083–9.

29. Casey RK, Damle LF, Gomez-Lobo V. Isolated fallopian tube torsion in pediatric and adolescent females: a retrospective review of 15 cases at a single institution. J Pediatr Adolesc Gynecol 2013;26:189–92.

30. Rody A, Jackisch C, Klockenbusch W, et al. The conservative management of adnexal torsion–a case-report and review of the literature. Eur J Obstet Gynecol Reprod Biol 2002;101:83–6.

31. Kokoska ER, Keller MS, Weber TR. Acute ovarian torsion in children. Am J Surg 2000;180:462–5.

32. Spigland N, Ducharme JC, Yazbeck S. Adnexal torsion in children. J Pediatr Surg 1989;24:974–6.

33. Galinier P, Carfagna L, Delsol M, et al. Ovarian torsion. Management and ovarian prognosis: a report of 45 cases. J Pediatr Surg 2009;44:1759–65.

34. Santos XM, Cass DL, Dietrich JE. Outcome following detorsion of torsed adnexa in children. J Pediatr Adolesc Gynecol 2015;28:136–8.

35. Poonai N, Poonai C, Lim R, et al. Pediatric ovarian torsion: case series and review of the literature. Can J Surg 2013;56:103–8.

36. Wang JH, Wu DH, Jin H, et al. Predominant etiology of adnexal torsion and ovarian outcome after detorsion in premenarchal girls. Eur J Pediatr Surg 2010; 20:298–301.

37. Aziz D, Davis V, Allen L, et al. Ovarian torsion in children: is oophorectomy necessary? J Pediatr Surg 2004;39:750–3.

38. Cass DL, Hawkins E, Brandt ML, et al. Surgery for ovarian masses in infants, children, and adolescents: 102 consecutive patients treated in a 15-year period. J Pediatr Surg 2001;36:693–9.

39. Celik A, Ergun O, Aldemir H, et al. Long-term results of conservative management of adnexal torsion in children. J Pediatr Surg 2005;40:704–8.

40. Oelsner G, Bider D, Goldenberg M, et al. Long-term follow-up of the twisted ischemic adnexa managed by detorsion. Fertil Steril 1993;60:976–9.

41. Guthrie BD, Adler MD, Powell EC. Incidence and trends of pediatric ovarian torsion hospitalizations in the United States, 2000-2006. Pediatrics 2010;125:532–8.

42. Ackerman S, Irshad A, Lewis M, et al. Ovarian cystic lesions: a current approach to diagnosis and management. Radiol Clin North Am 2013;51:1067–85.

43. Amies Oelschlager AM, Gow KW, Morse CB, et al. Management of large ovarian neoplasms in pediatric and adolescent females. J Pediatr Adolesc Gynecol 2016; 29:88–94.

44. Styer AK, Laufer MR. Ovarian bivalving after detorsion. Fertil Steril 2002;77: 1053–5.

45. Kurtoglu E, Kokcu A, Danaci M. Asynchronous bilateral ovarian torsion. A case report and mini review. J Pediatr Adolesc Gynecol 2014;27:122–4.

46. Abes M, Sarihan H. Oophoropexy in children with ovarian torsion. Eur J Pediatr Surg 2004;14:168–71.

47. Nagel TC, Sebastian J, Malo JW. Oophoropexy to prevent sequential or recurrent torsion. J Am Assoc Gynecol Laparosc 1997;4:495–8.

48. Weitzman VN, DiLuigi AJ, Maier DB, et al. Prevention of recurrent adnexal torsion. Fertil Steril 2008;90:2018.e1-3.

49. Fuchs N, Smorgick N, Tovbin Y, et al. Oophoropexy to prevent adnexal torsion: how, when, and for whom? J Minim Invasive Gynecol 2010;17:205–8.

50. Ayhan A, Bukulmez O, Genc C, et al. Mature cystic teratomas of the ovary: case series from one institution over 34 years. Eur J Obstet Gynecol Reprod Biol 2000; 88:153–7.
51. Hasson J, Tsafrir Z, Azem F, et al. Comparison of adnexal torsion between pregnant and nonpregnant women. Am J Obstet Gynecol 2010;202:536.e1-6.
52. Damewood MD, Hesla HS, Lowen M, et al. Induction of ovulation and pregnancy following lateral oophoropexy for Hodgkin's disease. Int J Gynaecol Obstet 1990; 33:369–71.
53. Simsek E, Kilicdag E, Kalayci H, et al. Repeated ovariopexy failure in recurrent adnexal torsion: combined approach and review of the literature. Eur J Obstet Gynecol Reprod Biol 2013;170:305–8.
54. Tsafrir Z, Hasson J, Levin I, et al. Adnexal torsion: cystectomy and ovarian fixation are equally important in preventing recurrence. Eur J Obstet Gynecol Reprod Biol 2012;162:203–5.
55. Crouch NS, Gyampoh B, Cutner AS, et al. Ovarian torsion: to pex or not to pex? Case report and review of the literature. J Pediatr Adolesc Gynecol 2003;16:381–4.
56. Rousseau V, Massicot R, Darwish AA, et al. Emergency management and conservative surgery of ovarian torsion in children: a report of 40 cases. J Pediatr Adolesc Gynecol 2008;21:201–6.
57. Zhai A, Axt J, Hamilton EC, et al. Assessing gonadal function after childhood ovarian surgery. J Pediatr Surg 2012;47:1272–9.
58. Bellati F, Ruscito I, Gasparri ML, et al. Effects of unilateral ovariectomy on female fertility outcome. Arch Gynecol Obstet 2014;290:349–53.
59. Agarwal P, Agarwal P, Bagdi R, et al. Ovarian preservation in children for adenexal pathology, current trends in laparoscopic management and our experience. J Indian Assoc Pediatr Surg 2014;19:65–9.
60. Maguire K, Westhoff C. The state of hormonal contraception today: established and emerging noncontraceptive health benefits. Am J Obstet Gynecol 2011; 205:S4–8.
61. Schindler AE. Non-contraceptive benefits of oral hormonal contraceptives. Int J Endocrinol Metab 2013;11:41–7.

Anesthesia for Common Pediatric Emergency Surgeries

Matthew C. Mitchell, DO[a],*, Ibrahim Farid, MD[b]

KEYWORDS

- Pediatric • Emergency • Anesthesia

KEY POINTS

- Many surgeries in the pediatric population are deemed emergent, requiring efficient preparation for the anesthesiology team.
- The preoperative assessment is critical in determining the proper management plan of the pediatric patient involved.
- Common emergent surgeries include airway/esophageal foreign body, appendicitis, intussusception, posttonsillectomy bleed, ventriculoperitoneal shunt, and facial fractures.
- Induction, maintenance, and postoperative care for the common pediatric emergency surgeries can vary.

The majority of surgeries performed in the pediatric population are planned. There are, however, a handful of surgeries that are true emergencies and require an immediate trip to the operating room. Many of these surgeries can be complicated for the anesthesia team for many reasons. It is imperative that the anesthesia team act quickly, formulating a preoperative plan for induction, maintenance, emergence, and postoperative care for the emergent pediatric patient. Seven emergency clinical scenarios seen often by anesthesiologists are discussed and reviewed in this paper. As with any elective procedure, an appropriate preoperative evaluation must be performed by the anesthesiologist before any emergency case begins. With the exception to traumas, even though cases are deemed emergent, there should be enough time to obtain consent and conduct a proper preoperative evaluation in an efficient manner. The preoperative evaluation should include, but not be limited to, a brief medical history, allergies and current medications, previous anesthetic exposure, NPO status, a thorough airway examination, and an anesthetic specific physical examination.

[a] Department of Anesthesia & Pain Medicine, Akron Children's Hospital, One Perkins Square, Room 4648, Akron, OH 44308, USA; [b] Department of Anesthesia and Pain Medicine, Pediatric Pain Center, NEOMED, One Perkins Square, Room 4648, Akron, OH 44308, USA
* Corresponding author.
E-mail address: MMitchell@chmca.org

Surg Clin N Am 97 (2017) 223–232
http://dx.doi.org/10.1016/j.suc.2016.08.014
surgical.theclinics.com

Consent can be an issue in the pediatric population, because most often the children will not understand the nature of the surgical procedure they are consenting to. Permission for medical care or surgery must therefore be obtained from the parents, guardians, or the courts, who does so with the child's best interest in mind. Typically, there is time to obtain consent for the surgical procedures, even in an emergency setting. Every effort to obtain consent and explain the risks and benefits of the anesthetic should be made.

PREOPERATIVE EVALUATION

During the preoperative period, the anesthesiologist should identify any potential diseases, physiologic/hemodynamic derangements, or congenital anomalies that could affect the anesthetic course. Most children are incapable of providing a detailed medical history; therefore, it is helpful if a parent is present to provide the child's history. Often, children are healthy and the history will be short. Other times, children can have complex diseases and parents may not be able to provide much information. Obtaining more information from medical records may be required in these situations. It is essential to question parents concerning premature birth, problems with the heart, lungs, nervous system, gastrointestinal tract, kidneys, endocrine system, or any other serious diseases/syndromes. Allergies to specific medications and current medication use should also be concluded. Many children have no history of anesthetic exposure; therefore, it is imperative that a family history of complications associated with anesthesia be elicited, with an emphasis on a history of malignant hyperthermia and succinylcholine apnea.

Preoperative fasting guidelines have been established to help prevent the aspiration of gastric contents during induction and maintenance of anesthesia. In 2011 new guidelines by the American Society of Anesthesiologists (ASA) Task Force were published. The guidelines recommend a fasting interval of 2 or more hours after the consumption of clear liquids, 4 or more hours after breast milk, 6 or more hours after infant formula, a light meal, or nonhuman milk, and 8 or more hours for solids ("2-4-6-8 rule"; **Table 1**).

The guidelines note that the ingestion of fried or fatty foods or meat may prolong gastric emptying time and recommend that both the amount and type of foods ingested be considered when determining an appropriate fasting period.[1] The ASA guidelines are intended for healthy patients undergoing elective procedures. The guidelines are not intended for children with conditions that may affect gastric emptying resulting in increased gastric volume. Fortunately, the incidence of perioperative pulmonary aspiration is rare; however, a large prospective study showed a greater frequency of aspiration in emergency procedures versus elective procedures.[2] Most patients who present for emergency surgery will be deemed to have full stomachs. An induction technique allowing for rapid securing of an airway device should be conducted, minimizing the risk of pulmonary aspiration.

With limited time in the setting of an emergency, the anesthesiologist should dictate the physical examination based on findings from the medical history gained. Even if no history was able to be obtained, the airway, lungs, and heart should always be examined. Observation of the child's color and the presence of respiratory distress should

Table 1 Guidelines for pediatric preoperative fasting			
Clear Fluids	Breast Milk	Nonhuman Milk or Formula	Solids
2 h	4 h	6 h	8 h

be monitored. Along with the physical examination, a current set of vitals should be monitored before proceeding to the operating room.

AIRWAY FOREIGN BODIES

According to the National Safety Council, suffocation from foreign body ingestion and aspiration is the third leading cause of accidental death in children younger than 1 year of age and the fourth leading cause in children between 1 and 6 years of age.[3] Foreign Body aspiration is a common emergent procedure in the pediatric population, occurring most frequently in children younger than 3 years of age. These cases can be some of the most challenging for the pediatric anesthesiologist. General anesthesia is usually necessary to help remove the foreign body by bronchoscopy. Most often, the foreign body aspiration is organic in nature, such as peanuts, seeds, or other small foods. Foreign bodies are embedded more commonly in the right main bronchus than in the left, and less frequently in the larynx and trachea.[4,5] Symptoms and signs associated with bronchial aspiration include coughing, wheezing, dyspnea, and decreased air entry in the affected side, whereas dyspnea, stridor, coughing, and cyanosis are more common with laryngeal or tracheal foreign bodies.[4] Removal of a foreign body may necessitate laryngoscopy, bronchoscopy, thoracoscopy, thoracotomy, or even a tracheotomy.[2] Most commonly however, a rigid bronchoscopy is the technique most often used for the removal of a foreign body.

Preoperative Assessment

In addition to the usual preoperative assessment, physical examination should focus on the location, degree of airway obstruction, and gas exchange. A review of the latest chest radiographs is helpful in determining the location of the foreign body and for evidence of secondary pathologic changes, such as atelectasis, air trapping, or pneumonia.[3] As always, a discussion with the surgeon detailing their primary approach and backup plans should be conducted. A peripheral intravenous catheter should be placed before arrival in the operating room. Other preoperative considerations are (1) cautious premedication to avoid worsening airway obstruction, (2) intravenous anticholinergic administration (such as glycopyrrolate) to decrease secretions and prevent reflex bradycardia during airway instrumentation, and (3) assessment of the risk for aspiration of gastric contents.[2]

Induction of Anesthesia

The type of induction used for foreign body aspiration must be individualized to the patient. All children should be monitored with the standard ASA monitors including a pulse oximeter, end tidal CO_2, electrocardiogram, thermometer, and automated blood pressure. A major controversy in the anesthetic management of patients undergoing bronchoscopy for foreign body removal is whether to control ventilation or to maintain spontaneous ventilation.[6,7] There are only few data available to dictate whether controlled versus spontaneous ventilation is better. The risk of controlled ventilation is to force the foreign body deeper into the small airways, and the risk for the spontaneously breathing patient is unexpected movement or cough.[8] Often, the child is preferred to be breathing spontaneously, and an inhalational induction with sevoflurane is performed.

Maintenance of Anesthesia

After induction, maintenance of anesthesia can be accomplished with a combination of an inhalational technique with boluses of propofol or a total intravenous anesthetic, consisting of propofol with or without opioids (eg, fentanyl, remifentanil). One advantage to total intravenous anesthetic is a consistent anesthetic that is not reliant on inhalation for depth of anesthesia. To decrease the chances of laryngeal irritation and laryngospasm during bronchoscopy, lidocaine 2% to 4% could be sprayed on the larynx. Often with bronchoscopy, one can ventilate through the side port of the rigid bronchoscope. It should be noted, however, that the side port does not allow for consistent tidal volumes and gas exchange, resulting in poor ventilation, leading to hypercarbia, hypoxia, and a light anesthetic plane. During the procedure, the anesthesiologist needs to be hyper vigilant, focused on the breathing of the patient, oxygenation, and CO_2 levels. The rate of increase in end tidal $Paco_2$ in apneic infants and young children is extremely high—approximately 9 mm Hg/min for the first minute.[9] It is imperative that the anesthesiologist communicate with the endoscopist/surgeon during the procedure. Once the foreign body is removed, a joint decision should be determined as to where the child should recover.

Postoperative Care

Laryngospasm, bronchospasm, hypoxia, and pneumothorax are all complications that can be associated with the removal of foreign bodies within the intraoperative and postoperative period. Steroids with potent glucocorticoid effects are beneficial in reducing airway edema and stridor, owing to their antiinflammatory actions. Dexamethasone (0.25–0.5 mg/kg to a max of 8 mg) given every 6 to 8 hours for 4 to 6 doses has been shown to be effective in decreasing airway edema.[10] Racemic epinephrine is also used to treat airway edema. The alpha-adrenergic effects of racemic epinephrine mediate mucosal vasoconstriction and its beta effects produce smooth muscle relaxation as well as inhibition of mast cell–mediated inflammation.[10] The child should be watched in the postanesthesia care unit (PACU) after racemic epinephrine for at least 2 hours owing to rebound upper airway edema.

ESOPHAGEAL FOREIGN BODIES

Often when foreign bodies are ingested, they go unrecognized by parents and typically have no long-term effects. When the foreign bodies become retained in the esophagus or stomach, it is necessary to remove them using endoscopy. The most commonly ingested foreign body is a coin, followed by food or bones. Other foreign bodies include buttons, batteries, pins, safety pins, thumbtacks, and small toys.[11] Symptoms and signs of upper esophageal foreign body include dysphagia, drooling, gagging, and vomiting. Airway compromise can also occur and the child may exhibit symptoms of coughing or choking.

Preoperative Assessment

In addition to the usual preoperative assessment, physical examination should focus on the location of the foreign body. A potential major hazard exists if the ingested foreign body is held in the hypopharynx, and coughing or choking causes the foreign body to slip into the larynx, occluding the airway. Chest radiographs should be reviewed to determine where the foreign body ingested is located. If the child is not dyspneic, and the object is not hazardous to the esophageal or stomach mucosa (eg, disk battery), surgery should be postponed 4 to 6 hours after last meal. Although this may not be possible, the anesthesiologist should prepare for rapid securement of an airway. A peripheral intravenous catheter should be placed before arrival to the operating room.

Induction and Maintenance of Anesthesia

Upon entering the operating room all children should be monitored with the standard ASA monitors (as discussed). Before induction, the patient should be well-sedated, with the exception of a child with dyspnea. A rapid sequence induction should be performed if the patient is suspected of having a full stomach. If no intravenous access has been established, a smooth inhalational induction should be performed with endotracheal intubation after deep sevoflurane anesthesia or propofol, with or without muscle relaxation. Maintenance can be performed with an inhalational anesthetic supplemented with opioids. Special attention should be placed on making sure the endotracheal tube is secure so the endoscopist/surgeon does not accidently remove it during removal of the foreign body.

Postoperative Care

Depending on the age of the child and any intraoperative complications, most of these children can be discharged home after their PACU stay. A prospective review involving more than 50,000 general pediatric anesthetic cases revealed that the incidence of postintubation croup after esophagoscopy was 20 times higher than that of the general pediatric surgical population during the same time period (Moro, Borland, and Motoyama, unpublished observations). Dexamethasone intraoperatively or postoperatively (0.25–0.5 mg/kg to a max of 8 mg) may decrease the incidence of postoperative croup along with reducing the size of the endotracheal tube used during the surgery.[12]

APPENDICITIS

Acute appendicitis is a common condition that affects children most often between the ages of 10 to 19.[3] Signs and symptoms of appendicitis can vary quite a bit, which can account for a relatively high incidence of negative appendectomy. Children often present with right lower quadrant pain that originates in the periumbilical region. Other signs consistent with appendicitis include nausea/vomiting, anorexia, and a low-grade fever. Ultrasound and computed tomographic imaging have been used to help diagnose appendicitis. Although there is some urgency in making the diagnosis and surgically removing the appendix, the operation is never so urgent that a proper review of the patient's medical history and physical assessment cannot be performed.[13]

Preoperative Assessment

Concerns involving the electrolyte and fluid status of the child should be addressed during the preoperative period. A peripheral intravenous catheter should be placed and an attempt to correct any electrolyte disturbances and dehydration should occur before moving to the operating room.

Induction and Maintenance of Anesthesia

Upon entering the operating room, standard ASA monitors should be placed while the patient is adequately volume resuscitated. Regardless of NPO status an intravenous rapid sequence induction should be performed using Sellick's maneuver. Maintenance of anesthesia can be managed with inhaled anesthetic with supplementation of opioids and muscle relaxants.

Postoperative Care

Patients who are hemodynamically stable can proceed to the PACU where they can be monitored. Typically these children stay the night in the hospital and are monitored. Postoperative pain can be monitored and treated with intravenous medications.

INTUSSUSCEPTION

Intussusception most often affects children less than the age of 1. Most often, it is idiopathic in nature, and children present with abdominal pain, bloody stools, and an abdominal mass. Intussusception can also manifest with neurologic findings (lethargy, apnea, seizures, hypotonia, opisthotonus) similar to a picture of septic encephalopathy.[14]

Preoperative Assessment

Many times, children with intussusception have diarrhea and vomiting, resulting in severe dehydration. It is imperative that a peripheral intravenous line be placed before surgery to adequately hydrate the child and correct any electrolyte imbalance that exist. Plain radiographs of the abdomen will likely show multiple fluid levels. A nasogastric tube should be placed before entering the operating room and left to freely drain to help reduce the chance of aspiration. Laboratory tests should be drawn and blood should be readily available before entering the operating room. Often times these children can present in shock, which should be treated before the induction of anesthesia.[13]

Induction and Maintenance of Anesthesia

A child presenting with intussusception should be considered at risk for aspiration of gastric contents owing to the intestinal obstruction. After standard ASA monitors are placed, a rapid sequence induction should be performed after adequately hydrating the patient. If the patient is hemodynamically unstable, the anesthesiologist should use an intravenous induction agent such as etomidate or ketamine. After induction and placement of the endotracheal tube, the child should be maintained on inhalational agents with intravenous supplementation of opioids and muscle relaxant. Nitrous oxide should be avoided because it can significantly increase the size of the bowel lumen causing difficulty for the surgeon and possibly increasing intraabdominal pressures and decreasing the ability to ventilate the child adequately.

Postoperative Care

After surgery, a decision should be established whether the child should go to the PACU or to the intensive care unit for further monitoring. Typically, these patients can be extubated and monitored in the PACU before going to the floor for further observation. Abdominal surgery, however, is associated with increased intraabdominal pressure, which can cause an increase in respiratory insufficiency. The anesthesiologist should make sure the patient is awake and breathing adequately with full reversal of muscle relaxant before extubating the child.

POSTTONSILLECTOMY BLEEDING

Adenotonsillectomy is one of the most common surgeries performed in the pediatric population, with approximately 250,000 tonsillectomies performed each year in the United States alone. Although a rare occurrence (0.5%–2% of cases), postoperative bleeding can be a potentially serious complication. There are 2 types of bleeding that occur: primary bleeding and secondary bleeding. Primary bleeding occurs within the first 24 hours and is usually associated with inadequate surgical hemostasis. Bleeding is usually brisk and easily identifiable. Secondary Bleeding occurs most commonly between 5 and 10 days postoperatively, but it can occur up to 28 days postoperatively.[12] The cause of secondary bleeding can be attributed to the sloughing of eschar tissue. Bleeding is usually slow and steady over a few days.

Preoperative Assessment

Hypovolemia from blood loss and decreased oral intake owing to pain is commonly seen in children presenting for posttonsillectomy bleed. On physical examination, children commonly present with tachycardia, tachypnea, and hypotension. Capillary refill prolongation with pale skin and dry mucous membranes are other commonly seen physical characteristics. Laboratory values might show decreased hemoglobin levels; however, if the patient is severely dehydrated a normal hematocrit value might reflect dehydration. A peripheral intravenous catheter should be placed before heading to the operating room. Appropriate fluid resuscitation should begin before induction of anesthesia. All patients should be considered to have a full stomach, regardless of their NPO status. Two laryngoscopes and 2 suctions should be available and ready for use.

Induction and Maintenance of Anesthesia

A child presenting with postoperative tonsillar bleed should be considered a high risk for aspiration, and a rapid sequence induction is indicated. Before induction, it is imperative that the child be appropriately resuscitated with crystalloids or packed red blood cells, depending on the clinical signs and laboratory values. The appropriate induction medication should be chosen. If hypovolemia is an issue, etomidate or ketamine can be used effectively. If hypovolemia is not an issue, propofol may be used judiciously. Muscle relaxants should include succinylcholine or rocuronium. A difficult airway with poor visualization should be expected. It may be helpful to have an assistant hold a Yankauer suction device in the oropharynx during intubation to aid in obtaining better visualization of the airway. Placement of a cuffed oral endotracheal tube will help to protect the airway from aspiration. The patient can then be maintained on an inhalational anesthetic agent. It is helpful to obtain another large-bore intravenous catheter in case blood needs to be transfused during the procedure. Upon completion of the surgery, the patient should be fully awaken before extubation paying close attention to any rebleeding.

Postoperative Care

Patients should recover in the PACU after an awake extubation. If they were diagnosed with primary bleeding, they will continue to be at risk for rebleeding in the postoperative period. Laboratory values including coagulation studies should be drawn. Intravenous fluid administration should be continued and postoperative pain controlled. Stridor, and wheezing should be evaluated and properly treated. A chest radiograph might be indicated if wheezing is suspected to be from aspiration. Hospital admission may be indicated depending on how the child does in the postoperative period.

VENTRICULOPERITONEAL SHUNT

Hydrocephalus, the most common pediatric neurosurgical condition, involves a mismatch of cerebrospinal fluid production and absorption, leading to increased intracranial cerebrospinal fluid volume. The majority of cases of hydrocephalus result from obstruction of cerebrospinal fluid flow or inability to absorb cerebrospinal fluid appropriately.[13] Hydrocephalus can be further classified into 2 categories based on whether cerebrospinal fluid can flow around the spinal cord in its usual matter. Nonobstructive/communicating hydrocephalus allows for this normal flow, whereas obstructive/noncommunicating hydrocephalus impairs or inhibits normal cerebrospinal fluid flow. Symptoms of obstructive hydrocephalus include lethargy, vomiting, cranial nerve dysfunction, and bradycardia. If not treated quickly, death can ultimately occur.

Unless the etiology of the hydrocephalus can be definitively treated, treatment entails surgical placement of a ventricular drain or ventriculoperitoneal shunt.

Preoperative Assessment

Concerns involving the neurologic status of the child should be addressed during the preoperative period. Many of these patients present with lethargy and an altered mental status. Vomiting often occurs, resulting in electrolyte imbalances and dehydration. A peripheral intravenous catheter should be placed in an attempt to correct any electrolyte disturbances and for preparation of a rapid sequence induction.

Induction and Maintenance of Anesthesia

The approach to patients with symptomatic hydrocephalus should be directed at controlling intracranial pressure and rapidly relieving the obstruction.[15] After the preoperative assessment, the patient should be brought to the operating room where the standard ASA monitors should be placed, and a rapid sequence induction performed. After placement of the endotracheal tube, hyperventilation to an end-tidal CO_2 of about 25 to 30 mm Hg should be instituted immediately to help decrease intracranial pressure. The patient can then be maintained on inhalational agents with intravenous supplementation of opioids and muscle relaxants.

Postoperative Care

After surgery, a decision should be established whether the child should go to the PACU or to the intensive care unit for further monitoring. Typically these patients can be extubated and monitored in the PACU before going to the floor for further observation. The patient's mental status should be monitored because of the possibility of the reobstruction of the shunt, leading to life-threatening hydrocephalus.[15]

FACIAL FRACTURES

Trauma to the facial skeleton may result in 1 or more fractures and may require surgical fixation. Typical facial fractures include zygoma fractures, Le Fort II, Le Fort III, mandible, orbital, nasal, and panfacial fractures.[15] Other injuries are commonly associated with facial trauma. In 1 study, 25% of patients diagnosed with facial fractures had associated injuries, including limb, brain, chest, spine, and abdominal injuries. Up to 10% of these patients had a brain injury.[16] Of concern is the fact that many of the brain injuries can be missed because many of these patients exhibit no signs or symptoms of having any brain injury. Facial fractures involving the midface commonly result in airway compromise because of the displacement of the midface posteriorly into the oropharynx.[17]

Preoperative Assessment

In addition to the usual preoperative assessment, a complete trauma assessment should be conducted with particular attention paid to any airway pathology. Blood and secretions should be identified because of their ability to further obstruct the airway. Patients should be believed to have full stomachs, which provides a challenge for the anesthesia team. Children not properly fasted require either a rapid sequence induction or a sedated fiberoptic intubation. All patients with suspected or known cervical injuries require cervical immobilization.[17] A peripheral intravenous catheter should be placed before entering the operating room to allow for any sedation or possible rapid sequence induction.

Induction and Maintenance of Anesthesia

Depending on the extent of the trauma and injury to the facial bones, the anesthesia team needs to determine how difficult intubating the patient might be. With a full stomach, a rapid sequence induction should be performed; however, if the intubation seems to be challenging, an awake fiberoptic intubation may be necessary. Blood and other secretions make a fiberoptic intubation very difficult, if not impossible with the limited visibility. It is a good idea to have an ear, nose, and throat surgeon at the bedside during induction in case a tracheostomy needs to be performed. After securing an airway, the patient can be maintained with inhalational agents with supplementation of opioids and muscle relaxant.

Postoperative Care

After surgery, a determination needs to be made whether the patient should be further monitored in the intensive care unit or the PACU. The patient should be fully awake before extubating with good grip strength and a sustained head lift.

SUMMARY

The anesthesiologist must be prepared on a daily basis to care for children who need emergency surgery. An appropriate perioperative plan must be formulated and executed to ensure successful management of the child. This article outlines how to prepare and effectively manage common pediatric emergency surgeries.

REFERENCES

1. American Society of Anesthesiologists. Practice guidelines for preoperative fasting and the use of pharmacologic agents to reduce the risk of pulmonary aspiration: application to healthy patients undergoing elective procedures. A report by the American Society of Anesthesiologists Task Force on Preoperative Fasting. Anesthesiology 2011;114:495–511.
2. Hagerman NS, Wittkugel EP. Preoperative fasting in the pediatric patient. In: Goldschneider KR, Davidson AJ, Wittkugel EP, et al, editors. Clinical pediatric anesthesia. New York: Oxford University Press, Inc; 2012. p. 63.
3. Landsman IS, Werkhaven JA, Motoyama EK. Anesthesia for pediatric otorhinolaryngologic surgery. In: Davis PJ, Cladis PF, Motoyama EK, editors. Smith's anesthesia for infants and children. 8th edition. Philadelphia: Mosby; 2011. p. 817.
4. Blazer S, Naveh Y, Friedman A. Foreign body in the airway: a review of 200 cases. Am J Dis Child 1980;134:68–71.
5. Cohen S, Pine H, Drake A. Use of rigid and flexible bronchoscopy among pediatric otolaryngologists. Arch Otolaryngol Head Neck Surg 2001;127:505–9.
6. Verghese ST, Hannallah RS. Pediatric otolaryngologic emergencies. Anesthesiol Clin North America 2001;19:237–56.
7. Chen L, Zhang X, Li S, et al. Risk factors for hypoxemia in children less than 5 years of age undergoing rigid bronchoscopy for foreign body removal. Anest Analg 2009;109(4):179.
8. Donlon JV, Benumof JL. Anesthetic and airway management of laryngoscopy and broncoscopy. St. Louis: Mosby; 1996.
9. Motoyama EK, Fine GF, Jacobson KH, et al. Accelerated increases in end-tidal CO_2 (Petco2) in anesthetized infants and children during rebreathing. Anesthesiology 2001;94:A1276.

10. Chidambaran V, Sadhasivam S. Foreign body in the airway. In: Goldschneider KR, Davidson AJ, Wittkugel EP, et al, editors. Clinical pediatric anesthesia. New York: Oxford University Press, Inc; 2012. p. 125–8.

11. McGahren ED. Esophageal foreign bodies. Pediatr Rev 1999;20:129–33.

12. Hein EA, Margolis JO. Tonsillar Bleed. In: Goldschneider KR, Davidson AJ, Wittkugel EP, et al, editors. Clinical pediatric anesthesia. New York: Oxford University Press, Inc; 2012. p. 142.

13. Hammer G, Hall S, Davis PJ. Anesthesia for general abdominal, thoracic, urologic, and bariatric surgery. In: Davis PJ, Cladis PF, Motoyama EK, editors. Smith's anesthesia for infants and children. 8th edition. Philadelphia: Mosby; 2011. p. 761.

14. Conway EE Jr. Central nervous system findings and intussusception: how are they related? Pediatr Emerg Care 1993;9:15–8.

15. Vavilala MS, Soriano SG. Anesthesia for neurosurgery. In: Davis PJ, Cladis PF, Motoyama EK, editors. Smith's anesthesia for infants and children. 8th edition. Philadelphia: Mosby; 2011. p. 736–7.

16. Thorén H, Snall J, Salo J, et al. Occurrence and types of associated injuries in patients with fractures of the facial bones. J Oral Maxillofac Surg 2010;68(4): 805–10.

17. Cladis FP, Grunwaldt L, Losee J. Anesthesia for plastic surgery. In: Davis PJ, Cladis PF, Motoyama EK, editors. Smith's anesthesia for infants and children. 8th edition. Philadelphia: Mosby; 2011. p. 839.

Index

Note: Page numbers of article titles are in **boldface** type.

A

Abdominal injuries
  in pediatric surgery
    clinical presentation of, 23–24
Abdominal trauma evaluation
  for pediatric surgeon, **59–74**
    background of, 60
    colon and rectal injuries, 67
    controversial topics, 70–72
      adult *vs.* pediatric trauma centers, 71–72
      FAST examination, 70–71
      negative workup, 71
    decision making related to, 68–70
    diagnosis of, 60–62
    diaphragm injuries, 68
    genitourinary injuries, 67
    imaging in, 64–66
      protocols, 68
    initial evaluation and stabilization of, 62–63
    introduction, 59–60
    laboratory studies in, 64
    liver and splenic injuries, 66
    modalities in, 63–66
    pancreatic injuries, 67
    presentation of, 60–62
    specific injuries, 66–68
    stomach and small bowel injuries, 66–67
    treatment in, 68–70
      solid organ injuries protocols, 68–70
Activity restriction
  after blunt solid organ injury during pediatric surgery management, 14
Acute traumatic injury
  laparoscopy in diagnosis and treatment of, 77–78
Airway(s)
  pediatric
    foreign bodies in
      anesthesia for emergency management of, 225–226
      aspiration for, 86–87
      clinical outcomes of, 89
      clinical presentation of, 86
      diagnostic and therapeutic procedures for, 86–87
      esophageal, **85–91** (*See also* Esophageal foreign bodies)

Surg Clin N Am 97 (2017) 233–247
http://dx.doi.org/10.1016/S0039-6109(16)52169-0
0039-6109/17

Moving?

Make sure your subscription moves with you!

To notify us of your new address, find your **Clinics Account Number** (located on your mailing label above your name), and contact customer service at:

Email: journalscustomerservice-usa@elsevier.com

800-654-2452 (subscribers in the U.S. & Canada)
314-447-8871 (subscribers outside of the U.S. & Canada)

Fax number: 314-447-8029

Elsevier Health Sciences Division
Subscription Customer Service
3251 Riverport Lane
Maryland Heights, MO 63043

ELSEVIER